27.50

Health Care Capital: Competition and Control

Editors
Gordon K. MacLeod
Professor and Chairman
Department of Health Services Administration
Graduate School of Public Health
University of Pittsburgh
Mark Perlman
The University Professor of Economics
University of Pittsburgh

Proceedings of
Capital Investment Conference
Sponsored by the
University of Pittsburgh
Graduate School of Public Health
and Supported under
Federal Contract No. HRA 230-75-0208

Ballinger Publishing Company • Cambridge, Massachusetts
A Subsidiary of J.B. Lippincott Company

This book is printed on recycled paper.

International Standard Book Number: 0-88410-521-0

Library of Congress Catalog Card Number: 77-22166

Printed in the United States of America

Library of Congress Cataloging in Publication Data

Capital Investment Conference, University of Pittsburgh, 1976.
  Health care capital.

  1. Health facilities—United States—Finance—Congresses. 2. Capital invest-
ments—United States—Congresses. I. MacLeod, Gordon Kenneth, 1929–II.
Perlman, Mark. III. Pittsburgh. University. Graduate School of Public Health. IV.
Title.

RA981.A2C28 1976	338.4'3	77-22166

ISBN 0-88410-521-0

❋

**STEERING COMMITTEE
CAPITAL INVESTMENT CONFERENCE
NOVEMBER 19-21, 1976**

Chairman

Nathan J. Stark, J.D.
Vice Chancellor of Health Professions
University of Pittsburgh
President of the University Health
    Center of Pittsburgh
Pittsburgh, Pennsylvania 15216

Members

Robert J. Blendon, Sc.D.
Vice President
Robert Wood Johnson Foundation
P.O. Box 2316
Princeton, New Jersey 08540

L. David Carley, Ph.D.
President
Medical College of Wisconsin
561 North 15th Street
Milwaukee, Wisconsin 53233

Frank J. Hoenemeyer
Executive Vice President

Prudential Insurance Company
Prudential Plaza
Newark, New Jersey 07101

Gordon K. MacLeod, M.D.
Chairman and Professor
Health Services Administration
Graduate School of Public Health
University of Pittsburgh
Pittsburgh, Pennsylvania 15261

Harry M. Malm
President
Lutheran Hospital

Home Society of America, Inc.
70 N. Fifth Street
Fargo, North Dakota 58102

Jack L. Melchor Ph.D.
Investment Consultant
Westwind Properties
170 State Street, Suite 210B
Los Altos, California 94022

Morton D. Miller
Vice Chairman of the Board
Equitable Life Assurance Society of
   the U.S.
1285 Avenue of the Americas
New York, New York 10019

Mark Perlman, Ph.D.
The University Professor of Economics
University of Pittsburgh
P.O. Box 7230

Oakland Station
Pittsburgh, Pennsylvania 15213

William J. Swanson
Financial Advisor
1860 Oak Knoll Lane
Menlo Park, California 94025

Kerr L. White, M.D.
Director
Institute for Health Care Studies
United Hospital Fund of New York
3 East 54th Street
New York, New York 10022

Bernard C. Ziegler
Chairman of the Board
B.C. Ziegler and Company
215 Main Street
West Bend, Wisconsin 53095

UNIVERSITY OF PITTSBURGH
FACULTY SUPPORT

George A. Huber, J.D.
Lecturer, Health Services Administration
Graduate School of Public Health
University of Pittsburgh
Special Assistant to the President for
   Legal Affairs
University Health Center of Pittsburgh
Pittsburgh, Pennsylvania 15261

FEDERAL ADVISORY GROUP

Kenneth M. Endicott, M.D.
Administrator
Health Resources Administration
U.S. Department of Health,
    Education and Welfare
Room 1005, Parklawn Building
5600 Fishers Lane
Rockville, Maryland 20852

Harold Margulies, M.D.
Deputy Administrator
Health Resources Administration
U.S. Department of Health,
    Education and Welfare
Room 1005, Parklawn Building
5600 Fishers Lane
Rockville, Maryland 20852

William A. Lybrand, Ph.D.
Associate Administrator
Health Resources Administration
U.S. Department of Health,
    Education and Welfare
Room 1005, Parklawn Building
5600 Fishers Lane
Rockville, Maryland 20852

Daniel Zwick
Associate Administrator
Office of Planning, Evaluation and
    Legislation
Health Resources Administration
U.S. Department of Health,
    Education and Welfare
Parklawn Building
5600 Fishers Lane
Rockville, Maryland 20852

Thomas McCarthy, Ph.D.
Deputy Associate Administrator
Office of Scientific Affairs
Health Resources Administration
U.S. Department of Health,
    Education and Welfare
Parklawn Building
5600 Fishers Lane
Rockville, Maryland 20852

Contents

Foreword

Nathan J. Stark

The University of Pittsburgh bids you welcome. It is good to have you with us for these three days. I am Nathan Stark, your conference chairman. When I am not working on assignment from the Health Resources Administration and from my good friend, Dr. Ken Endicott, I work at being the vice chancellor for the six Schools of the Health Professions at the University of Pittsburgh and as president of the University Health Center of Pittsburgh with its seven hospitals. In either case, I am very much concerned with the health industry, and the focus of this conference is crucially important in that area.

In considering the subject of capital investment in the medical industry, I think that we should be mindful of five key objectives or guidelines.

The first is *integrity that involves both analysis and synthesis.*

As you are aware, this conference is sponsored by the University of Pittsburgh—a university that shares a general tradition with all academic institutions but also aspires to its own particular forms of excellence. Integrity is part and parcel of the academic tradition as we see it. While we are concerned with what is popular and political and practical, we are also concerned with the whole truth—not the expedient aspects of the truth. In other words, we seek not only to *analyze* aspects of the truth for their logic and insight, but also to *synthesize* the parts to make a comprehensive "whole truth." Doing both for so complex a thing as a multi-billion dollar industry is no small goal.

The second key objective is *choice, or the balancing of short-term cost-efficiency with the flexibility of the system.*

We should explore the capital financing considerations that can bring soundness to the modalities of the health care systems as they exist or as they are likely to develop in this country. And we should point out the areas of critical choice in the development of the medical care industry. How we handle these choices can improve the short-term cost-efficiency of the entire system, including operating and capital costs, while also allowing for flexibility within the system.

The third key point is that *there are four kinds of capital investing to be studied.*

A steering committee has been working on the organization of this conference since June 1975. We have had several meetings, and we have thoroughly discussed one extensive working paper. From that discussion, I identify these four kinds of capital problems:

A. *Bricks and mortar*, involving the location and construction of medical indus-try facilities. These facilities range from hospitals to clinics, from research centers and laboratories and schools to administrative offices where plans and costs are processed.

B. *Equipment procurement and replacement.* Here we have a very important problem. It is the problem of distinguishing depreciation from obsolescence. In a simple world, it is possible to pass on to the ultimate consumers their share of the cost of equipment's wearing out. In the technology of this in-dustry, however, the rate of obsolescence that involves technological replace-ment seems to outpace planned rates of depreciation. We are critically interested, therefore, in how our economy can provide rapid technological change where the costs of that change are great and where the time necessary to depreciate equipment is unpredictable.

C. Then there is the question of *human capital.* Investment in medical person-nel, both by public and private sources, is an old American tradition. The latest chapter in terms of the public contribution is the Health Professions Educational Assistance Act of 1976. But what kinds of professional person-nel should we train? Old rules about substituting more cost-efficient for less cost-efficient personnel seem to be denied in this industry. The proliferation of guilds of emerging new health professions which, rightly or wrongly, seek self-governance, limits flexibility still further. We know that a highly skilled, broadly trained person can be replaced at much less cost by one who is trained in a narrow specialty. But patients resist that change. And the diffi-culty for less trained personnel to defend themselves from patient propen-sities to sue has slowed down the processes of substitution. Moreover, shortages of creative, skilled administrative personnel seem to have slowed down the introduction of recently developed health care modalities into various locations where they are needed.

D. Finally, there is the problem of *working capital.* The problem has grown along with the rising costs of medical care. The problem has grown along with the role of capital equipment. The problem has grown since the time when workers in the field were willing, for religious or other societal reasons, to live close to the subsistence level. The problem has grown along with the cost of construction capital. When the interest rate was close to 2 or 3 percent, it was no major undertaking to finance institutions between the time that they incurred costs and the time that they were reimbursed. Now, the problem of maintaining pools of capital to support medical care institutions in their production periods has emerged as a principal challenge to capital investment in this industry.

We come now to the fourth key objective that I want to convey: the *avoidance of ideological debate.*

Throughout its discussions, the steering committee was concerned with two quite different approaches to the solution of these capital consideration problems. One solution relies upon the interaction between the desires of competing parties; the other approach is to plan fully, before the event, the allocation of all resources. The rubric for the former approach is "competitive market allocation." The rubric for the latter approach is, of course, "national or regional planning." This conference should not be an exercise in ideological exposition. We are concerned with specific questions, and we are seeking answers that will be effective both in the short-run and in the long-term future.

Finally, there is the fifth key point, a phrase that goes back to Dr. Merriam: *Experts on tap, not on top.*

It is timely to recall that the national election is now in the past. We at this conference seek to provide an integrated discussion of the ways in which the capital financing of the medical care industry can best be handled. Yet, it is not for us to make the final choice. Indeed, it is important to remember that it is not even for the executive branch of the federal government to make the final choice. Rather, it is for us to provide a discussion which the two houses of Congress can use to fashion legislation and which the executive branch can use to negotiate with the Congress.

To point out that we will not make the final decision is in no sense to denigrate the opportunity we have here. We are a national group, meeting under the auspices of an old and large university, listening to papers and criticisms prepared by individuals with considerable expertise. If we do our job properly and produce the kind of integrated document that we are capable of developing, the Congress should be appreciative, the executive branch should likewise be aided, and the general American community should be grateful.

Preface

Over a period of eighteen months, the steering committee for this conference on capital investment for health care met to evaluate Hill-Burton funding and its relationship to other approaches to health facilities funding.[1]

At the request of the Health Resources Administration, Nathan J. Stark, J.D., vice chancellor of Health Professions at the University of Pittsburgh, agreed to chair the conference steering committee. In addition to Mr. Stark, committee members were Robert J. Blendon, Sc.D., vice president of the Robert Wood Johnson Foundation; L. David Carley, Ph.D., president of the Medical College of Wisconsin; Frank J. Hoenemeyer, executive vice president of the Prudential Insurance Company; Gordon K. MacLeod, M.D., professor and chairman of the Department of Health Services Administration at the University of Pittsburgh Graduate School of Public Health; Harry M. Malm, president of the Lutheran Hospitals and Homes Society of America; Jack Melchor, investment consultant; Morton D. Miller, vice chairman of the Board for the Equitable Life Assurance Society of the United States; Mark Perlman, Ph.D., the University of Pittsburgh professor of economics; William J. Swanson, investment consultant; Kerr L. White, M.D., professor of health care organization, Johns Hopkins University; and Bernard C. Ziegler, chairman of the board for B.C. Ziegler and Company. James Shanks and Theodore C. Haaser of the Rosslyn Foundation, and Edward J. Burger, M.D., of the National Science Foundation, were also quite helpful during the steering committee proceedings.

Throughout its activities, the committee was aware of the growing concern that the health care industry was overcapitalized, particularly with respect to inpatient services, especially when compared to health maintenance organizations. Further, it was aware of the frequently expressed concern that most public hospitals—and even some private community hospitals—could not be totally supported by existing income, with or without philanthropic support. It also recognized the rapid rate of technological change without the parallel ability to ensure its appropriate use or to pay for the depreciation of diagnostic and monitoring equipment and facilities prior to their obsolescence. It was also concerned with the question of productivity resulting from the tremendous spurt in the number of health professionals entering the health care field since World War II.

The initial impetus for the conference was supplied by Kenneth M. Endicott, M.D., administrator of the Health Resources Administration, whose active lobbying was largely responsible for the stimulation of congressional interest in the project. His energy and encouragement were invaluable throughout all stages of planning.

Gratitude is expressed for the assistance and advice of Harold Margulies, M.D., William Lybrand, Ph.D., Daniel Zwick, Thomas McCarthy, Ph.D., and Marian Fox, all of the Health Resources Administration. Also, from the federal government, Harry Cain II, Ph.D., Clifton R. Gaus, Ph.D., and Stanley Wallach, Ph.D., were helpful in generating both public and private interest in the conference.

Conference participants came from all parts of the country and elsewhere in the world, and from a multitude of organizations within and without the health care industry. Sincere thanks are extended to all participants and to their respective organizations for their time and contributions.

Preparation for the conference was undertaken by the Department of Health Services Administration at the University of Pittsburgh. The dedication of department members and their eagerness to contribute to the team effort were greatly appreciated. Special thanks are extended to Janet S. Phillips and Barbara T. Lynn of the department's administrative staff for their contributions.

NOTES

1. The conference was supported through a project contract (HRA–75–0208) between the Health Resources Administration, United States Department of Health, Education and Welfare, and the University of Pittsburgh.

Project Faculty Staff
Gordon K. MacLeod
Mark Perlman
George A. Huber

Chancellor's Welcome

Wesley W. Posvar

I am here to welcome you with great respect, humility, and admiration, as you are outstanding leaders, scholars, thinkers, businessmen, and government officials who are concerned with the problems of health care and the costs of health care. As a matter of fact, I am having a meeting of my executive committee of the university Board of Trustees elsewhere in this building at the same time, and I have to leave to rejoin them and report to them in a couple of minutes, so that some of them might have the opportunity to audit the sessions of this meeting this afternoon. Their interest in the subject is very high, indeed, as is their responsibility for the subject.

I should say, for myself, that while you are concerned with the macro aspects of the problem—the cost of health facilities—at this level and at the level of higher education nationally, cost is one of my principal concerns and principal problems. I just came, in the last week, from two major meetings, one of the Association of American University Presidents and another of the Presidents of the State Universities of America. Both of these have very active committees, of which I am a member, on health manpower and health care. We have been actively working, lobbying, and advocating the interests of health care in Washington in recent months, and we intend to do a great deal more in the future. I can say nothing to this group that will inform you about the subject that you are facing, except to make the brief observation, obvious to us all, that we are dealing with fundamental and conflicting forces. We are in a period of rising expectations; the people have Cadillac tastes without the nation having the means to pay for them. We are confronted with the possibility of spending another $50 or $100 billion a year for health care in this country, and many studies show that whatever that money may provide, it probably will not provide much better health care.

We are facing demands for more sophisticated methods and facilities and advanced research. Health care equipment and facilities rapidly become obsolete; the economic life of our equipment and of our facilities does not match its cost. Threats of malpractice make practitioners all the more eager for the most modern and the safest kind of care. Of course, in addition to all of this, insurance has distorted the marketplace for health care, and has altered the attitudes of patients and hospitals and doctors toward health care in terms of its true and its apparent cost.

Our models of ownership and construction and capital investment are diverse: public ownership, corporate investment and mixed systems, such as we have here in Pittsburgh. As you well know, the cost of our medical care in this country is already up to $140 billion a year. It is one of the giant sectors of our society and it has not yet come in for the kind of analytical treatment that we have focused on defense, and are now focusing on energy and transportation. This conference represents an important advance in bringing about that analysis. It is a commitment on the part of the university, of our funding agency, HEW, and of all of you to become deeply involved in this task. I shall be involved in it as well. I would like to compliment Nathan Stark and Gordon MacLeod for the tremendous effort that they have put forth to make this conference possible. I wish you a very happy time here, and I welcome you again.

✳ *Chapter 1*

Marketplace and Regulatory Trade-offs

Gordon K. MacLeod

The University of Pittsburgh Conference on Capital Investment, held November 19-21, 1976, represented the culmination of numerous steering committee meetings and small group sessions of authors, session chairmen, federal officials, and staff from the Graduate School of Public Health at the university. The conferees were asked to evaluate health care capital financing trade-offs, experience, and trends in the United States in an effort to determine available options, whether in the government or the private sector, for harnessing the extraordinary projected rise in capital costs, unique in medical care history. At the same time, consideration was given to preserving an appropriate level of medical care as it is viewed by both consumers and providers, to containing the trend toward higher prices, and to decreasing the rate of encroachment by health on the Gross National Product.

As the conference took shape, its title: "The Evaluation of Other Approaches Than Hill-Burton Funding to the Capital Financing of Health Facilities" could have been paraphrased to read "A discourse on the balance between increasing reliance upon citizen choice with regard to the modality of health service and a growing dependency upon governmental standards to contain the cost of delivery of health care services." While each of the papers was to show both perspectives, the topics chosen for examination at the conference were readily grouped into four categories. The first covered both the recent history of health care financing and the current trade-offs between the free market and regulatory mechanisms. The second examined the effect of human resources and health maintenance organizations on capital formation. The third explored the history and experience of philanthropy and of private corporate investment in the health care industry. And the fourth inspected present and future capital markets for the health care industry.

1

Each of the authors and discussants was asked to cover specific capital areas such as (a) the fixed cost requirements for the construction of hospital and all other health care facilities—e.g., clinics, nursing homes, surgicenters, etc., including public, private and proprietary organizations; (b) equipment costs; (c) the cost of human resources; and (d) operating costs.

Because of the growing vested interest of all levels of government in health care it was also important to scrutinize the impact of federal legislation on citizen choice of health care modalities. The steering committee also deemed it necessary to review the impact of state regulation upon operating capital through rate setting boards and through certificate of need legislation.

We faced, then, a series of issues from regulation to free choice. On the regulatory side, we looked at the issue of earnings from Medicare payments as an essential source of initial and growth capital and we raised specific questions about the adequacy of straight-line depreciation allowances based on historical costs through Medicare and about the possibility of regionally pooled capital payments for depreciation. We also considered options such as tax exempt local bonds, prospective reimbursement, and reimbursement of institutional fiscal needs by insurance carriers. Few of these problems emanating from financing issues were addressed in the National Health Planning and Resources Development Act (P.L. 93-641) which established federal guidelines for the health systems agencies.

On the side of free choice, the United States is unique among nations in offering an opportunity to express a preference between two distinct patterns of health care delivery to a small but growing number of citizens: between the traditional fee-for-service reimbursement pattern or an alternative prepayment plan now commonly called a health maintenance organization. This alternative differs from fee-for-service payment, not only in cost, utilization and outcome, but also in consumer participation in governance. Also, these two patterns manifest differences over issues of full disclosure of financial status, of professional organization, and of ensuring accessibility and availability of comprehensive health care services including preventive care.

While each of the authors presenting papers at this conference was advised to address the interaction between regulation and freedom of choice, the discussants for each paper were given the opportunity to present their perception of how well the author covered the assigned topic. All of the papers were reviewed by project staff from the University of Pittsburgh prior to the conference; additions and changes were suggested and made by the authors wherever appropriate.

Mr. Wolkstein was asked to examine the principal legislation affecting health care facilities capital financing since the 1940s. He described the shift from philanthropic support, through government subsidy, to meeting capital requirements from third party reimbursement. Dr. Enthoven spoke strongly about the need for free choice among competing systems of care which would be self-regulating. He rejected the idea that government actions contain incentives for decision makers to make the amount and kinds of investment that will supply the socially desirable amount of hospital services. Dr. Merriam called attention to the importance of continuing and assured sources of payment for services as a basis for capital funding and to the need for legislation authorizing funding of research and experimentation on methods for health care reimbursement.

Mr. Joe, Mr. Needleman, and Mr. Lewin pointed out the need for future federal policy initiatives which combine the positive elements of the free market with those of public regulation. They called for limiting the risk to investors for facilities subsequently identified as unneeded. One of the features of their approach is to place providers at some risk for poor management and for investment in unneeded facilities and equipment. Professor Havighurst recognized the importance of permitting meaningful competition to stimulate and guide cost containment, arguing that tax incentives which discourage cost cutting, as well as legal and professional restraints on private cost control efforts, should be removed, so that more lower cost alternatives can be made available to consumers who have reason to economize. Dr. Evans sought the root cause of the factors which make hospital costs so high and those which underlie the current escalation of costs such as underoccupancy, overcapitalization, overcapacity, excessive gadgetry, and unnecessary procedures being performed on patients, including enormously expensive "heroic medicine" for short-term life support. He observed that cost containment is also income containment and that policies directed at controlling cost increases must limit either the number or the income of providers.

Dr. Ginzberg highlighted the lack of effective legislation for meeting the diverse social goals and public policies relating to health care services. He referred to the apparent lack of a resource-economizing motive driving health manpower legislation. He cited the fact that investments in health manpower, substituting new health workers for higher level professionals, have seldom made even modest gains in resource efficiency although other studies have suggested the opposite. Dr. Rosett pointed out that despite the seemingly chaotic state of the health care industry, it may be efficiently producing health care in just about the amounts that the public wants to buy. He argued that the very multiplicity of programs, suggesting inefficiency, may produce just the reverse through competition among various programs. The concern remains, however, that the shift from the private to the public sector may rob the future of productive capacity and individual liberties. Dr. Lampman concurred with the input-output analysis of Dr. Ginzberg. While a tripling of inputs of labor, capital, and intermediate products (e.g., supplies and materials) is comparable to the nation's output of health services, relatively small changes have occurred in the stock of such key items as acute care hospital beds and physicians. But, he is not persuaded that the health care industry has overinvested in physical and human capital.

Mr. Vohs and Mr. Palmer pointed out that under the Kaiser-Permanente capital financing policy, total debt is limited to net worth. Economies are achieved through large-scale operations. Earnings are an essential source of long-term capital. They proposed that government, through reimbursement mechanisms, include in its payment for services an appropriate level of earnings in addition to cost. Mr. Brindle strongly endorsed the hospital-based prepaid group practice plans and compared the capital expenditure experience from a number of prepaid group practice plans. He suggested liberalization of HMO support from all levels of government and insurance companies, as well as reclassification of the tax status of HMOs so that charitable foundations, organizations, and individuals might also contribute to their support. Mr. Sibery's paper, read by Mr. Berman, emphasized the capital formation problem and the need for some mechanism better than the existing planning agencies to direct the right amount of capital to the right place. Reform of the financing system is needed so that each class of purchaser must pay, at a minimum, its own unique economic cost.

Mr. J. Hill pointed out that investor-owned hospitals have received inequitable treatment under existing legislation, which tends to favor the more traditional form, nonprofit organizations. He suggested seven policy areas for review: the problem of regulation; the rate of return for investor-owned hospitals; present tax law inequities; financing of high technology equipment; industrial revenue bond financing; malpractice insurance; and the cost-effectiveness of building codes. Dr. Feldstein believes that we do not need more investment in hospital care, but, rather, more emphasis on extensive coinsurance for middle and upper income households. Ms. Wrenn stated that the record, the size, and the proven managerial capability in investor-owned hospitals make it feasible to channel private risk capital into them in the form of equity investment.

Mr. Terenzio reported on a survey that he conducted on philanthropy as a source of capital for the needs of the health care field. In the present economic atmosphere, he points out, the loss of tax revenue from philanthropy is the only significant cost to government. Dr. Lipset concluded that the historical cultural sources of support for philanthropy and voluntary associational activity in America still have vitality for philanthropy. Mr. Hernandez implied that the relative importance of philanthropy to meet capital needs will continue to diminish, but he observed its potential importance as venture capital for high risk modalities.

Mr. Clapp and Mr. Spector studied the American capital market and its relationship to the capital needs of the health care field. They observed that the shift of funding from private capital to public funds occurred mostly at the state and local level. Even so, institutional providers of health care are now depending less upon philanthropy and the federal government and more upon debt financing. Mr. R. Williams, reading Mr. Bays' paper, discussed the idea that health care institutions must improve the management of their financial positions to achieve lower costs of capital and an adequate share of funds in the public capital markets. Also, leasing capital may be a viable alternative to competing for funds in the capital market. Dr. Bosworth concluded that a capital crisis is not a significant problem for the health care field. But if, indeed, the health care industry has excess capacity, then future investment should not be encouraged through credit subsidies such as loan guarantees, interest subsidies, and increased reliance on tax-exempt bonds.

Mr. Kelling and Mr. Williams do not foresee a "capital gap" for bricks and mortar construction of community hospitals within the next five years, but are concerned that the ability to attract investment capital may be inadvertently impaired by federal and state cost control efforts. Mr. Cathcart cautioned public policymakers to recognize that health care facilities are not incurring substantial new fixed costs; administrators are further confronted with government proposals to place a ceiling upon any increase in federal payments for hospital services. Mr. L. Hill warned state government not to limit or to stop capital resources for hospitals through certificate of need legislation. He also warned against state regulation of hospitals that would render them financially risky by making it difficult for them to live within interest rates set by state agencies.

In summary, the following concerns were identified at the University of Pittsburgh Conference:

1. Private debt financing is playing an increasingly important role in satisfying capital requirements. There is great concern that debt financing may be in jeopardy since the certainty of income flow upon which debt financing depends is subject to mounting public criticism about the ineffectiveness of current reimbursement mechanisms in controlling health care costs.
2. Large amounts of capital are needed in the formation and growth of HMOs. The paper describing the financing of the Kaiser Foundation Health Plan documented for the first time the capital investment policies of that most successful type of HMO. The authors stressed the need for such a nonprofit organization to be allowed to include provision for creating and servicing debt capital in their net income.
3. Great concern was raised over the current network of regulation, tax exemption, and public subsidy which has shaped the recent growth of the health care industry. One participant was particularly interested in demonstrating the inequity and inefficiency associated with current tax regulation. He specifically noted that most of the population pays for medical services with untaxed dollars through fringe benefit arrangements whereas others buy services with taxed dollars. For example, foreborne tax revenue by virtue of employer and invidivual tax deductions for health insurance premiums may amount to at least a $6 billion "loss" in tax revenue to the federal government.
4. Current regulations do not provide incentives for cost-efficiency. One view from the perspective of investor-owned health care institutions specified the particular regulations which were felt to stifle the growth of private enterprise. Another view is that the existing regulations have to be modified in order to make the industry more effective (i.e., increasing service to presently neglected groups while at the same time not significantly diminishing the service it

offers to others). New means by government together with the private sector must be found to slow the rate of cost and price increases. The conferees believe that federal regulation alone is not going to be able to control the costs of the health care industry.

5. There was a clear call for physicians to improve the organization of practice and to contain the number of services. There was a belief that all sectors of society, including the financial community, are concerned about the poor quality of health financing information, the need for health outcome measures, the rapidly increasing number of physicians, the inequitable distribution of men, women, and minorities within the health professions, and the confusion over cost/benefit issues. Attention was also focused on public and professional unwillingness to substitute new health workers for high level professionals.

The conference seemed to accomplish what it set out to do. It was designed to reveal the changing patterns of capital funding of the health care industry in the United States and to explore alternative patterns of capital formation. A unique assemblage of new and old voices presented their views on health care financing and addressed current and future trends in capital formation, patterns of equity funding and tax policy; they also reviewed the impact of health maintenance organizations, reimbursement mechanisms, and human capital. In addition to the authors and discussants, the conference brought together a wide range of professional and health insurance interests, along with commercial and investment banking interests and others who had not previously been participants in this kind of discussion but who are recognized for their imaginative insights. The prepared papers and the general discussion touched upon the entire spectrum of capital formation, most of which, if not all, must be considered in developing policy related to health care financing.

✳ *Chapter 2*

The Impact of Legislation on Capital Development for Health Facilities

Irwin Wolkstein

Capital development for health facilities in the United States has gone through three stages. Originally, hospitals, for which some two-thirds of facility construction expenditures are made, were supported primarily by philanthropy for private institutions and by government investment in its own facilities. In view of this history, it is not surprising that the preservation of philanthropy in health has had a high priority, and the ability to donate has always been protected against progressive income and estate taxes.

The second stage of health capital development emerged after the Great Depression and after World War II has put a virtual stop to hospital construction for some fifteen years. At the same time, the revolution in technology in health care began to affect greatly the perceptions of how much health capital was needed, and private sources seemed incapable of meeting this need. Meanwhile, a great debate over national health insurance took place and the move to expand the welfare system gained strength. While national health insurance was defeated, it seemed quite natural, under the prevailing economic circumstances, for the federal government to provide funds to both private and government sponsors for making adequate hospital facilities available to everyone and to try to make sure that such facilities existed throughout every congressional district, even in rural ones. This seemed a proper political decision for the time.

The priority given to direct government support for health capital development gradually receded, and payment for patient care and funds for operations became increasingly important in capital development giving rise to the third and present stage in the process of capital development in which operating funds, including those paid for care through Medicare and Medicaid, played a large part in meeting capital needs.

Presently, the criticism is increasingly being made that an excessive emphasis is being given to expensive investment in new technology. The concern about the need for restriction of cost increases and for setting priorities on development suggests that we may be entering a fourth stage of capital development and that this stage may be characterized by efforts that will be made to control capital expenditures.

SOURCES OF CAPITAL

The analysis of capital development for health facilities has to begin with identification of the sources of such capital. In this paper I shall, therefore, discuss these sources, describe the kinds of actions that government has taken to affect capital development relating the actions to the sources affected, and then discuss the specific legislation that has been enacted and its consequences. I shall deal primarily with investment in facilities and only briefly with investment in human capital.

The primary sources of capital may be alternately described as being of two types, public or private, or of five types, some of which are mixed public and private. These five are:

1. Investment by government in facilities which it owns.
2. Philanthropy.
3. Government grants-in-aid for capital development of nongovernmental facilities.
4. New equity investment (i.e., equity from funds developed outside of the facilities).
5. Funds from operations (i.e., internally generated funds).

While, historically, first philanthropy and then government grants-in-aid for construction have provided major portions of the total investment in the physical plants of health facilities, in recent years funds from operations have become the principal source of new capital. Hospital depreciation costs alone amounted to about $1 1/2 billion in 1974. While about two-thirds of medical facility capital consists of hospital plant, depreciation in other parts of the health industry constitutes a substantial addition to the total depreciation expense incurred, which probably totals over $2 billion a year. Funds from operation—internally generated funds—consist of net income plus depreciation, plus funds from assets that are sold, so that internally generated funds that may be used for capital purposes exceed depreciation costs by a significant amount. Of these, not all net revenues are retained internally; some are paid out to investors.

Of the two ways that internally generated funds can be used for capital purposes—(1) a prospective approach through the accumulation of reserves to finance future investment in capital facilities, and (2) a retrospective approach through which operating funds are used to pay interest and to retire debt that is incurred when purchasing capital—the retrospective approach has become the method of choice. The data show this to be true for hospitals, and, in my opinion, throughout the health field generally. The result is that the reinvestment of funds that are received in reimbursement of depreciation expense does not merely keep the plant assets at their previous levels, but, rather, is a major source of funds for expanding plant. With funds from operations as the major contributor to capital development, with debt becoming such a major factor in health facility investment, and with funds from reimbursement by third parties for health services being the major source of hospital income, the specifics of reimbursement have become vital not only to capital development, but to the very survival of hospitals.

Long-term debt is now equal to one-fourth of the assets of short-term hospitals. If reimbursement does not meet the sometimes heavy requirements for debt repayment, the result is default. The principal role of philanthropy and grants has become that of helping to provide down payments that are needed for borrowing funds and to provide a chance for community input. The amounts of philanthropy and grants that are involved are relatively small, but their actual or potential leverage is large, as I shall illustrate later.

Borrowing is not a primary source of capital, although it now plays a very important role in capital development. Interest on borrowing must be paid and the amount borrowed must be repaid from some other source. Normally, loan payments are made from internally generated funds. The source of funds for loan payments is then the primary source of the generated capital, and borrowing is a secondary source, a mechanism for facilitating, generally for speeding, capital generation and, over a period of years, equalizing the amount of funds that must be raised.

Internal generation of funds is also a key to the investment of new equity. Equity capital will not be invested without expectation of an appropriate return. Internally generated capital provides this return through its net revenue component. For nonprofit facilities there is little, if any, difference in the uses of net revenues as compared with the uses of depreciation.

Operating funds in hospitals are derived primarily from reimbursement for care, which, because of its nature, makes financing of capital additions somewhat different in the health field than in most other industries. Capital additions in other industries, for example, are normally supported to a greater degree than they are among hospitals through the excess of income over cost. A second difference is that competition is a greater restraint in other industries than it is among hospitals on the extent to which capital costs can be included in total costs and reflected in prices. Hospitals can sometimes entirely finance capital additions by increasing their gross operating incomes without the need for additional profit as part of the financing. When a hospital makes an investment in additional plant, its operating income may rise automatically, either through cost reimbursement or through charges that are set in relation to cost, thereby covering its new interest and depreciation costs and enabling it to finance debt.

Because the hospital industry has a strong tendency to grow, debt instruments with minimum down payments to permit early investment are more attractive than is a slower accumulation of reserves for construction. Reserve accumulation not only slows investment, but the hospital also foregoes considerable income when it delays investment and when income is related to costs that rise when the investment is made. This, I believe, has been an important factor in changes in capital development in the health field ever since third party payments became prevalent in the health care system.

The development of capital in the health care system has taken some drastic turns over time. The change in capital development started with the relatively recent accelerated growth of scientific medicine which gave rise to much higher costs of care and much greater need for capital, both of which were accompanied by a surge in demand for those new services that were perceived as being able to sustain or prolong life. These were among the forces that produced the third party payment system for care, including both private insurance and government programs that pay for care in private hospitals.

In the days when a hospital was the equivalent of an almshouse, or little more, philanthropy and government investment in its own facilities accounted for essentially all capital investment in health care. The change in the nature of hospital care occurred at the same time as did a large rise in the income of patients who then became capable, through prepayment mechanisms, of financing much of the more expensive care that came to be provided. While there are scant financial data for very early periods—and even the data for later years are not fully satisfactory—it is significant that in fiscal year 1929, of the $209 million estimated to have been spent on construction (not including investment in capital equipment when no construction was involved), about half came from government funds spent on government hospitals and most of the other half from philanthropy. Construction investment almost disappeared during the depression, and during World War II investment was small, and made primarily by the government for military purposes. After World War II, the backlog resulting from some fifteen years of depression and wartime restriction, and the impetus of new medical technology, gave rise to a boom in the construction of health facilities, especially private general hospitals, many of which received government grants. In FY 1950, of the $737 million invested in construction of medical facilities, $522 million came from government funds much of it in the form of grants-in-aid.[1]

The government's share of medical facility construction expenditures has since fallen sharply, but it is still large. In FY 1975, of the $4.5 billion in construction expenditures, about 40 percent was appropriated for this purpose by the government, but, of the government share, two-thrids was invested directly in government-owned hospitals.[2]

As the funds from government diminished, borrowing instruments became more and more important in capital plans although it is not clear which is cause and which is effect—i.e., the reduction in government money may have resulted, in part, from the availability of other sources and, conversely, the reduction in grants may have produced a need to seek money elsewhere. At the same time, the growth in health insurance and the enactment of Medicare and Medicaid resulted in a degree of assurance of a reliable hospital income flow that made loans to hospitals appear to be safe and, therefore, attractive to financial institutions.

An estimate for 1962 is that 12 percent of new hospital plants was financed by borrowing.[3] By 1969, some 40 percent of the funds for construction of non-profit hospitals was borrowed, and 63 percent of construction funds for investor-owned facilities came from borrowing.[4] In 1974, debt comprised two-thirds of the construction funds for nonprofit hospitals as well as for investor-owned hospitals (Table 2-1). Internally generated reserves added 15 percent to the non-profit funds, so that funds from operations will probably account for over 80 percent of the total of 1974 hospital construction funds when prospective and retrospective payments are both taken into account. As a result of increased borrowing over a period of years, long-term debt in short-term, nonfederal hospitals in 1974 amounted to some $10 billion, about 25 percent of the total assets of those hospitals.[5]

TYPES OF GOVERNMENT ACTIONS

Table 2-2 shows the basic forms of actions that government takes to affect capital development and the capital sources which each action affects. I have identified seven types of government actions: (1) direct investment; (2) grants; (3) tax actions; (4) loan provisions; (5) reimbursement provisions; (6) conditions applied in relation to other governmental action; and (7) conditions applied to all facilities. As Table 2-2 indicates, some actions can affect all sources of capital while others are quite limited in result. The first two of these types of actions—investments and grants—constitute direct action by government to provide capital funds, while hospital loan and reimbursement provisions involve a kind of indirect contribution by government to capital. Taxes and conditions imposed on facilities involve attempts to affect the decisions of individuals and/or organizations on whether to invest and, if so, in what areas.

It should be understood that there may be a difference between the effect that is intended by an action and the effect that is achieved. One reason is that once money is fed into a system its final use cannot always be controlled. Take, for example, an institution that budgets $10 million in expenditures, of which $8 million would go for services to patients who pay their way, $1 million for charity care, and $1 million for capital additions. If patients who pay their way are expected to pay $9 million, the institution will fully meet its budgeted requirements if it receives grant funds of $1 million, whether that million is said

Table 2-1.   Distribution of Sources of Funds for Community Hospital Construction Begun in 1974

Hospital Classification	Total Funding (millions)	Percent				Borrowing			
		Total	Grants and Appropriations	Philanthropy	Reserves and Owner's Equity	Total	Tax Exempt	Government Guaranteed	Other
Total	$2,943	100.0	13.8	10.6	14.2	61.4	29.9	10.9	20.6
Nongovernmental, nonprofit	2,212	100.0	5.4	13.2	14.9	67.1	28.6	13.4	25.1
Investor-owned	52	100.0	4.5	0.4	29.3	67.1	32.3	0.0	34.8
State and local government	679	100.0	41.6	2.8	10.9	45.9	37.6	3.4	4.9

Source: Sallie Manley, "AHA Research Capsules No. 19, Sources of Funding for Construction," *Hospitals*, December 1975, p. 108.

Table 2-2. Types of Government Actions Affecting Capital Development in Health by Capital Source Affected

Government Actions	Source Affected				
	Investment by Government in its Facilities	*Philanthropy*	*Government Grants*	*New Equity Investment*	*Funds from Operations*
Government investment in its facilities	X				
Government grants			X		
Tax provisions		X		X	X
Loan provisions				X	X
Reimbursement provisions	X	X	X	X	X
Conditions applied to all facilities*	X	X	X	X	X
Conditions applied to grants, loans and reimbursement		X	X	X	X

*Including franchising for new facilities and rate review.

to be intended for charity care, capital, or is divided between two purposes. Another reason why the effect of any action to add to funds is not fully known and controllable is that funds may be created that substitute, in part, for funds that could otherwise have come from another source. A third reason is that the conditions under which the funds are given may raise the cost of the project involved so that part of the contributions pays for this added cost.

Numerous laws have been enacted in an effort to put into effect the actions which have been discussed. The motivations for such legislation are not always clearly recorded. Even when they are, the written words may be mere rationalizations and not the results of true conviction. Seldom does interest in advancing the causes of a congressman's own district and constituents creep into the record, yet such motivations are often present. Moreover, the record seldom reveals any doubts about the expected result. This omission may occur, not because lawmakers are always certain that they have made perfect decisions, but because most explanations of law are recorded in committee reports and floor statements that precede votes and are part of the campaign to gain support necessary for passage. As a result, the true opinions of the sponsors of a bill cannot always be determined.

It is also hazardous to guess the consequences of any given action. Causes are hard to identify when so many events occur at the same time. For example, the factors that affected health care changes after World War II included, in addition to the legislation that was enacted, the greatly depleted supply of resources at the outset of the period, the expansion of medical technology, a period of un-precedented prosperity, a particularly significant social and economic change in some of the poorest agricultural areas, and a great increase in coverage of private health insurance. In addition, several different government programs were in operation simultaneously. The consequences of any one legislative action are very difficult to isolate either from other legislative results or from the social and economic setting.

THE EVER-PRESENT PROGRAMS FOR CAPITAL DEVELOPMENT

Government Facility Investment

One of the most important actions of government in capital development has been, and continues to be, government investment in its own facilities. In 1974, about one-half of all of the 1.5 million hospital beds, 29 percent of the 1 million short-term beds, and over 90 percent of the half-million long-term beds were government owned. There were 136,000 federally-owned beds and over 600,000 beds owned by state or local governments.[6] The federal government spent an estimated $319 million on the construction of federal facilities in fiscal year 1974; the greatest part, $246 million, was for the modernization and replacement of hospitals and for environmental improvements although other construction funds went for new hospitals, for long-term care, for ambulatory care, and for health research facilities.

The three major federal agencies involved in construction are the Department of Defense (DOD) and the Veterans Administration (VA), each spending over $115 million in that year, and the Indian Health Service, which spent at some-what less than half the level of each of the other two. While expenditures on defense and veterans facilities have risen, they have declined, in significant part, as a factor in health care because the constituency for these facilities has been shifted through the Civilian Health and Medical Program of the Uniformed Ser-vices (CHAMPUS) and other programs, to privately-owned facilities.[7] Perhaps the primary characteristic of the programs that sponsor federal hospitals is that each is intended for a specific constituency. A minor step away from caring for only a specific constituency was taken in the case of the veterans hospitals when, under very limited circumstances, they were allowed to share certain specialized facilities with private hospitals. The case of the Indian Health Service is somewhat different from that of the DOD or the VA and may be more nearly the equivalent of local government hospitals that have acted as the last resort of the poor. There are grounds for argument that federal hospitals with single constituencies run contrary to the concept that underlies planning—an integrated single system of health care for all people—and seem to pose a potential contradiction to federal planning policies. Political relationships with the constituency involved may be a consideration in the retention of separate systems. However, the reality of federal support of planning, or other moves toward effectiveness, may be doubted if federal facilities do not mesh well with the planning programs or the Professional Standards Review Organization (PSRO) system.

Federal hospitals constitute an exception to the normal system of reimbursement. They do not receive significant reimbursement from third parties and very little directly from patients. There is little, if any, internal generation of capital in these facilities. As a consequence, the controls instituted by third party reimbursers generally are not applicable to federal facilities.

State and local government constitue a much larger factor than does the federal government in ownership of health facilities and their construction. In fiscal years 1974 and 1975, approximately $1 billion a year was spent on construction of facilities owned by state and local governments.[8] While beds owned by such governments have declined sharply—from a little over 900,000 in 1965[9] to a little over 600,000 in 1974[10]—they still comprise some two-fifths of all beds, with long-term beds making up two-thirds of the state and local government total. Long-term facilities are often quite inadequate because long-term care is underfinanced, although the rapid growth in nursing home beds suggests that capital is not short for at least some types of long-term care facilities. There seems to be a general tendency, not limited to the United States, to underfinance the treatment of patients whose primary need is for care rather than cure, i.e., for ministration to illnesses that are not amenable to cure. Very little long-term care is covered by health insurance.

State and local government short-term hospitals include a wide variety of institutions, comprising some whose operations differ hardly at all from private community hospitals, some that are closely affiliated with medical schools, and some whose primary function is to serve the poor. Government long-term hospitals generally serve a population that is unable to pay. Isolating the poor from other income classes, as often occurs in state and local government hospitals, would seem to be counterproductive in planning an integrated health system, and seems also to be questionable from other points of view—acceptability to patients, consistency with theories on how society should treat its less fortunate members, and the probable effect on adequacy of care when services and facilities are designed exclusively for persons who cannot pay. The decline in importance of state and local government hospitals that occurred, in part because of improvement in treatment of psychiatric illness and tuberculosis and in part because of a decline in the number of poor who must use these facilities of last resort, is a welcome trend.

Tax Provisions

The longest standing provisions for government aid to health organizations have been provided through the tax system. The forms of tax aid fall into the following categories:

1. Tax provisions related to deductions for philanthropic giving
   a. Personal income tax
   b. Estate tax
   c. Corporation income taxes
   d. Tax on foundations
2. Exemption of philanthropic giving from gift tax
3. Exemption of nonprofit organizations from tax
   a. Corporate income tax
   b. Property tax
4. Proprietary organization capital investment allowances
   a. Investment tax credit
   b. Accelerated depreciation deductibility for tax purposes
5. Exemption from income tax of interest on state and local government bonds that are issued for the financing of nonprofit health facilities
6. Exemption of employer payment of employee health insurance premiums from personal income tax and income tax deduction for health insurance premiums.

The tax provisions have a number of different functions. First, they support philanthropic contributions for health purposes, which totaled about $4 billion in 1974. While three-quarters of a billion dollars was provided for the express purpose of constructing health facilities,[11] the effect of the total donations on the capacity of the health industry to develop capital, as opposed to meeting other needs or reducing prices, is less clear because the ultimate effect of giving on capital development is likely to be greater than are the funds designated specifically to support construction. I make this assertion because if donations fully cover the patient bad debts of an institution, it is likely to be in a good position to make capital investments even if it receives no donations earmarked for capital. The tax provision that has the most marked effect on philanthropy is the one that makes charitable donations deductible for persons itemizing deductions on their personal income tax returns. Martin Feldstein estimated that eliminating this charitable deduction would reduce individual giving to hospitals by 50 percent.[12]

The importance of philanthropy today is associated less with the size of the total contributions than with the major points of its concern:[13]

1. Venture-capital support for the formulation of new projects or ideas.
2. Projects that go beyond the limits of current governmental funding policies.

3. Underwriting the losses of hospitals and clinics that serve low-income patients without adequate coverage.
4. Support of out-of-hospital medical care programs.

The importance of philanthropy in capital development may go well beyond the effect of the dollars contributed because frequently the philanthropic giver influences the expenditures of internally generated funds that may be many times larger than the philanthropy. In other words, philanthropy may, and sometimes does, exercise leverage. The area planning agencies that are considered to be most effective have referred to the acceptance of their recommendation by major donors as being an important source of their power because, without the donations, the projects became impossible.[14]

The second function of some tax actions is to reduce the costs of the organizations that are involved or to increase the cash flow to the organization. If costs are reduced, the institution may either lower its charges or increase its net revenues. Increased net provides a base for capital development. The net revenues of nongovernmental, not-for-profit, community hospitals amounted to $455 million in 1974.[15] If this net revenue were taxed under rules applying to profit institutions, it would be subject to a tax rate of nearly 50 percent. It should be noted that taxing the net revenues would not necessarily reduce these revenues to half their present total because hospitals might well increase charges, and reimbursement provisions might be changed to compensate for tax costs. If revenues were not adjusted to compensate for such taxes, hospitals would find themselves less able to provide services on which they absorb losses and less able to develop new capital. In other words, the operating margin of nonprofit hospitals is so small—only about 2 percent on an overall national basis in 1974—that compensating steps might be required to maintain the margin if income taxation were applied to nonprofit hospitals.

Additional property taxation certainly would be reflected in reimbursement and would, then, largely be passed through to reimbursers and patients.

Another government action to reduce nonprofit hospital costs is the provision under which hospitals are able to develop loan funds through state or local government tax-exempt bonds which bear a lower interest rate than do equivalent taxable bonds.

The third function of tax action in health is to increase the incentive to purchase health insurance. The most significant action taken in this connection was to make employer payments of their employees' health insurance premiums not taxable to the employees. The health insurance benefits are also not taxable. Thus, health insurance coverage through plans financed totally or in large part by employer contributions is attractive to employees. If employees forego wages to obtain such coverage, they forego income that is subject to tax and gain an equivalent that is tax free. This stimulant to obtain health insurance may be an important factor in accounting for health insurance as it exists today and, in turn, for much of the current importance of internal generation of capital among health facilities.

THE POST-WORLD WAR II STAGE—THE
POLICY OF INCREASING RESOURCES

Government Grants

While, during the depression and World War II period, agencies like the Federal Works Agency, the Public Works Administration (PWA), and the Works Progress Administration (WPA) assisted with a substantial number of hospital projects,[16] the first federal legislation to provide a regular program of grants-in-aid for health facility construction was the Hospital Survey and Construction Act—the so-called Hill-Burton program—enacted in 1946. The original law was applicable only to public and other nonprofit hospitals and public health centers. It put the federal government into the business of aiding private and state and local government facilities. Hill-Burton was, to all intents and purposes, a hospital construction act, but with the construction intended to be based on plans developed from surveys of resources. It was intended further that the bill would have the effect of increasing the care to be provided.[17] There was no question at that time of the need for, and value of, the addition of more health facilities and services. In effect, a decision was then made for the first time that the federal government should take very direct action to help solve a private capital shortage by contributing its funds, by using grants, to encourage private actions which would provide matching funds.

The law provided for the distribution of funds among states on the basis of population and income, with lower income states receiving a greater per capita share than higher income states. Considerable support was given to the construction of many small community hospitals in rural areas, a concept that is now widely considered to have been erroneous. The grant for any given project was, generally speaking, limited to one-third of its costs. A number of conditions were applied to states and to projects for which a grant was sought. The law set up ratios of beds to population above which additions to the supply of beds would be considered unnecessary, but lesser ratios were authorized to be established administratively.[18] Since the original law was enacted, the Hill-Burton program has been the most significant federal program providing specific construction support for health care facilities. In recent years, Hill-Burton has provided some 70-80 percent of the federal grants-in-aid for private hospital construction.

It is not possible to determine with certainty the quantitative effects of this legislation and its subsequent amendments which later provided grants for modernization, shared services, ambulatory and preventive care, long-term care, and rehabilitation facilities. There have been attempts to use regression analysis to ascertain some of the consequences, the most noteworthy study being that of Judith and Lester Lave.[19] However, even though the growth in beds by state is shown by statistical test to have been correlated significantly with the Hill-Burton funds per capita granted in a state, the regressions do not prove a cause-and-effect relationship. Most of the money for the construction which received Hill-Burton support came from private sources, and the question is to what degree, in the absence of the Hill-Burton funds, other capital sources would have produced the observed growth. Nevertheless, the Laves concluded from their analysis that the program did serve to increase the number of beds, but they did not say by how much.

No attempt was made, as part of the Hill-Burton program, to apply a test of need in awarding funds for a project, i.e., no priority was given to aiding health care institutions that would otherwise have been incapable of developing necessary capital. (Grants—by reducing borrowing requirements—have the potential for making residual needed loans supportable from available cash flows.) Nor did the program give any priority to supporting institutions that had performed effectively or whose plan for use of funds seemed likely to improve the effectiveness of care, so that the planning process provided no significant incentives for efficiency or for lower costs.

The Hill-Burton program started out with the primary objective of helping to remedy a shortage of supply. There were limits to the amount of capital made available and, therefore, a plan for distributing the fixed sum was needed. That may be why planning first came to be used under federal law. Such control mechanisms will be discussed later.

It should be understood that the Hill-Burton Act and its amendments, despite the importance of that Act, do not constitute the totality of grant efforts. Other principal federal grant programs[20] include:

—Health Professions Educational Facilities Program
—Nurse Training Facilities Construction Program
—Allied Health Facilities Program
—Community Mental Health Centers Construction Program
—Mental Retardation Facilities Construction Program
—Health Maintenance Organization Program
—Developmental Disabilities Program
—Economic Development Agency Grant Program
—Appalachian Regional Commission
—Neighborhood Facilities Program

The first of these ten programs provide grants for the construction of facilities for training. However, grants for construction are only a small fraction—about one-eighth—of the $1.6 billion in federal support for the development of human capital through training in 1974. Even the $1.6 billion federal support figure does not include the amount of training cost that was paid for by Medicare or Medicaid as part of their reimbursement for hospital services. These two programs help to support training of interns and residents, as well as many hospital programs that train ancillary personnel through the operating income of hospitals. For most training, however, operating income is not as significant a factor as it is for patient care, and the same basis for displacement of grant programs by internally generated funds has not developed. About one-fourth of federal training funds come from the Department of Defense and the Veterans Administration, in an attempt to recruit and train staff for their facilities.[21]

The largest human capital program was developed under the Comprehensive Health Manpower Training Act. The legislation was intended to expand the supply, extend capacity, and improve distribution of personnel while also stabilizing the finances of educational institutions. While the numbers of those trained have increased since the enactment of these programs, the distribution of personnel by specialty of physician and by geographic location continues to be wanting.[22] The number of physicians and their specialties seem to be important determinants of the amount of expenditures on care, not only on expenditures for physicians' services but for the services which the physicians prescribe. An increase in the number of physicians almost inevitably results in an increase in the use of hospital service and, given a reluctance to allow queuing for services, also increases the demand for plant capital.

The last seven on the list of grant programs were designed to assist in the development of types of patient care that seemed to have a particularly high urgency. In the case of mental health, mental retardation and the Developmental Disabilities Program, the programs were intended to increase attention, which seemed quite inadequate, to the diseases involved.

In the case of the Appalachian region, Economic Development Agency and neighborhood health facilities, the target group was the indigent and, in the cause of the HMO program, the aim was to improve the effectiveness of care at a faster rate than would otherwise have occurred without aid to this organizational form. The very number of independent programs on the list, in addition to the various provisions of the Hill-Burton program, suggests that one important process in capital development involves the allocation of funds to the various programs in operation. There is no evidence of the development of a rational method of fund allocation among the federal programs according to priority of need. Nor are there any systems for coordinating federal and state grant programs. While state grants for the construction of privately owned health service facilities are estimated at only $16 million in FY 1975,[23] state support may be important for some facilities—for example, some medical schools.

Loan Provisions

The government action on loans for health facilities has two principal purposes: (1) to aid facilities in obtaining loans with smaller down payments and (2) to reduce the cost of borrowing. The implementation of Medicare and Medicaid in 1966 is widely considered to have produced an important breakthrough in making lenders receptive to borrowers who provide health services.[24] This implementation represented a substantial addition to the already large percentage of hospital revenues paid by third parties, thereby making these revenues sufficiently dependable to support revenue bonds. Loan funds became much more widely available because hospitals were regarded as secure borrowers.

Government programs that participate in lending generally do not appear to make money available for many borrowers who would have been considered such poor risks that they could not have borrowed privately in the absence of these programs. However, the programs tend to make it possible for borrowers to secure larger loans, lower interest costs, and longer terms of repayment. The Hill-Burton loan provisions were adopted as part of a move to reduce government expenditures from the level that occurred when grants were made. The change from grants to loan provisions does not appear to have had the effect of reducing the amount of construction.

The most important of the government lending programs are: Hill-Burton loan guarantees with interest subsidies, FHA insured mortgage loans, and the previously mentioned state or local government tax-exempt revenue bonds. The last comprise the largest element in current borrowing (Table 2-1). Tax exemption constitutes what is known as a tax benefit since the government, in effect, makes a contribution—a sort of interest subsidy—of the income it foregoes by the noncollection of taxes on the interest income.

These government programs tend to increase the percentage of a project's cost that can be borrowed and to reduce down payments. This means that the flow of funds that are made available from reimbursement for depreciation and interest starts at an earlier date because the down payment can be accumulated more quickly. Of course, larger debts mean higher operating costs. Interest is an increasing factor in hospital costs, and debt arrangements can make a significant difference in the total costs of an institution. In 1974, interest on long-term debts of hospitals amounted to half a billion dollars, although the interest rate averaged only about 5 percent of debt, reflecting the fact that much of the debt was incurred in periods of lower interest rates than at present.

THE PREPAYMENT ERA—CAPITAL FROM OPERATING FUNDS

Reimbursement Provisions

Because the greatest part of funds now being developed for capital purposes is internally generated, government provisions for reimbursement are very important factors in capital development. One reason is that the upper limit on borrowing is determined by the degree to which lending to the facility is considered secure, and government programs play an important role in determining the security of the loan. This security depends, in part, on the certainty of the continuity of flow of income and, in part, on the amount of expected cash flow—the expected excess of the facility's income over operating needs.

Cash flow in hospitals is largely determined by the reimbursement provisions of third party payment programs. Reimbursement provisions of federal programs have an important effect, not only in their own right, but because their features often serve as models for states and for nongovernment programs. In fiscal year 1974, government programs paid some $34 billion for personal health care, while private health insurance paid $23 billion of the total of $90 billion spent on personal care. Of the year's total hospital care expenditures of $41 billion, some 90 percent came from either government programs or private health insurance.[25] In other words, all but one-tenth of the hospital operating funds that support most of their capital development comes from third party reimbursement. And hospital plant comprises the greater part of the health capital of the country.

Federal programs comprise a very sizable factor in reimbursement. Medicare and Medicaid are the dominant government programs, having paid $22.5 billion in benefits in 1974. Maternal and child health services benefits amounted to another half a billion dollars. All other federal programs paid out about $2 billion in additional benefits, $800 million under the federal employees health insurance program and about $500 million through CHAMPUS. Of federal reimbursement expenditures, almost 90 percent came from Medicare and Medicaid. The major state reimbursement program—other than that involved in the state share of the already mentioned public assistance subject to federal grants-in-aid— is workmen's compensation, for which the states spent some $1.4 billion in 1974.

Medicare sets the tone for government reimbursement for hospital care. For nursing home care, Medicaid is the principal program, and reimbursement to nursing homes under that program is largely in the hands of the states. Medicare pays hospitals through a cost reimbursement system. The only specific payment by Medicare towards net revenues is in the form of a return on equity capital of investor-owned facilities. The return paid on equity capital of proprietary facilities is one and one-half times the average rate of return earned on investments in federal bonds purchased by the Medicare trust fund.

Other capital-related features of the reimbursement formula include payment of depreciation, essentially on a straight line basis, and payment of interest on borrowed funds. Depreciation of all depreciable assets is reimbursed, including what is purchased with the aid of Hill-Burton grants, i.e., depreciation is paid on assets that are purchased with grant funds, apparently on the time-proven assumption that such grants would not recur and depreciation would supply replacement funds. However, under a 1972 provision applying not only to Medicare but to the Medicaid and to Maternal and Child Health programs as well, when a capital expenditure is disapproved by a state planning agency, depreciation, interest on borrowed funds, and a return on equity capital will not be payable.

Other provisions of Medicare reimbursement also affect the amount of internal generation of funds that may be used for capital development purposes. These include a provision for covering the bad debts of hospitals deriving from failure of beneficiaries to pay Medicare deductibles and coinsurance. However, Medicare does not cover any of the other hospital costs that are unreimbursed because of bad debts.

Pertinent Medicare provisions also relate to the program's treatment of various forms of income from other sources. Under Medicare, hospitals are permitted to retain for their own use, without suffering a reduction in Medicare payments, any funds generated from patient extras (private rooms, telephones, television, etc.), service not considered related to patient care (parking lots, gift shops, rental of office space to physicians, etc.), general donations, or income earned on endowments or depreciation reserves. Thus, while Medicare pays no more than the costs of the services that it covers, Medicare patients contribute to the net income of some institutions.

The Medicare policy also took into account the effect of timeliness of payment on capital resources by providing for "current financing" that was intended to make up for the lag between the provision of service and reimbursement for this service. This current financing provision was curtailed recently as part of an effort to reduce the federal budget.

The 1972 amendments to the program added a provision for the establishment of limits on the amount of reimbursement that would be considered reasonable and payable. It was hoped that the publication of the limits would have the effect of inducing high-cost hospitals to lower their costs to avoid losses. The initial application of this provision did not affect many hospitals and, so far, it has had no significant effect on capital. However, the stringency of application of this provision was increased in its second year and it has the potential for producing reductions in cash flow in connection with Medicare services in a significant number of hospitals.

The intent of the Medicare law was to leave the health care system largely unchanged. However, the very existence of coverage may have widespread effects on health care and its delivery. For example, program coverage may contribute importantly to capital development if it provides sufficiently comprehensive benefits for a group previously experiencing difficulty with bill payment. The new coverage, in such a case, significantly reduces losses previously experienced in providing care so that expansion becomes more affordable.

The 1935 Social Security Act had a notably significant impact on nursing homes by virtue of its coverage provisions. Because the county poor farm and similar almshouses operated by state or local governments were regarded as totally unacceptable to those who framed the Act, the welfare grant provisions prohibited the use of federal matching funds for cash assistance to persons residing in public institutions. Substantial responsibility is attributed to this provision for the rapid change from the public poorhouse to the largely investor-owned nursing home industry as we now know it. The 1935 law created a demand for modest private homes that welfare recipients could afford from their small cash assistance payments since, originally, no special provision was made for medical assistance. Over the subsequent years, the proprietary boarding houses that comprised a large part of the initial ventures to meet the need for domiciles for the aged poor who could not live at home, assumed to an increasing degree the responsibility for meeting the personal and nursing needs of their aging residents.[26]

Similarly, it was never believed that Medicare would be an entirely neutral factor in the health care system. It was thought, for example, that Medicare coverage of the aged might induce an increase in supply. This possibility was not a source of concern at the time of Medicare's enactment. However, there was little feeling that any serious capital shortage existed in health care in 1965, although it was acknowledged that appropriate kinds of nursing homes were not available and that there was a general shortage of home health services. The latter, however, did not involve capital issues. ·

A number of Medicare provisions were expected to raise quality levels, and the rise in quality was associated with improvement that, in some cases, required capital. The initial Medicare reimbursement policy provided for payment of a 2 percent factor added to costs as well as for accelerated depreciation. Even these two provisions in support of capital development were later dropped.

The posture of Medicare vis-à-vis affecting the health system has changed over the years, and the change is reflected in the 1972 amendments to the program,[27] with much more emphasis being placed on control of growth in 1972 than in 1965.

While it is difficult to assess with certainty the degree to which Medicare has, in fact, departed from neutrality in its effects on capital development, there are some fairly reliable data on the dollar growth of hospital assets before and after Medicare's enactment. However, the data on assets are affected by changes in hospital accounting—more complete recording of asset values; by the effects of inflation, which was different in the period before Medicare than afterwards; and, of course, by the various non-Medicare factors impacting on hospitals. The data are shown in Table 2-3, and reflect a tapering-off in the rate of expansion of assets between 1947 and 1965. An increase back to the 1950-1955 level in the years since Medicare was enacted indicates an improvement in the ability of hospitals to develop capital and suggests that Medicare may have contributed to this ability.

Cost-related reimbursement as employed in Medicare is the primary method that is used by the government in paying for hospital care, but physicians' services are reimbursed on the basis of charges and Medicaid's payments to nursing homes—which accounted for over 90 percent of government nursing home payments in 1974—have often been on a fixed rate basis. When charges are paid, a contribution to net revenues is normally included in the payment. There are no data on the amount of capital invested by physicians in their offices, including

Table 2-3. Total Hospital Assets and Rate of Increase by Five-Year Period
1950-1974

	Total Hospital Assets (in millions)	5-Year % Increase
1950	$7,791	N.A.
1952[1]	9,418	60
1955	11,986	54
1960	17,714	48
1965	24,502	38
1970	36,159	48
1974[2]	51,706	54

Sources: Hospital Statistics, 1975 Edition, American Hospital Association, p. 3, and *Hospitals, Part Two,* August 1, 1964.
1. Hospital assets in 1947 totaled $5,881 million.
2. Hospital assets in 1969 totaled $33,547.
N.A. = not available.

some rather elaborate radiology units and pathology laboratories. Very likely these resources have grown greatly, but, for the most part, the major investment in plant that physicians use in the course of their practice is made by hospitals.

There are little data on capital investment in nursing homes, but, obviously, the industry has flourished in recent years, with beds in homes that provide nursing care almost quadrupling, growing from 319,000 to 1,107,000 between 1963 and 1973.[28] This despite the general belief that the rates paid for nursing home care are quite low and often insufficient to support a very large expansion of resources in short order. Some measure of the size of investment can be derived from the fact that total construction expenditures for medical facilities in 1975, including hospitals, nursing homes, medical clinics and medical research facilities, was $4.5 billion, while hospital construction begun in 1974 was estimated to be nearly $3 billion (Table 2-1). Most of the remaining $1.5 billion was probably invested in nursing homes. There are, of course, many differences between the nursing home situation in 1963 and that of hospitals at that time or now, so that it should not be deduced that payment of a fixed rate or of charges to hospitals would result in capital growth similar to that which occurred in nursing homes.

Up to this time there has been no apparent increase in hospital failures resulting from the use of internal generation of capital to support debt as a means of capital development. However, facilities with large debts are quite vulnerable to changes in reimbursement, and any changes in reimbursement should be made only after taking carefully into account the flow of funds that are required to support debt repayment. Otherwise, widespread defaults could occur.

THE DEVELOPING FUTURE—THE ERA
OF CONTROLS?

Conditions on Payments

The government has obviously contributed in various ways to the development of capital funds in the health service industry. However, conditions have generally accompanied the contributions. A statement of the approval by the American Hospital Association of the bill that became the Hill-Burton Act welcomed the planning control aspects of the law.[29] The planning provisions of that law became a device for distributing the appropriated grant funds, which were allocated by formula among states but according to state plans within the states. Standards of construction were also applied, and prevailing wages had to be paid. The prevailing wage requirement, of course, increased the cost of construction. There was also a Hill-Burton requirement for the provision of care to those who cannot pay. Conditions such as these have been encompassed in almost all government loan or grant programs.

Even those who believe that Hill-Burton planning activity was quite effective find a number of faults with its performance. These include: (1) unclear goals and objectives (a fault of other planning programs that have since been instituted); (2) an excessively technocratic planning process, relying on numerical measures that were only vaguely related to the true objective; and (3) an absence of influence over projects for which no federal funds were provided.[30]

Another form of control is applied in Medicare. That program requires, as a condition of hospital participation, the meeting of quality standards quite similar to those used in the hospital accreditation process, as well as the implementation of a utilization review program in each hospital. Medicare also requires financial records to support the reimbursement that it pays.

Furthermore, participation in Medicare was, and continues to be, conditional on the desegregation of institutions, a condition that was enforced under the Civil Rights Act and was implemented immediately after Medicare's enactment. The Civil Rights Act was considered applicable to hospitals because of Medicare reimbursement.

More recently, payment of capital-related components of Medicare reimbursement has been tied to planning. Under the 1972 amendment of the Social Security Act, depreciation, interest, or returns on equity capital may not be paid in the case of a construction project disapproved by a state planning authority. A recent study of this process concluded that while thus far this control had not had great success in preventing unnecessary capital investment, several states had performed quite well, and there was promise that exporting the methodology used by these states would produce substantial improvement. The recent assessment by Lewin and Associates also commented that the absence of clear-cut goals was a severe handicap to this planning process.[31]

Conditions on All Institutions

The original provisions applying conditions that hospital or other health facilities must meet in order to operate were enacted in the form of state licensing laws. Conditions that must be met in order for a facility to operate comprise forms of ultimate controls on capital investment. State licensing of hospitals is an activity of relatively recent origin. At the end of World War II, less than a dozen states had comprehensive licensing laws and some of these were not enforced. The Hill-Burton legislation, which required that hospital standards be established, provided an impetus for the extension of licensing throughout all states.[32] The 1950 Social Security Amendments did the same with respect to nursing homes and reinforced the Hill-Burton incentives to enact hospital licensing laws.

From this early effort at establishing minimum standards for health facilities, some states have gone to quite comprehensive efforts to regulate quality standards, and some have proceeded from regulating quality standards to regulatory review of reimbursement rates for hospitals and to applying planning controls, including certificate of need legislation.

Some of the impetus for rate review came from the feeling, in some states, of the need to establish additional controls on Medicaid expenditures because market controls were inadequate. In New York State, control on increases in Blue Cross premiums was also a concern that gave rise to rate review legislation. The rates determine, of course, the degree to which operating income can support capital development.

At the federal level there have been three attempts to remedy some of the defects in the Hill-Burton planning legislation as a device for rationing the limited resources available for capital development in the health field. The first attempt consisted largely of encouraging more comprehensive planning activities but without enforcing the decision. This federal reform effort was made through the Regional Medical Program, which was intended to develop integrated regional programs related to the treatment of heart disease, cancer, and stroke and related diseases.[33] A more direct approach to incorporating hospital planning in a broader planning program was next taken under another law, enacted in 1966,[34] which provided grants-in-aid for comprehensive health planning activities. Not long after these laws were enacted they began to be described as adding little more than confusion to the situation, and they have now been succeeded by a third step, the planning legislation which became P.L. 93-641, enacted in 1974, placing all planning activities within a health service area under the jurisdiction of a single agency. This law also includes a provision making state enactment of certificate of need legislation a condition which must be met if federal grants are to continue to be made available to any state. Thus, the program is planned to have sharp teeth.

It should be understood that government franchising of health facilities has a side effect. Certificate of need has sometimes been considered a benefit to existing hospitals since it gives them a measure of assurance of a share of the market for services. This factor tends to make lenders consider hospitals with the right to operate better risks than they would be in the absence of the certification process.

There has not been sufficient time to get the new planning program into operation, much less to measure its results. Nevertheless, President Ford's 1976 Budget Message, while proposing to require the states to carry out planning activities, proposed, in effect, to repeal P.L. 93-641. President Ford's plan did not meet with much enthusiasm by the Congress. Moreover, both the president and the Congress support the need for planning controls in growth, and grant and loan support by the federal government has been sharply curtailed. The current policy seems to be to control growth, although its implementation has not had any significant observable effects thus far.

SOME CLOSING COMMENTS

Operating income accounts for the great bulk of the funds that are now being raised for capital purposes and borrowing, repaid from such income, is the predominant mode of capital development. Philanthropy and grants, while much smaller in amount, can exercise a great deal of leverage in determining the distribution of capital investment funds, so that the wise use of philanthropy and grants continues to be very important. Donations and grants have a special mission in relation to hospitals that provide substantial services to medically needy persons whose care is not covered by any third party payment program, for health education facilities that are not benefited by patient payments, and for innovative projects that might not otherwise be supported. Their success depends significantly on the degree to which the agencies making donations or grants are able to make well-informed judgments.

Recently, increasing concern has been expressed that the present system has given rise to an excessive investment in technology, contributing not only to the rise in health costs (primarily not through capital costs but for the operating costs that follow) but, paradoxically, to a lowering of the level of health because of a maldistribution of resources.[35] The main instruments of government for dealing with this problem are planning and certificate of need applied not just to federal activities but to the entire industry and, increasingly, to the future development of health facilities.

To what degree the new system of controls on capital expenditures that is established under P.L. 93-641 will be more successful than efforts of the past remains unclear. Broadening the planning activity and giving it teeth seem to promise greater success. However, planning faces some serious obstacles that may not be readily overcome. It must be able to implement order for the public good in a system that has been historically dominated by narrower interests. To be successful, the planning system must sometimes refuse to allow the private owner to spend his own money as he wishes, thus infringing, at least to some degree, on private property rights. Furthermore, restrictions on the availability of a facility in a hospital may interfere with the ability of its physician staff to use the best resources to care for their patients where they have hospital privileges. To succeed, planning must, therefore, have strong backing from the community, and to have such backing it will need to operate in support of goals with wide acceptance. Such goals have not yet been well developed, and considerable public education would be required to make them viable.

One aid that some have suggested for increasing the power of planners is a better and more complete integration of planning and reimbursement activities, so that reimbursement will not, on the one hand, provide capital development funds whose expenditure the planning agencies may, on the other hand, find it necessary to deny.

For this reason, depreciation pooling has found some favor in the past to assure that seed money is available where needed, and to reduce the pressure of resisting private property rights where expenditures are questionable. However, in many hospitals the flow of depreciation reimbursement has become essential to the repayment of debt, commitments that will have to be met. Nevertheless, the setting of priorities in the development of further capital remains critical in achieving a proper reflection of public interest needs in its distribution.

In any event, it seems that good planning requires a consensus of understanding of the issues by all those involved in the planning decisions. These consist not only of members of the planning agencies, but, also, those who operate the facilities—physicians, philanthropic donors, government grantors, reimbursement programs, and the public generally. It was the thought of the American Hospital Association committee that developed the AHA's approach to national health insurance that the Association should back the creation of Health Care Corporations (HCCs), umbrella agencies that would have coordinating authority over all the elements that provide care in a specified geographic area. They theorized that the existence of HCCs would reduce the conflict between the interests of individual health service units and broader, areawide interests.

The basic question in capital planning is the level of cost for which we should aim. It will need to be addressed repeatedly, along with numerous other interrelated questions, as we seek to shape the health care system of the future. Even after we reach conclusions on basic issues, however, we will need to learn how to moderate or accelerate the flow of funds to meet our goals, to decide what combinations of direct and indirect governmental intervention will best suit us, and to direct the funds to the appropriate places. Our history suggests that we have found a number of ways to increase the flow of funds, but reducing its flow is a new—and a far more complex—question. We have scarcely begun to identify alternative answers, but the time seems to be approaching when we will find it increasingly difficult to postpone resolutions.

NOTES

1. Barbara S. Cooper, Nancy L. Worthington, Mary F. McGee, *Compendium of National Health Expenditures Data* (Washington, D.C.: U.S. Department of Health, Education and Welfare, Social Security Administration Office of Research and Statistics 1976), pp. 8–11.

2. Marjorie S. Mueller and Robert M. Gibson, "National Health Expenditures, Fiscal Year 1975," *Social Security Bulletin*, February 1976, p. 7.

3. J.B. Silvers, "How Do Limits to Debt Financing Affect Your Hospital's Financial Status?" *Hospital Financial Management*, February 1975, p. 32.

4. David E. Marine and John A. Henderson, "Trends in the Financing of Hospital Construction," *Hospitals*, July 1, 1974, p. 56.

5. Unpublished data of the American Hospital Association.

6. *Hospital Statistics 1975 Edition*, American Hospital Association, pp. 4–5.

7. L.B. Russell, Blair B. Bourque, Daniel P. Bourque, and Carol S. Burke, *Federal Health Spending 1969–74* (Washington, D.C.: Center for Health Policy Studies, National Planning Association 1974), pp. 83–93.

8. Mueller and Gibson, "National Health Expenditures (FY 1975)."

9. *Hospitals, Guide Issue, Part Two, Journal of the American Hospital Association*, August 1, 1966, p. 442.

10. *Hospital Statistics 1975 Edition*, American Hospital Association.

11. *Giving USA, 1975 Annual Report*, American Association of Fund-Raising Counsel, Inc., p. 38.

12. Martin S. Feldstein, "Estimating Separate Price Elasticities by Income Class," *Guide to Sponsored Research of the Commission of Private Philanthropy and Public Needs*, 1975, p. 27.

13. Robert J. Blendon, "The Changing Role of Private Philanthropy in Health Affairs," *New England Journal of Medicine*, May 1, 1975, pp. 947–48.

14. Robert M. Sigmond, "Hospital Planning in Allegheny County," *Group Practice* 13, 6 (June 1964).

15. *Hospital Statistics 1975 Edition*, American Hospital Association.

16. *Hospitals, Journal of the American Hospital Association*, April 1946, p. 102.

17. "Statement by the President," *Hospitals*, September 1946, p. 37.

18. P.L. 79–725. Sec. 613–Sec. 622.

19. Judith P. Lave and Lester B. Lave, *The Hospital Construction Act, An Evaluation of the Hill-Burton Program, 1948–1973* (Washington, D.C.: American Enterprise Institute for Public Policy Research), pp. 29–37.

20. Russell et al., *Federal Health Spending 1969–74.*

21. Ibid.

22. Committee on Labor and Public Welfare, *Health Professions Educational Assistance Act of 1974*, Senate Report No. 93–1133, p. 52.

23. Mueller and Gibson, "National Health Expenditures (FY 1975)."

24. *A Guide to Capital Financing for Hospitals* (Eastdil Health Funding, Inc., 1974).

25. Nancy L. Worthington, "National Health Expenditures, 1929–1974," *Social Security Bulletin*, February 1975, pp. 3–20.

26. Glenn R. Markus, *Nursing Homes and the Congress: A Brief History of Developments and Issues* (Congressional Research Service, Library of Congress, November 1972).

27. Irwin Wolkstein, "Medicare 1971: Changing Attitudes and Changing Legislation," *Symposium on Health Care: Part II, Law and Contemporary Problems,* Duke University School of Law, 1970, pp. 697–715.

28. *Health Resources Statistics, 1975* (Washington, D.C.: U.S. Department of Health, Education and Welfare, National Center for Health Statistics), p. 365.

29. George Bugbee, "Auspicious Start for S. 191," *Hospitals,* February 1945, pp. 42–43.

30. Symond R. Gottlieb, "A Brief History of Health Planning in the United States," in Clark C. Havighurst (ed.), *Regulating Health Facilities Construction,* (Washington, D.C.: American Enterprise Institute, 1974), pp. 7–25.

31. Lewin and Associates, Inc., *Evaluation of the Efficiency and Effectiveness of the Section 1122 Review Process* (Washington, D.C.: Prepared for Health Resources Administration, DHEW, Sept. 1975), pp. 3–4.

32. Anne R. Somers, *Hospital Regulation: The Dilemma of Public Policy,* Princeton, New Jersey: Princeton University Press, 1969, p. 102.

33. P.L. 89–239.

34. P.L. 89–749.

35. Howard H. Hiatt, "Protecting the Medical Commons: Who Is Responsible?" *The New England Journal of Medicine,* July 31, 1975, pp. 235–41.

Discussion of
The Impact of Legislation on Capital
Development for Health Facilities

Alain C. Enthoven

To assess the impact of legislation on capital development for health facilities, one needs a point of view or a set of criteria that can help us to relate each law to the public interest.

I propose to approach the impact of legislation on capital development for health facilities by comparing it with the workings of a rational capital market. My criterion will be the efficient allocation of resources to, and within, the health care industry. My analysis will proceed along the following lines. First, despite the existence of many significant imperfections, in fields other than health care, the competitive industrial market economy does provide firms with incentives to produce roughly the amount and kinds of output desired by society at minimum cost. Are there, or could there be, similar incentives at work in the market for health care services?

Certainly, as presently constituted, the market for health care services does not fit the competitive market model at all well. This is because of certain inherent characteristics of health services, and it is exacerbated by third party reimbursement insurance. Thus, none of my criticisms of government actions should be taken as a plea for laissez faire or as a defense of the status quo. But a review of the legislation outlined by Mr. Wolkstein shows that, for the most part, it does not provide incentives to motivate a socially desirable amount of investment in health facilities. So I go on to explore some ways in which public action might help to restructure the market for health care services so that it will generate an appropriate amount of capital and allocate it efficiently. Capital costs are roughly 10 percent of the total costs of health care services, and it is the total benefits and costs that are of interest to society. To make sense of the health facilities capital market, therefore, one must consider the whole market for health services.

In a competitive industrial economy, firms have a powerful incentive to match their productive capacity to the amount of their product that society demands. If a firm builds too much capacity, it suffers reduced profits. If it builds too little capacity, it suffers foregone profit opportunities and perhaps a loss to competitors of valuable market position. Moreover, firms seeking to increase profit have an incentive to make the amount and kind of capital investments that will enable them to produce their output at minimum cost. If demand for the product increases, its price is bid up. This increases profits, permitting firms to retain more earnings and to borrow or raise new equity capital to finance expansion. And, if demand decreases, competition drives prices down, the attractiveness of new investment is reduced or eliminated, and firms are motivated to invest their capital elsewhere.

This is not to say that the system works perfectly. There are monopolies and oligopolies, externalities (e.g., noise and pollution), and even deception. Public action is required to preserve competition (antitrust), or to regulate natural monopolies, to correct private costs (e.g., by effluent taxes) where they do not reflect social costs, and to correct deception, all in order to create conditions in which the private market economy will produce socially desirable results. Moreover, the private market does not always produce an income distribution that meets our society's ethical standards. Public action is required to reduce inequality and help the less fortunate. And even when this is done, there will be mistakes in private-sector decision-making. But, in a competitive economy, mistakes are systematically and inexorably punished by impersonal market forces. Firms that persist in inappropriate investment decisions lose money, are unable to grow, and fail. Investors lose money and managers are replaced. But, roughly speaking, in the long run, the system moves firms to produce the output that is desired by society at minimum cost.

It is well known that, as presently organized, the markets for health care services in general and hospital services in particular do not fit this model. Without attempting a complete catalogue of market imperfections in health care, let me mention a few that are of particular relevance to hospital capital financing. First, the consumer and the physician who decide on the use of hospital services do not bear the marginal cost of their decisions. In Fiscal 1975, 92 percent of expenditures for hospital care was paid by third parties.[1] Therefore, the decision to use hospital services does not reflect a marginal valuation equal to society's marginal cost. The price of hospital services, thus, bears no systematic relationship to society's valuation of them. Moreover, the third party insurer is not in a position to shop around and bargain for reduced prices. To attempt to do so would interfere with the doctor-patient choice of hospital and the individual's choice of physician. The insurance system has been organized primarily by provider interests to assure that their costs and fees are paid without controls or interference by the reimbursement agency. Second, information on the efficacy of treatment is extremely imperfect and very costly for the consumer to acquire. The consumer must rely heavily on the physician who has a huge information advantage. Physicians make the decisions about use of costly technology. The utilization of health services is mainly determined by "provider variables" such as physician organizations and financial incentives.[2] Hospitals compete for physicians—who brings in the patients—by providing the equipment and facilities that the physicians use to earn income. Physicians usually earn more income from employment of more costly technology, and the hospitals can pass on the higher costs of excess capacity and high technology equipment to the third party payers. There are then, no incentives to promote an efficient allocation or equitable distribution of resources.

Failure of the private market (as presently constituted) suggests a need for corrective action by government. But one cannot safely assume that government action is always in the public interest. There is such a thing as "market failure" in the public sector, too. To assess the impact of legislation, one must look in detail at specific government actions and see whether their actual effect is to make things better or worse. Let us then review the seven types of government action identified by Mr. Wolkstein and ask:

1. Do they contain incentives for decisionmakers to make the amount and kinds of investments that will supply the socially desirable amount (and quality) of hospital services (i.e., where marginal value equals marginal cost) at minimum cost?

2. Do they help correct, or do they exacerbate, the distortions in resource allocation that are caused by the imperfections of the health services market and the third party financing system?

GOVERNMENT INVESTMENT IN ITS OWN FACILITIES

Do government investments in its own hospitals correspond closely to the needs of the populations that are served? I have been unable to find evidence that they do. And what reason would there be to expect it? The discipline of competing demands on the budget might lead one to expect that hospital investments would have to be justified on the basis of need. But provider and other powerful and well-focused political interests are at least as effective as considerations of need. Short-term general beds owned by state and local government have been a significant contributor to the national surplus in that category; their occupancy rates are below those of private, not-for-profit hospitals. The difficulties in closing Public Health Service hospitals and county hospitals in overbedded areas provide evidence of the political strength of their constituencies. Moreover, a local government is likely to find that an expansion of hospital operations will lead to an increase in employment and income in its area, as well as improved services that are paid for by Medicare and other third parties who draw their money mainly from outside the area. Understandably, local governments are not immune from the financial incentives that motivate voluntary not-for-profit hospitals, and they are far more vulnerable to constituent pressures for jobs and contracts.

At least by civilian standards, the Defense Department operates and fills far too many beds. While the 1974 occupancy of 74.2 percent was not far out of line, especially considering the many small installations, the per capita utilization of hospital beds was extremely high. For example, in Fiscal 1974, hospital days of care for active duty military personnel, 95 percent of whom are males 18-44, was 1,887.[3] The Military Health Care Study compared this to 611.5 days for noninstitutionalized American males age 15-44, 204.8 days for Kaiser Northern California, and 559.4 days for nonactive duty beneficiaries of the Military Health Services System. Of course, much of this must be explained by the particular conditions of military life, and I doubt that the military and civilian utilization data refer to exactly the same thing. Nevertheless, much of the difference is explained by longer stays for the same diagnosis.[4] As the Military Health Care Study tactfully phrased it, "the incentives in workload-based programming may encourage relatively heavy use of inpatient care."[5] The point is that the budgeting system, like many in the public sector, based on workload rather than on capitation, gives to physicians incentives with respect to utilization that are similar to those provided by fee-for-service.

GRANTS

In 1946, Congress created the Hill-Burton program under which the Surgeon General was empowered "to prescribe the number of general beds required for adequate hospital services for each state, not to exceed 4.5 beds per thousand population, except in sparsely populated areas."[6] The program has been very successful in achieving its goal and, at the outset, doubtless deserved much of its widespread public support because there had been little construction during the depression and World War II. But, thirty years later, we have achieved the original goal—inflexibly adhered to—only to discover that it was excessive. It is now a widely held view that 4.5 beds per 1,000 is too many, and a significant contributor to rising health care costs. For example, in a Policy Statement on Controlling the Supply of Hospital Beds, an Institute of Medicine committee concluded:

> ... the evidence clearly indicates that significant surpluses of short-term general hospital beds exist or are developing in many areas of the United States and that these are contributing significantly to rising hospital care costs.

and it recommended

> that a national health planning goal be established ... to achieve an over-all reduction of at least 10% in the ratio of short-term general hospital

beds to the population within the next five years and further significant reductions thereafter. This would mean a reduction from the current national average of approximately 4.4 non-federal short-term general hospital beds per 1000 population to a national average of approximately 4.0 in five years and well below that in the years to follow . . . [7]

The program was responsive to a widely perceived need for more, and more equitably distributed, health services which found expression in the political process. The main problem with the program appears to have been its inflexibility. As Lave and Lave observe, "If there are too many beds today or too much reliance on inpatient care, the problem is due to the original act and the failure to change it, rather than to the operation of state and federal agencies."[8] Such rigidity is not surprising. Such a law creates vested interests and expectations of gain on the part of persons who will fight hard to prevent the program from being reduced in size. (This includes physicians who gain from having the use of larger and better-equipped workshops, with no risk or direct capital contribution on their part.)

Moreover, such a subsidy program is likely to encourage overbuilding by lowering the marginal cost of the project to the sponsoring community. There is no generally accepted standard of "need" for hospital beds. The problem of how much is enough is better conceived as one of balancing marginal benefits against marginal costs. As the number of beds is increased, the extra health benefits from adding more will be reduced. A program that reduces the marginal cost, as perceived by decisionmakers, below the cost to society, will induce them to overinvest.

As Mr. Wolkstein noted, ". . . the planning process provided no significant incentives for efficiency or lower costs." On the contrary, Hill-Burton became just one more federal program to encourage health care spending whose cumulative effects we are now finding excessive.

THE TAX LAWS

Martin Feldstein has shown that, because employer contributions to health insurance are not taxable to the employee, and because, within limits employee premium payments are tax deductible, the tax laws motivate Americans to buy more health insurance coverage than they would otherwise find in their best interest. The tax aspect makes first-dollar coverage economically attractive to many who would otherwise prefer a policy with a higher deductible. Thus, the tax laws motivate Americans to consume more medical care than they would if they weighed the marginal benefits against the true marginal costs, not distorted by the tax laws (i.e., more than if they had to pay for it themselves).[9]

Perhaps the first thing to note about the tax laws, insofar as they affect charitable giving, is that they are uniform across the board with respect to eligible charities, and not specifically related to the needs for, or benefits from, additional hospital facilities. Charitable giving is related closely to the tax status of the donor. And the percentage of total giving that goes to hospitals (1.7 percent on average) rises sharply with the gross income of the donor: persons with gross incomes between $15,000 and $20,000 direct 1.5 percent of their giving to hospitals; persons with $50,000 to $100,000 direct 5.9 percent of their giving to hospitals.[10] The effect is that most hospital philanthropy is by the wealthy. I do not have data on the subject, but there is plenty of reason to believe that such donations are related to personal factors rather than to systematic evaluation of community needs. In a study of the role of capital financing in hospital resource allocation, Paul Ginsburg concluded, "The substitution of philanthropic equity capital for ownership profit-seeking capital is to a large extent responsible for lower correlation between consumer demand and total hospital investment than would occur in an idealized market."[11] For what it is worth, private giving for medical facilities construction did not decline as the nation approached the goal of 4.5 beds per 1,000. On the contrary, from 1960 to 1972, it increased by an average of $50 million per year to $960 million in 1972.[12]

Mr. Wolkstein observes, "Philanthropy and grants, while much smaller in amount, can exercise a great deal of leverage in determining the distribution of capital investment funds, so the wise use of philanthropy and grants continues to be very important. . . . [T]heir success depends significantly on the degree to which the agencies making donations or grants are able to make well-informed judgements." The problem is not one of wisdom or information; the problem is one of differing objectives. Private philanthropy accomplishes some very important and valuable things, but it is not systematically related to the need for health facilities capital.

LOAN PROVISIONS

It would be a complex matter to trace out all the effects of an interest subsidy in a system in which the hospital can pass on practically all of its costs to third parties. The decision to finance with tax-exempt bonds will mean lower costs or charges—hence, lower costs to Blue Cross and Medicare, and lower income tax revenues. I doubt that the overall effect on resource allocation is large. Apparently, the main reason why a not-for-profit hospital management cares whether its interest rate is 6 percent or 9 percent, when it can pass either on to third parties, is that the lower rate helps it to get in under the Medicare cost ceilings. What broad social purpose is served by favoring hospitals that happen to qualify for tax-exempt financing over those that do not? In any case, the hospital still needs a down payment in order to be able to borrow.

Twenty years ago, hospitals had poor access to capital markets because private lenders regarded lending for such special purpose facilities as very risky. In that context, a loan guarantee could give to a hospital access to markets which it would otherwise not have had. A loan guarantee might be considered superior to complete reliance on grants because it forced a hospital to consider financial feasibility in the light of an obligation to repay. However, in today's context, with loans much more readily available to hospitals having sound financial prospects, and with over 90 percent of costs being reimbursed by third parties, loan guarantees have become equivalent to grants in the sense that they reduce the amount of capital that the hospital has to have to start a project (i.e., lenders can accept a smaller or no down payment if the loan is guaranteed). They are promised streams of (contingent) payments that have expected present values, and their effect on real economic activity is the same as that of a grant.

A government loan guarantee circumvents one kind of market discipline for the borrower, another for the government. The borrower can borrow larger amounts at better terms than would otherwise be the case, for he and his lender know that the government will make the payments if he cannot. This reduces the penalty for default and enables the hospital to take greater risks, i.e., to invest in projects of even more uncertain need. On average, this will increase the number of unneeded facilities.

For the government to guarantee a loan is merely to push a present cost off to future budgets. It would be accounted for as a present expenditure on the income statement and an increased liability on the balance sheet if the government used accrual accounting. By assuming the risk, the government assumes the contingent obligation to make payments in the future whose expected present value it does not have to report as expenditures today, even though the economic impact is the same as that of a grant which would be reported as expenditure today. So the substitution of loan guarantees for Hill-Burton grants in today's context is a fiscal trick that enables the government to understate its true (i.e., accrual basis) deficit and further to weaken the discipline of the budget. This is the kind of financial policy for which New York City has become justly famous and that got it to its present unenviable position.

There is no reason to suppose that loan subsidies and guarantees improve the allocation of resources; quite the contrary.[13]

REIMBURSEMENT PROVISIONS

Medicare seems fully committed to the cost reimbursement approach, which obviously rewards hospitals that incur greater costs with greater revenues, thus encouraging cost increases. Cost overruns and inflation have been the universal experience of cost reimbursement systems, so it is not surprising, for example, that projected Fiscal 1977 Medicare outlays are 48 percent above their Fiscal 1975 level. Yet Congress appears to be unable to make fundamental changes in the way that the government pays for hospital services, despite numerous acknowledgements in committee reports of the cost-increasing effect of cost reimbursement.[14]

With respect to capital costs for not-for-profit hospitals, Medicare reimbursement is based on straight-line depreciation and historical costs. This is too much for a hospital whose services are not needed and it is too little for a hospital whose services are needed. In the former case, it merely helps the unneeded hospital to perpetuate itself, while, in the latter case, the Medicare formula fails to make allowance for inflation, technological advance, or the accumulation of net worth to finance growth. Moreover, the Medicare formula does not reward greater efficiency in the use of assets. It does not enable the more efficient hospital to accumulate funds for expansion by doing a better job in serving the needs of Medicare beneficiaries. There is no "invisible hand" here, no built-in incentive to reward or motivate socially desirable behavior.

Mr. Wolkstein's discussion of reimbursement provisions completely misses this important point. He seems to be trying to suggest that Medicare and Medicaid pay for the capital costs of the services which they cover. He refers to ". . . the present stage in the process of capital development in which operating funds, including those paid for care through Medicare and Medicaid, played a large part in meeting capital needs." He observes that ". . . while Medicare pays no more than the costs of services it covers, Medicare patients contribute to the net income of some institutions" (through patient extras, services not related to patient care, donations, etc.). He observes that the increase in the rate of expansion of hospital assets "in the years since Medicare was enacted, indicated an improvement in the ability of hospitals to develop capital and suggesting that Medicare may have contributed to this ability." The plain fact is that Medicare does not pay the capital costs of the services that it covers on a realistic basis. In the case of not-for-profit institutions, it pays no net income, and its (straight-line) depreciation allowances are based on historical cost. But building costs and the requirements of new technology are increasing faster than 9 percent per year, so that depreciation based on *historical* cost soon becomes a mere fraction of depreciation based on *replacement* cost. Mr. Wolkstein's appeal to the growth in total hospital assets as an indicator of the adequacy of Medicare's capital cost reimbursement provisions reminds me of the story of the man who had one hand on a hot stove and the other on a block of ice, but who announced that "on the average" he was comfortable. Medicare reimbursement contributes to a paradox of too much and too little. It will pay part of the capital cost of a thousand unneeded facilities, but it will not pay its full share of the capital costs of one needed facility. Perhaps you have heard the story of the man who drowned in a river with an average depth of one foot. I understand that he died because his overbedded community had no emergency room.

FACILITIES REGULATION

Having generated a costly excess of hospital facilities by inappropriate incentives, the federal government has been seeking for years to correct the damage it has done by deeper involvement through detailed regulation of facilities (i.e., Health

Systems Agencies, Certificate of Need programs, and Section 1122 programs). It seems ironic that we should be plunging head-long into hospital regulation just at a time when research on the effects of economic regulation in other industries has shown that it protects producers, retards cost reducing innovation, provides subsidies to politically favored interest groups, reduces efficiency and increases cost to the consumers.[15]

Roger Noll, a leading student of the subject, put it this way:

Either regulation performs no function at all . . . or regulation succeeds, not in lowering prices so that profits will resemble those in competition, but instead in raising costs so that the potential profitability of monopoly pricing is eroded away. . . . Regulatory agencies often set prices designed to prevent low cost firms or industries from capturing business from high cost competitors. . . . Regulatory agencies have delayed or prevented many beneficial technological innovations, and have promoted or permitted many others that were not justified. . . . The presence of regulation, by altering the incentives faced by firms, also damages the efficiency of their operations. . . . Thus, if the pattern extends to public utility regulation of hospitals, the following results could be expected to obtain: (1) resistance by regulators to medical care delivery systems (such as prepaid group health plans) regardless of their merit; (2) substantial consumer cross-subsidization and producer protectionism in the price structure, and (3) persistent upward drift in prices toward monopolistic levels in order to finance subsidies and inefficiencies created by regulation.[16]

So far, the evidence seems to be that Certificate of Need and Section 1122 controls are not effective in preventing overbedding. For example, a recent study by Lewin and Associates found that:

Nearly 75% of the sample states and areas [i.e., states and areas having such controls for which complete data could be obtained] approved hospital beds in excess of 105% of their published need projections for five years hence. Fourteen of these began the period overbedded [by their own published need projections] and approved additional beds; five others became overbedded during the period studied as a result of the projects they approved. Only five states and areas began with more than 105% of the projected need for long-term care beds. However, all of these approved still more beds and six other jurisdictions approved additions to bed supply that made them overbedded. . . . In our view, it is clear from the evidence produced by this study that, as presently administered, [these] controls do not perform effectively in preventing unnecessary capital investment in health facilities and services and, thus, are not an effective means of containing health costs.[17]

Of course, there is nothing incompatible between ineffectiveness in controlling total bed supply and a high degree of effectiveness in, for example, (1) blocking growth of hospital-based prepaid group practice plans (or forcing them to buy facilities in excess supply at above-market prices), (2) refusal to permit surgi-centers to enter the market ("because they are not needed"), and (3) retarding or stopping the growth or entry of investor-owned hospitals. Lewin and Associates found that "there is strong evidence that CES (i.e., Certificate of Need and Section 1122) review agencies systematically discriminate against for-profit providers of all types, particularly hospitals."[18] In fact, such behavior is exactly what would be predicted by the hypothesis that the regulatory agencies are captured by the dominant not-for-profit voluntary hospital industry.

One of the main reasons to expect facilities regulation to be ineffective is that there exist no defensible or generally accepted standards for bed needs, not to mention costly items of high technology equipment. For example, the Institute of Medicine Committee on Controlling the Supply of Short-Term General Hospital Beds in the United States labored for about five years on the subject of controlling short-term general hospital beds and was not able to agree on a standard of bed need, though it was able to agree that the supply should be reduced to substantially below 4 per 1,000. We simply do not *know* what is *the right* or *best* age-specific utilization rate. In fact, there is no such thing. On the contrary, there are very wide variations in per capita utilization rates for comparable populations with no discernible difference in resulting health status.

Nobody has a basis for *proving* that a rate is right or wrong, so I do not believe that regulators will be able to develop defensible standards. For example, in 1973, Kaiser Permanente Northern California had a hospital utilization rate of about 552 days per 1,000, when age adjusted to the U.S. population, compared to a national average of 1,238.[19] At 80 percent occupancy in both cases, this would mean a requirement of 1.89 beds per 1,000, as compared with 4.24 for the United States as a whole. Who is to say that one is "right," or that the average between it or some other number is "right"? After all, the Kaiser Northern California membership includes many educated middleclass people who elected Kaiser as a matter of free choice, while a larger number of similar people chose insurance and fee-for-service. Presumably, in the judgment of those who chose Kaiser, the added benefits of a higher per capita rate of hospitalization were not worth the higher costs. (And, considering the possibility of unnecessary surgery or iatrogenic illness, there may be no added net benefits.) Others, however, may see it differently. What if N women per 1,000 in Community A want to follow their physicians' recommendations and have hysterectomies, as compared to one-half N in Community B? What is the right utilization rate? The answer ought to be based on informed judgments weighing all of the costs, risks, and health benefits of the alternatives, with the marginal costs appropriately internalized, and not by an appeal to some arbitrary standard.

It is very unlikely that Health Systems Agencies will attempt to cut the supply of facilities in an area below the current level of utilization. It would be politically untenable. They may eliminate excess capacity, but they will not cut capacity to the point where doctors cannot hospitalize some patients for lack of beds. And they will not refuse another CT scanner to a community when all the ones in that community are running twelve hours a day. The major issues of cost are in *utilization,* not in excess capacity. The big difference, for example, between the Kaiser bed ratio of around 1.5-1.6 per 1,000 and the national average of about 4.4 is accounted for by large differences in age-specific utilization rates and some difference in age composition, but not by much difference in occupancy rates. To eliminate utilization of low or uncertain or no net marginal value, it will be necessary to address the organization and financial incentives of medical practice. It cannot be done by Health Systems Agency planners.

The likely political economy of the Health Systems Agencies will be captured by the not-for-profit hospital industry and the medical profession. In fact, one might say that the hospitals have an "economic need for regulation."[20] It is little wonder that the hospital associations are among the leading proponents of Certificate-of-Need regulation. "Consumers" on the HSA boards are not likely to be effective in representing the public interest. Where will they get information about hospitals? From whom will they feel pressure? Why should they resist additional facilities in their area—bringing jobs and more service—when the money to pay for them will come largely from nationwide reimbursement agencies?

One reason for pessimism concerning the ability of health facilities regulation to control cost is the fact that so much *government* action has been a significant barrier to the growth of prepaid group practice—which is, apparently, the most efficient form of delivery system on the American health care scene. For example, as of February 1972, more than twenty states had legal bars to prepaid group practice.[21] A recent report by the Comptroller General of the United States provides ample evidence to support the view that the Health Maintenance Organization Act of 1973 and HEW's implementation of it have done as much to retard as to help the growth of HMOs.[22] And, today, because of its reliance on cost reimbursement, Medicare systematically pays what is, in effect, a large subsidy to beneficiaries who choose the more costly fee-for-service over prepaid group practice. A recent study by the Social Security Administration showed, for example, that Medicare paid 37 percent more per capita on behalf of fee-for-service beneficiaries than on behalf of beneficiaries who had chosen five hospital-based prepaid group practice plans.[23] It is hard to see the basis for optimism that health facilities regulation will not become yet another tool to serve established physician and hospital interests.

Yet another danger in the regulation of health facilities is rigidity—perhaps worse than what Lave and Lave attributed to the Hill-Burton program. Planning for health facilities construction is filled with uncertainties. Conditions affecting need can change suddenly and unpredictably, and a very important part of effective economical planning is flexibility and continuous adaptation. Since the approval process is typically long and slow, institutions must ask for, and build, facilities that they "might need" just to be sure that they have them. Once a facility is approved, a vested interest is created, and unneeded facilities may be built simply because they have been approved.

LACK OF INTEGRATION OF PUBLIC ACTIONS

An important aspect of these government actions which Mr. Wolkstein failed to mention is their lack of integration or sensible relationship one to another. The situation reminds me of the famous army captain in Vietnam who remarked, after the Tet offensive, "We had to destroy this town in order to save it." In this case, Certificate of Need and the National Health Planning and Resources Development Act are justified on the grounds that "we have to control these hospitals to prevent them from doing what we are paying them to do."

Section 1122 of the 1972 Social Security Amendments was a step toward integration of approval of need and reimbursement. Somehow, we ought to create a system that ties capital generation to need as well as to effective performance.

IN SEARCH OF A RATIONAL MODEL

What can be done for a better alignment of the interests of individual decision-makers and society's welfare in the hospital capital market?

Lave, Lave, and Silverman have proposed that hospitals be paid a fixed prospective rate based on a formula relating costs to hospital characteristics and case mix (complexity), with an agreed upon allowance for general inflation. Reimbursement for an individual hospital would depend on the costs of a group of similar hospitals, and not on costs incurred by that individual hospital. Thus, a hospital that has lower than (adjusted) average costs would be able to keep (half, in their proposal) the savings and apply them to capital formation. A hospital that has above average costs would realize losses, be forced to cut back expenses relative to revenues, and be unable (or less able) to accumulate capital. Competition would work to drive costs down. The efficient could expand while the inefficient would be unable to.[24]

There is much to recommend this proposal. For example, under the present Medicare formula that reimburses incurred operating costs fully and capital costs inadequately, economically justified labor-saving capital investments are unattractive to hospitals, while, under the Laves' proposal, they might become attractive. I believe that it would be an important step forward, and ought to be tried.

However, in my judgment, the Laves' proposal has an important short-coming. I believe that most of the waste, and the potential for saving, is in the area of utilization. That is, society could save very large amounts of money if we were to cut back on utilization with low, zero, or very uncertain (and possible negative) net marginal value to the well-being of the patient. Wide variations in the per capita consumption of health services with no apparent resulting difference in health status suggest that there is a great deal of "flat of the (benefit-cost) curve medicine" being practiced. For example, in his studies of small area variations in health care delivery in Vermont, Dr. John E. Wennberg found that the probability of a person having a tonsillectomy by age twenty-four varied from 0.07 in one area to 0.62 in another; the probability of a woman having a hysterectomy in her lifetime varied from 0.26 to 0.52; the rate of surgical procedures per 1,000 per year varied from 36 in the lowest to 69 in the highest. And, he observes, "There is no evidence that the latter have greater medical need, or indeed, that more health is produced . . . [In] terms of their health status, it is not possible in my opinion to argue that Vermonters in more expensive areas are better or worse for the effort."[25] One might make similar observations about the variations in surgery rates between fee-for-service and prepaid group practice beneficiaries. The same conclusion is suggested by the high rates at which recommendations for surgery are not confirmed by a second opinion.[26] Physicians control utilization.

The shortcoming of the Laves' proposal is that it does not tie in the doctors. Under their scheme, a hospital could prosper as the most efficient producer of unnecessary CT scans, hysterectomies, etc. In fact, the medical staff might be encouraged to build up the volume to help lower the unit cost. To reduce unnecessary utilization, I believe that one must give the physicians a central role in the form of organizational and financial responsibility for maintaining appropriate utilization and hospital cost as is done, for example, in hospital-based prepaid group practice plans. This implies, in my opinion, capitation financing for comprehensive physician and hospital services.

Another possibly useful step worth exploring might be called "regulation with incentives." As noted earlier, Health Systems Agencies will be under pressure from hospitals, hospital workers, physicians, construction companies, unions and others, to approve expansion proposals. Why should they resist when practically all of the money to pay for them will come from outside of the area, i.e., from Medicare, Medicaid, Blue Cross, Blue Shield, and commercial insurers (assuming that the latter are experience rated on an area wider than the Health Services Area)? The problem is that the people in the Health Services Area correctly see little or no relationship between their payroll taxes, premiums and benefits, and the cost and utilization of facilities in their Area. The financing system relieves them of the marginal costs entailed by the decisions that are made in their Area. The resulting bias would be corrected if, in effect, each third party would experience rate each Health Services Area. Under such a scheme, for example, Medicare would pay the adjusted (actuarially and for price and wage level) national average per capita cost on behalf of each beneficiary in an Area. If the Area's costs vary from the average, the cost sharing would be adjusted to keep Medicare's contribution fixed. Then, beneficiaries in an Area with above average costs would feel the difference through, e.g., higher deductibles or copayments, and have an incentive to apply their pressure on their Health Systems

Agency for most cost reduction. (It would be appropriate for the Social Security Administration to include in the announcement of higher cost sharing an explanation of the reasons and the name and address of the director of the beneficiary's Health Systems Agency.) Similarly, to the extent that experience rating of groups by the Blues and the insurance companies reflected variations in cost from one HSA to another, then, at the margin, the money to pay for expanded and more costly services in a Health Services Area would not come from the outside. Marginal cost implications of facilities investment decisions would be internalized within each Health Services Area.

Could we create a rational capital market for health facilities comparable to that in the competitive industrial economy? Since facilities are only one factor of production, and capital costs are only about 10 percent of the total cost of physician and hospital services, one can speak of a rational capital market only in the context of an economically rational market for health care services. I believe that, at least in principle, one can conceive of an economically rational structure for the health services industry. (Whether we can get there from here politically is, of course, another question.) I recently outlined such a system as follows:

> A rational incentive system would rest on two principles: groups of physicians accept responsibility to provide *all* necessary health services for members of a defined population for a fixed per capita payment (based on age, sex, and other factors) set in advance; and consumers exercise free choice from among competing systems of care, but if they elect a more costly system, they pay the difference themselves. Physicians control the lion's share of health care expenditures. They are by far the best qualified to make the difficult judgments about need and cost effectiveness. So it makes sense for them to accept the main responsibility for keeping health care costs within the limits desired by society. In such a system, the physicians as a group do not get more money for providing more or more costly services. They have an economic incentive to provide appropriate cost effective care.
>
> These principles are at work every day for the 6 million Americans who receive their medical care through Health Maintenance Organizations (HMOs). Many organizational forms can and do exist in such a framework, including Foundations for Medical Care in which the individual physician continues to practice on a fee-for-service basis in his own office, but in which he and his colleagues agree to work within a fixed per capita total; hospital-based Prepaid Group Practice (like Kaiser and Group Health of Puget Sound); Prepaid Group Practice without a hospital (like Group Health of Washington, D.C.); and many other possibilities. Individual family doctors could continue to practice in rural areas in association with one or another of these organizations. University and other "tertiary care" referral centers would continue to exist for the treatment of especially ill patients. The HMO referring the patient acts as his agent and can negotiate

with alternative referral centers for favorable terms. Typically, prepaid group practice plans hospitalize their members about half as much as fee-for-service physicians, and provide comprehensive care for 20 to 30 percent less cost.

Competition among HMOs is an essential part of this framework. Like their fee-for-service counterparts, HMOs make mistakes, keep their patients waiting, sometimes waste money, and are sometimes badly managed. As in any business, competition is necessary to keep them under constant pressure to find ways of providing better service at lower cost. (In some areas, the market is too small to permit effective competition. But benefits and costs of HMOs in those areas can be judged by standards set by those in competitive areas.)[27]

I believe that there is reason to be more optimistic about the ability of consumers to choose between competing *systems* of care than to make judgments about the nec sity and probable outcomes of specific procedures. Consumers can judge on the basis of reputation, on the basis of the experience of their friends, as well as their own experience, on formal qualifications of the physicians, convenience, service, etc. I do not want to suggest that consumers would be perfect, or even necessarily very good judges of what health services are in their best interest; my contention is merely that, in most cases, the consumer is the *best* qualified judge.

In a world of competing organized systems of care like HMOs, the ones that do a better job of widening the difference between what consumers are willing to pay for their services, and what they pay for inputs to produce them, i.e., those who can increase their net incomes, would be able to accumulate a greater net worth with which they could finance growth. Organizations that could not earn a net income, either because of lack of need for their services or because of inefficiency, would not be able to finance growth. In such a system, physicians would have incentives to provide the care that is necessary and beneficial, and to do so efficiently. Persistent provision of inadequate care would cause their organization to lose members, and might mean higher costs for late care. Excessive care or excessively costly care would reduce net income and, in the long run, be likely to mean reduced income for physicians. In a competitive environment, hospital-based organizations would have an incentive to match facilities to need, just as in the competitive industrial economy. If they persist in buying unneeded facilities, they suffer reduced net income. If they buy inadequate facilities, they will lose dissatisfied members. Nonhospital-based organizations have an incentive to shop around for the most economically provided hospital services. Here, the HMO is acting as a well-informed and appropriately motivated agent on behalf of its members. Both have an incentive to buy services outside of their plan when it is more economical to do so—thus contributing to the regionalization of costly specialized services.

Such an economic system would not be completely self-regulating. There would be a need for government regulation or other intervention with respect to some aspects. For example, some organizations might be tempted to try to succeed by enrollment procedures designed to select only health members. Government action would be needed either to assure that HMOs took a representative cross-section of members, or to subsidize the extra cost of high risk people. Some might be tempted to achieve a short-term success by underserving members. Government might correct this by such devices as (1) requiring full disclosure of sources and uses of funds; (2) restricting the ability of sponsors to take short-term profits out of the business (in the long run the competitive market would discipline the persistent underservers); and (3) limiting the percentage of Medicaid beneficiaries on the grounds that quality and accessibility would then not be less than that enjoyed by employed middle class consumers. I believe that such controls would have a far greater chance of achieving their purpose than, for example, price and facilities investment controls in fee-for-service cost-reimbursement economy. It would be much easier to police bias in membership selection than, say, "unnecessary surgery" or utilization in general.

If this is an attractive model, how can we get there from here?

A good place to start would be Medicare. The law should be changed to include a genuine "HMO option" whereby any beneficiary can have his actuarial equivalent cost paid on his behalf to the HMO of his choice in the form of a fixed capitation payment set in advance. The present Medicare law has a very complex provision for paying HMOs (Section 1876), but, in effect, it is a cost-based system with the wrong incentives.[28] If the law were so changed, HMOs would be able to use their lower costs to attract more Medicare members either by offering benefits not covered by Medicare or by reducing premiums. The clear implication of the Corbin and Krute and the Goss studies that were cited earlier is that the federal government is offering what are, in effect, large subsidies to beneficiaries who choose the more costly fee-for-service, cost reimbursement system. While that is understandable politically as a response to pressure by the dominant interest groups, it is neither equitable nor economically rational.

Medicare is important because, in the United States, people who are sixty-five and over account for 34 percent of total short-term hospital days.

Some Medicaid programs have experimented with HMO options with mixed results. California's now notorious entry was hasty, unwisely motivated, and poorly managed. The state administration was apparently interested only in saving money, and contracted with almost any organization that would offer it a money-saving arrangement, with little attention to qualifications. Moreover, as families cycled in and out of Medicaid eligibility, they were cycled in and out of HMO membership, creating major administrative problems and disrupting the continuity of care. In addition, the state permitted very serious marketing abuses. However, the failures should not blind us to the fact that some HMOs have apparently done a good job in serving Medicaid populations,[29] and that there have been equally serious Medicaid abuses on fee-for-service. A sensible public policy with respect to Medicaid would strongly encourage a shift to capitation financing with adequate controls to prevent fraud and other abuses.

A national health insurance system compatible with these principles might be modeled after the Federal Employees Health Benefits Program. The government would make an actuarially adjusted per capita payment on behalf of each beneficiary, who would have a free choice from among alternatives, and would pay the extra cost himself if he chose a more costly plan. That would give the beneficiary a personal incentive to consider carefully whether the extra benefits provided by his plan were worth the extra cost.

Returning to the questions raised at the beginning of this paper, do the government actions identified by Mr. Wolkstein contain incentives for decision-makers to make the amount and kinds of investments that will supply the socially desirable amount of hospital services at minimum cost? The answer is "no." Do they help correct, or do they exacerbate, the distortions in resource allocation that are caused by the imperfections of the health services market and the third party financing system? For the most part, they exacerbate them. Most of the programs reduce or eliminate the marginal cost to the consumer or community of his/its decision to buy, build or use a more costly system of medical care. Their cumulative impact is the excess utilization and cost that has now become such a major concern.

The achievement of acceptable cost, effectiveness, and equity in the use of health services resources will require more carefully conceived legislation designed to create a system of rational economic incentives in the market for health services and the health facilities capital market.

NOTES

1. Marjorie Smith Mueller and Robert M. Gibson "National Health Expenditures, Fiscal Year 1975," *Social Security Bulletin,* February 1976, p. 14.

2. See, for example, Diana B. Dutton "A Causal Model of the Use of Health Services: the Role of the Delivery System," Ph.D. dissertation, MIT, February 1976; George N. Monsma, Jr., "Marginal Revenue and the Demand for Physicians' Services," in Herbert E. Klarman (ed.), *Empirical Studies in Health Economics,* Baltimore: Johns Hopkins Press, 1970.

3. *Report of the Military Health Care Study Supplement: Detailed Findings,* DOD, DHEW, OMB, December 1975, p. 599. (Data reported in patient bed days per 1,000 people per year.)

4. *Report of the Military Health Care Study,* DOD, DHEW, OMB, December 1975, p. 40.

5. Ibid, p. 6. Despite the study team's efforts, there may be significant elements of noncomparability in the data. There are also differences that might be explained by the needs of the military institutions, and population (presumably healthier). Nevertheless, the evidence of overutilization appears strong.

6. Judith R. Lave, and Lester B. Lave, *The Hospital Construction Act, An Evaluation of the Hill-Burton Program, 1948-73* (Washington, D.C.: American Enterprise Institute, 1974), p. 9.

7. *Controlling the Supply of Hospital Beds,* A Policy Statement by the Institute of Medicine, National Academy of Sciences, Washington, D.C., October 1976, pp. ix and 16.

8. Lave and Lave, *Hospital Construction Act,* p. 7.

9. See Martin Feldstein, "The Welfare Loss of Excess Health Insurance," *Journal of Political Economy,* 81, 2 (March/April 1973), pp. 251-280, and papers to which he refers.

10. *Giving in America.* Report of the Commission on Private Philanthropy and Public Needs, John H. Filer, Chairman, 1975.

The following table was constructed from data on page 61 for 1970.

Adjusted Gross Income	Average Yearly Giving		Percent to Hospitals
	Hospitals	Total	
$5,000 and under	$ 0	$ 89	0
5-10,000	1	202	.5
10-15,000	2	284	.7
15-20,000	6	389	1.5
20-50,000	25	688	3.6
50-100,000	119	2,020	5.9
100-500,000	615	9,182	6.7
500-1,000,000	5,546	72,025	7.7
1,000,000 and over	14,688	257,276	5.7
Average all incomes	4	233	1.7

11. Paul B. Ginsburg, "Resource Allocation in the Hospital Industry: The Role of Capital Financing," *Social Security Bulletin,* October 1972, p. 27.

12. Ralph L. Nelson, *Private Giving in the American Economy, 1960-72,* January 1975, prepared for the Commission on Private Philanthropy and Public Needs.

13. For an excellent critique of loan guarantees, see the Lave and Lave, *Hospital Construction Act,* pp. 52-54.

14. See, for example, *Social Security Amendments of 1971,* Report of the Committee on Ways and Means on H.R. 1, May 26, 1971, pp. 89-90; Senate Report 92-1230, *Report of the Committee on Finance to Accompany H.R. 1, the Social Security Amendments of 1972,* p. 224.

15. Roger G. Noll, "The Consequences of Public Utility Regulation of Hospitals," *Controls on Health Care* (National Academy of Sciences, 1975).

16. Ibid., pp. 33-41.

17. Lewin & Associates, Inc., *Evaluation of the Efficiency and Effectiveness of the Section 1122 Review Process,* Washington, D.C., 1975, pp. 1-25. See also, for example, Fred J. Hellinger, "The Effect of Certificate-of-Need Legislation on Hospital Investment," *Inquiry,* June 1976.

18. Ibid., pp. 5-19.

19. Kaiser data from *The Kaiser Permanente Medical Care Program, A Symposium,* Anne R. Somers (ed.), Appendix A Tables Revised as of November 1975, with 1974 data converted to 1973 on the basis of the Region's decline in utilization by 5 percent from 1973–74. U.S. data from *Health United States 1975,* U.S. DHEW, HRA, p. 309.

20. See George Stigler, "The Theory of Economic Regulation," *The Bell Journal of Economics and Management Science,* Spring 1971.

21. This statement is taken from Judith R. Lave and Lester B. Lave, "The Supply and Allocation of Medical Resources: Alternative Control Mechanisms," in Clark Havighurst (ed.), *Regulating Health Facilities Construction* (Washington, D.C.: American Enterprise Institute, 1974). The source they cite is, "Over Twenty States Have Legal Bars to Group Practice," *Group Health and Welfare News,* February 1972, as reported in *Medical Care Review,* March 1972.

22. *Factors that Impede Progress in Implementing the Health Maintenance Organization Act of 1973,* Report to the Congress by the Comptroller General of the United States, September 3, 1976.

23. See Steve Goss, "A Retrospective Application of the Health Maintenance Organization Risk Sharing Savings Formula for Six Group Practice Prepayment Plans for 1969 and 1970," Actuarial Note Number 88, DHEW Pub. No. (SSA) 76–11500 (11-75). This is an update to reflect final settlements of the study, "Some Aspect of Medicare Experience with Group Practice Prepayment Plans," by Mildred Corbin and Aaron Krute, *Social Security Bulletin,* March 1975. The weighted (by number of Medicare enrollees) average incurred per capita cost for the five hospital-based prepaid group practice plans was 73 percent of the adjusted average per capita cost for non-PGP members.

24. Judith R. Lave, Lester B. Lave, and Lester P. Silverman, "A Proposal for Incentive Reimbursement for Hospitals," *Medical Care,* March-April 1973. See also Lave and Lave, "The Supply and Allocation of Medical Resources: Alternative Control Mechanisms," in Clark Havighurst (ed.), *Regulating Health Facilities Construction* (Washington, D.C.: American Enterprise Institute, 1974).

25. Statement of John E. Wennberg, Waterbury Center, Vermont, in "Getting Ready for National Health Insurance: Unnecessary Surgery," Hearings before the Subcommittee on Oversight and Investigations of the Committee on Interstate and Foreign Commerce, House of Representatives, July 15, 1975, pp. 74–81.

26. See, for example, Statement of Eugene G. McCarthy, Professor of Public Health, Cornell University Medical College, in "Getting Ready for National Health Insurance: Unnecessary Surgery," pp. 108–11.

27. Alain C. Enthoven, "Medical Care Costs: Where to Go From Here?" *National Journal,* No. 30 (July 24, 1976), pp. 1054–55.

28. For a more detailed critique of Section 1876, see Alain C. Enthoven, "Prepaid Group Practice and National Health Policy," keynote Address to the 1976 Group Health Institute, to appear in *Proceedings, 26th Annual Group Health Institute,* June 14, 1976.

29. See, e.g., Clifton Gaus, Barbara Cooper, and Constance Hirschman, "Contrasts in HMO and Fee-for-Service Performance," *Social Security Bulletin,* May 1976.

Discussion of
The Impact of Legislation on Capital
Development for Health Facilities

Ida C. Merriam

Mr. Wolkstein has given us an overview of the types and specific pieces of legislation that have impinged on capital formation for health facilities—primarily hospitals—in the past four decades. The impact of that legislation, not only on capital formation but on the entire health delivery system, should be a matter for discussion and analysis throughout the remainder of this conference, but a few general comments can usefully be made at the start.

First, we need to keep in mind that capital expenditures are a relatively small part of total health expenditures—construction of medical facilities about 4 percent in recent years and other capital expenditures perhaps the same amount.[1] Their importance, both in relation to adequacy and quality of care and in relation to cost inflation, stems from the scope of the services that they make possible and the expanded labor and other operating costs which they entail. Social policy relating to capital development for health facilities can be formulated only as part of a broader policy for the system as a whole.

As one reviews the developments of the past thirty years, it becomes clear that an assured source of payment for services—quite aside from the method of reimbursement—has been a factor of overwhelming importance in the availability of capital for construction, for modernization and for technological updating of health facilities. During the past ten or fifteen years, medical technology has been changing rapidly and, with it, perceived capital needs. More and more physicians, including those still practicing entirely on an independent fee-for-service basis, have been trained to rely heavily on the technology and resources that the hospital provides. As we turn now to problems of cost containment and a more rational and socially justified allocation of health resources, it is again evident that one has to look beyond technical mechanisms of capital funding and look for the motive force and effectiveness of any controls in the structure and organization of the total health delivery system.

The Hill-Burton Act of 1946 was, itself, a response not only to shortages that had developed during the depression and war years, but, also, to the pressures and concerns that were generated by the debate on national health insurance which came to a climax in the Truman Administration. One of the arguments of the opponents of health insurance was that there were simply not enough hospital beds available to permit the assurance of needed hospital care to all persons. Careful studies made by the Social Security Board undercut this argument, but they also assumed corrective action to expand resources in deficit areas as effective demand increased.[2] Federal grants for hospital construction had been seriously discussed in 1938 as part of a national health program and were included in the Wagner health bill of 1939. The legislation which became the Hill-Burton Act was perceived by most of its major supporters as one part of a broader health program which, most important, would include a system of prepayment of medical costs. (The other three components of Truman's proposed program were the expansion of federal-state public health, maternal and child health services; federal grant-in-aid for medical education and research; and cash sickness insurance.) When the broader program faltered, hospital construction was both a legatee of the more general concern and a safe alternative.

Hospitals were constructed in many areas and did help bring doctors to them. By the time the impetus of construction grants had lost some of its initial force, third party arrangements had begun to provide the needed source of assured payment for services. With the adoption of Medicare and Medicaid, over 90 percent of all hospital care expenditures are now covered by third party payments. Mr. Wolkstein brings out very clearly the way in which such assured payment for services had made it possible for hospitals and nursing homes to turn to borrowing as a source of capital. The particular developments that have occurred are closely related to specific methods and formulas of reimbursement under Medicare and other programs.

The fact that an assured source of payment for services makes capital investment feasible does not necessarily mean that the reimbursement monies should cover capital costs. Particularly when a large part of the funds for both consumption and capital development come from the same source—i.e., tax revenues— a separation of the two flows of funds may lead to greater accountability and more informed public decisions and planning controls. I must admit that, currently, this issue has largely disappeared from sight, but it could be revived as more attention is directed towards capital funding for noninstitutional care. It is interesting that while most of the major national health insurance proposals which were introduced in the 94th Congress would reimburse hospitals and other institutional providers on a basis that would cover capital costs, and the Ullman bill (H.R.1), supported by the American Hospital Association, is very specific as to the hospital costs to be covered, for the Health Service Corporation which it could establish to provide comprehensive and coordinated health services, the Ullman bill calls for "a special study of the capital needs of health care corporations and related organizations to examine methods of replacing traditional sources of capital financing with a national funding program."[3] As Mr. Wolkstein points out, if any change in methods of reimbursement of hospitals were made now, it would have to take into account the large amount of existing debt and provide for some type of transitional arrangements. Such change is not impossible.

There is another side to the story of the growth of third party payments for hospital care, and that is the resulting encouragement of overhospitalization and—primarily because of the lack of comparable insurance support and of organized methods of service delivery—the underutilization of outpatient and ambulatory services. Although the method of organizing and paying for services is the critical factor, a conference on capital funding should not neglect the question of the capital needs of noninstitutional service delivery programs. While the capital construction needs of outpatient facilities, clinics, home health programs or HMOs are of a different order of magnitude than those of hospitals, their needs for some construction monies, for equipment and for working capital are real and important. Unless these needs are satisfied, it will be difficult to overcome the imbalance in the present health delivery system. Furthermore, it is in this area that we may find the most hopeful approaches to cost control linked to improvements in the quality of care. I wish that Mr. Wolkstein had given a little more attention to the implications of expanded outpatient services.

He does describe a number of pieces of legislation that make some provision for the construction of facilities for outpatient or ambulatory care. As early as 1954, the Hill-Burton Act was amended to provide funds for the construction of diagnostic and treatment centers, rehabilitation centers and facilities for long-term care. While the bulk of the Hill-Burton monies continued to go for the construction or modernization of short-term hospitals, in recent years sizable grants have been made for these other types of facilities. Mr. Wolkstein lists ten relatively new federal grant programs that provide some funds for health facility construction. As he points out, the training programs are of a different character than those providing health services, and construction has a somewhat different role. Of the other programs which he lists, three represent attempts—not markedly successful—to direct more attention and resources to problems of mental health and mental retardation or other developmental difficulties. Three are directed towards low-income population groups and areas, and one—the Health Maintenance Organization program—is intended to encourage a method of organizing service delivery. In all cases, grants for construction are a subsidiary aspect of the program although they are seen as necessary to make possible a desired expansion in services. Grants for equipment, for working capital, and for covering operating deficits for a number of years may be more important. Grants to cover operating deficits for an initial period will, however, run out. The question of continuing support will then become critical.[4]

Looking ahead, it may be of some interest to ask what the major national health insurance proposals would do to encourage out-of-hospital services. The major bills, though differing significantly in the scope of the benefits provided, in the use deductibles and coinsurance, in methods of administration and funding and in other important aspects would, nevertheless, all provide assured support for a broader range of outpatient care than is common under existing health insurance. Several include special provisions, among them construction grants, to encourage the development of organized ambulatory care services. The general pattern is that of provision for federal grants or loans and loan guarantees, for planning, construction, medical equipment, etc., together with funds to cover deficits for a reasonable period (three to five years). The organization that would be the primary vehicle for development of noninstitutional care systems would be Comprehensive Health Care Centers under the Burleson-McIntyre bill (H.R. 5990 and S. 1438, supported by the Health Insurance Association of America), and Health Care Corporations under the Ullman bill and the largely identical Staggers bill (H.R. 2049) which also uses the term health maintenance organizations. Under the Corman-Kennedy Health Security Act (H.R. 21, S.3) both health maintenance organizations and other specified types of group practice organizations could receive financial assistance. That bill establishes a Health Resources Development Fund, supported, initially, by 2 percent and, eventually, by 5 percent of the total income of the national health insurance program that would give "priority to improving services on an ambulatory basis as part of a system of comprehensive care."

Consideration of needed and desirable expansion of out-of-hospital services—as presently perceived—brings us back to the question of how we can control overfunding and cost escalation, not only for hospital care but for all types of medical service. I am not sure that anyone has the answer to that question. Presumably, multiple answers to different facets of the problem will have to be developed.

Mr. Wolkstein sees the developing future as one of controls. Primarily, he discusses planning and reimbursement controls as related to capital funding. I think that it somewhat confuses the issue to refer, as he does, to licensing laws or standards of construction, fire and safety laws, and other efforts to regulate quality of care in the same context as planning and controls directed at the supply of capital funds and containment of costs.

The original Hill-Burton Act provided grants to states not only for the construction of hospitals, but, first, for surveys of need and for the development of state plans to assure appropriate allocation of construction grants within states. The formula which determined the amounts going to each state was based on a measure of presumed need and ability to pay, but, for individual hospital grants a closer measure of community needs, interest and effort was required. Standards of adequacy prescribed by the Surgeon General provided general but not specific guidance. All subsequent planning legislation has faced the same difficulties of measuring need—in the light of changing medical technology and standards of performance—of appropriately weighing community concerns and interest group pressures, of considering all significant aspects of a proposal without inordinate delay in the process, of being flexible but still tough. Over the years, planning has become more comprehensive in scope, and with stronger sanctions to enforce at least negative decisions.

The growth of state certificate of need legislation, the Medicare reimbursement requirements in the 1972 Social Security Act amendments, and the provisions of the 1974 National Health Planning and Resources Development Act are potentially strong controls. Several of the major national health insurance proposals would require either a certificate of need or approval by a state planning agency of substantial capital expenditures as a condition of provider participation in the program. Several others include only the less stringent control of exclusion of reimbursement of disapproved capital expenditures that is now contained in the Medicare reimbursement formula.

The question is how such planning controls are being used or can reasonably be expected to operate. Experience to date is not very encouraging. Mr. Wolkstein refers briefly to the Lewin and Associates study of the effectiveness of certificate of need and Medicare reimbursement controls.[5] I think that it is worth summarizing their findings in a little more detail. In a review of the disposition of some 3,000 proposals, they found that states approved more than 93 percent of all projects and 90 percent of the dollar expenditures proposed. Interestingly, new facilities were a small proportion of the hospital proposals received and had a lower approval rate than did proposals for the expansion of existing hospitals. Proposals to purchase equipment and add new services were always approved. The difficulties that state agencies have in turning down requests for approval of expenditures on high technology equipment are confirmed in another recent study.[6] In the Lewin survey, nearly 75 percent of the sample areas studied approved hospital beds in excess of 105 percent of their published need projections for five years hence; five states began with more than 105 percent and approved still more beds. One may assume that more sophisticated measures of hospital capacity would also have shown an excess supply in most of the areas. The significant point is the way that state agencies behaved in relation to their own established standards.

In explanation of this situation, the study emphasizes the lack of generally agreed-upon standards, data, and techniques for need projections in most states, the lesser commitment to cost containment and the kinds of interest group pressures that operate with particular strength at the local and state levels. While the Medicare section 1122 requirements and, perhaps more important, the funds for planning activities that are channeled to the state agencies under this program have strengthened the review capacity of state planning agencies, much more is needed. Among the factors associated with good performance (defined to include efficiency and fairness as well as adherence to need standards) the

Lewin study identified well-developed review criteria covering a broad range of services and facilities, assignment of certificate of need functions to a special agency and comparatively high salaries and low turnover among agency directors. Clearly, there is opportunity for improved performance and more sophisticated analysis, interpretation and projection of need in the planning process. The Lewin study sees hope in the diffusion of methods and techniques that have worked in a few states. They urge DHEW to enforce the provision in the National Health Planning Act that states must require statistical and other reports from all health providers. With this requirement one could not disagree.

But I suspect that the more significant finding is that it is in those states that have a prospective reimbursement system for hospitals that certificate of need and planning legislation really work. The imperatives of cost-plus reimbursement are stronger than any planning intentions.

The question of prospective rather than retrospective reimbursement is distinct from the issue of the treatment of capital costs. In either case, such costs can be taken account of to a greater or lesser degree—or handled separately. The advantages of prospective reimbursement and the disciplines which it introduces are becoming more and more widely recognized. Prospective reimbursement is, however, an umbrella term; it covers a variety of specific methods and techniques, some of which may be more effective or more adapted to particular situations than to others. This is not the appropriate time or place to attempt a detailed review or evaluation. I would observe that effective controls on hospital costs clearly have to go beyond the hospital itself to the health system as a whole. The methods of reimbursement of doctors, as well as the availability and organization of noninstitutional services, are critical factors. It is impossible to shut down hospitals or to control expansion unless other alternative modes of care are available in a community. And, since it is physicians who send people to hospitals, they should have financial as well as organizational incentives to control utilization and cost.

One type of legislative provision that Mr. Wolkstein does not mention is the authorization and funding of research and experimentation related to methods of health care reimbursement. Two years after Medicare was adopted, the 1967 Social Security Act amendments, recognizing a problem of cost escalation, made provision for incentive reimbursement experiments. The early experiments were not very meaningful or productive. The 1972 Social Security Act amendments, however, broadened significantly the scope and funding of the research. Studies and experiments now under way on various types of prospective reimbursement for hospitals—budgeting, budgeting by exception, negotiated rates, formulas using case mix, occupancy and intensity of care, diagnostic specific rates, and others—as well as studies related to alternative methods of reimbursement of physicians, physician extenders and health maintenance or other prepaid group practice organizations, hold real promise. Such SSA-supported studies complement, and in some cases mesh with, studies concerned more with the organization of health service delivery, experiments with state rate regulation and the development of uniform systems of reporting and classifying data on health care providers and health costs mandated and supported under the National Health Planning and Resources Development Act of 1974.

In an excellent study on reducing hospital capacity which is soon to be published, Walter McClure makes the point that we already have the technical tools to do many of the things that need to be done; what we have still to develop are the political and organizational skills to use the techniques for consistent policy purposes. While there is a large measure of truth in that judgment, there are still many questions to which we do not know the answers, and many areas in which further analysis and research could help clarify policy goals and improve our understanding of the way that the health system does, and might, operate.

Later in this conference we shall be discussing two aspects of this broader field—the supply of medical manpower and the potential contributions of HMOs. The whole question of public understanding and attitudes towards health and a clearer distinction between medical care and health outcomes deserves to be mentioned. In the end, the degree of comprehensiveness, balance and coordination in the delivery of all types of health services will largely determine what kind of health care we have and what capital requirements we must provide.

NOTES

1. Marjorie S. Mueller and Robert M. Gibson, "National Health Expenditures, Fiscal Year 1975," *Social Security Bulletin,* 39, 2 (February 1976): 3–21.

2. *Medical Care Insurance.* Report from the Bureau of Research and Statistics, Social Security Board, to the Committee on Education and Labor, U.S. Senate, 79th Congress, 2nd Session, Senate Committee Print no. 5. (Washington, D.C.: U.S. Government Printing Office, 1946).

3. *National Health Insurance Proposals.* Provisions of Bills Introduced in the 94th Congress as of February 1976 Compiled by Saul Waldman. DHEW, SSA. ORS (Washington, D.C.: U.S. Government Printing Office, 1976), pp. 44. This compilation was used in all the analyses of proposed health legislation in this paper.

4. For an analysis of the consequences for education and the arts, as well as for health, of adequate seed money followed by starvation, see Bruce C. Vladeck, "Why Non-profits Go Broke," *The Public Interest,* No. 42 (Winter 1976): 86–101.

5. Lewin and Associates, Inc., *Evaluation of the Efficiency and Effectiveness of the Section 1122 Review Process* (Washington, D.C., Sept. 1975). Prepared for Health Resources Administration, DHEW.

6. Abt Associates, Inc., *Incentives and Decisions Underlying Hospitals' Adoption and Utilization of Major Capital Equipment,* Executive Summary, Sept. 1975. Prepared for Health Resources Administration, DHEW.

Discussion

Mr. Hernandez: It has been mentioned that the primary sources of capital in recent history have been retained earnings and debt. I think that Mr. Wolkstein's paper makes the point that debt has increased in relation to all other portions of capital in the balance sheet of aggregate hospitals in the country. Now, that means that there has been either too little reimbursement for capital related items, causing an increase in debt or, alternatively, that the planning mechanism which regulates the capital expenditures has not been working properly, or a combination of both.

As far as the guaranteed and subsidized borrowing programs operated by the government are concerned, the significant default experience seems to indicate that there have been investments in unneeded facilities, if one uses default and unutilized facilities as criteria. These factors seem to require further explanation.

Mr. Wolkstein: I might say that the percentage of debt to total assets of an industry varies from industry to industry—some have very high debt, some have very low debt. Nobody has decided what percentage of debt is appropriate in the hospital field. In the public utility field, they use very high debt; they use two-thirds debt. I would not say that the existence of a certain percentage of debt is, by itself, indicative of anything in terms of whether reimbursement is right, wrong, too much, or too little.

Mr. Hess: I think that the historical review on the relationship of the depreciation provision and planning deserves a little bit more comment, because I think that, for better or for worse, our reimbursement system is going to be committed to pumping money to providers in recognition of depreciation.

Obviously, it would drive the hospitals mad if you pooled all of their depreciation, but it is possible to take a percentage of depreciation, and Dr. Merriam suggested the possibility of separating the depreciation policy from the reimbursement policy. You could begin to use some of that funding so that the hospitals that do not really need it and do not need to stay in the business do not get the same amount of depreciation as those which can justify their need.

But to whom is all this justification going to be directed? Is it to the payment agency, the planning agency, to consumers? In some way or other this depreciation, if there is going to be planning, has to express public policy. One of the reasons why we did not get stronger teeth in the relationship between reimbursement and planning is that nobody had any confidence that the planning agencies were prepared to make that kind of decision. I think that this relationship between depreciation reimbursement and plans for capital investment is something that we want to pay more attention to as time goes on.

Mr. Needleman: What is a rational capital market in the health care sector? You spoke about consumer preference and, currently, about 42 percent of the funds for personal health care services in the country are being paid by government. The fact of the matter is that government programs represent a major subsidy to providers of health care services. One way to deal with the problem of addressing consumer preference is to turn it over, in some way, to the individual involved to spend in his own way. But, to the extent that people are making consumption decisions, they will be making marginal consumption decisions rather than first dollar consumption decisions.

Dr. Enthoven: I do believe that we have reached the point where we have to consider consumer preferences. In this country today, we are spending about $600 per capita per year for medical care. Can you picture a family of four on Medicaid being told that the only type of medical care which they can have costs $600 per year per capita? The head of that household might come in and say, "Well, I would rather have $200 per year style medical care and let me have the $400 a year per capita to spend on better food and housing for my kids, and I can find a lot of experts to testify on my behalf that that will be better for the health of my family."

Mr. Needleman: In a sense, we are talking about income redistribution; we are prepared to give people food stamps, which you cannot cash. At the same time we are willing to say that we are prepared to spend so much to be sure that people get the health care they need, as part of an income redistribution concept. Unless and until society is prepared to say that we are going to give every person the full $5,000 which is needed to maintain a minimum standard of living and let him spend it as he wishes, we are going to have trouble in not letting people cash in their health benefits.

Mr. Wolkstein: There are some peculiar experiments with regard to what people are willing to spend on health care. At the University of Pennsylvania some time ago, there was a test by a now-deceased health economist on whether people would pay the larger premium for a high health cost policy that really was not worth it, or save the money for a lower cost one that was more nearly worth it. After a full explanation, the faculty of the University of Pennsylvania elected the higher cost policy. Apparently, people have not reached the maximum of what they are willing to pay.

Dr. Blanpain: In connection with that experiment in Philadelphia, I would like to refer to the Australian experiment with compulsory insurance which is now taking place where the consumer has been given the option either to contribute 2 percent of his income to the government insurance plan and then be eligible for the whole wide range of the package, or to figure out for himself, within his income, whether he will opt out of that system and then buy a limited package of services through private insurance.

Dr. Enthoven: Ultimately, if we want to get back to a satisfactory result, we have to produce a system which involves competition and in which various consumer groups bear the cost implications of the decisions that they make. If they choose a more costly system, then they should bear the consequences.

❋ *Chapter 3*

Health Care Capital Financing: Regulation, the Market, and Public Policy

Thomas Joe
Jack Needleman
Lawrence S. Lewin

INTRODUCTION

The purpose of this paper is to explore issues related to capital financing of health care, with special emphasis on "market" versus "regulatory" strategies for influencing capital allocation decisions. Too frequently, this debate has been phrased in terms of dichotomy between a deregulated free market health care industry and an industry controlled by government regulation. Given the current mix of health care financing and its likely future, this dichotomy is too theoretical and bears little relation to reality. Government now pays 42 percent[1] of the total health care bill and further influences capital allocation through the availability of tax-free bonds, loan guarantees, and its reimbursement formulae. National health insurance may change the mechanisms by which government distributes its medical care funds but, almost certainly, it will not reduce the proportion flowing through government and is likely to increase it.

If the debate between "market" and "regulation" is to be relevant to public policy, it must be recast to reflect the fact that government involvement in health care financing is a dominant feature of the current scene. Regulation is already extensively established. The critical questions for capital policy are, therefore, not whether to have complete or no regulation, but how is regulation likely to affect capital availability and allocation and utilization decisions; how can the existing tendency toward overcapitalization best be controlled; and how extensively can market mechanisms be developed within an environment of government financing.[a] To address these issues, this paper will:

[a](Phrasing the issue in this manner underscores the fact that a functional market must be created by design and will not be achieved by merely reducing regulatory efforts.)

1. Provide a brief background analysis of the characteristics and critical problems of the health industry that have created the current need to examine the way in which the industry functions;
2. Describe efforts by government and others to influence capital allocation decisions in the health industry;
3. Analyze the likely impact of these efforts on the availability of capital; and
4. Discuss a strategy for policy initiatives which utilize government regulation but introduce market elements into the capital financing system.

It must be strongly emphasized that the availability and allocation of capital in the health care industry is an important issue. This importance stems first from the fact that the distribution of capital sets limits on the distribution of health care services. An inadequate supply of capital or its maldistribution (geographically or in the mix of services created) can reduce the availability of necessary services. The importance of capital transcends this and encompasses the relationship of capital allocation decisions to the way we examine and structure the health care system in this country. The availability and allocation of capital cannot, and should not, be considered apart from the related issues of health care financing, delivery, administration, and manpower. This conference cannot be so narrowly focused that it views capital policy either apart from other issues in health care or as dominating them to the point where other issues are viewed as subordinate to it.

Capital policy must be tied to a broader health care policy. While we do not have sufficient knowledge about how the different factors affecting the health care system interact with each other, we do know that unnecessary capital expenditures, both in terms of overused hospital and nursing home beds and expensive equipment and technology, have contributed significantly to the high cost of medical care. Moreover, if we can develop a policy on capital financing, we should be able to make some headway toward controlling health care costs in general. There has been a tendency in the past to consider the policy issues of capital financing as an adversary argument between two theories, two philosophies and two mechanisms—that is, a private free market opposed to public control and accountability. The challenge of this conference is to bring together both concepts to address the issue of so managing capital financing as to optimize the entire health care system.

PROBLEMS IN THE HEALTH CARE INDUSTRY

The most acute problem affecting health care in this country today is our inability to control costs. The cost control issue is related to all aspects of the structure—incentives and financing of health care in general—and, specifically, to policies that affect the formation and allocation of capital. The rapid growth in health care expenditures and prices is a relatively recent phenomenon that began with the expansion of third party coverage under private health insurance programs following World War II and accelerated dramatically with the enactment of the Medicare and Medicaid programs in 1965.[2] The federal government, although clearly desirous of controlling costs under Medicaid and Medicare, has, itself, never been able to establish and implement effective policy in this area and has, instead, relied largely on jawboning the private third party insurers which function as fiscal intermediaries. From FY 1965 to 1975, per capita health expenditures in the United States rose from $170 to $476 and total personal health care expenditures rose from 5.9 percent to 8.3 percent of the GNP.[3] In addition, the rate of increase in the cost of health care throughout the decade has consistently been above the inflation rate in the economy as a whole.

Walter McClure has done an excellent job in analyzing the structure of the health care system and how its incentives lead inevitably to the increased costs that we are now experiencing. He concludes that there is an inexhaustible "demand" for health care services and that, so long as the health care industry is dominated by third party payers, specialized physicians, hospitals which are dependent on physicians for their patients, provider-induced demand, and reimbursement policies based on reasonable costs and charges, health care services will continue to consume greater and greater portions of the GNP.[4] As a result, we are currently in a situation where the need for controls on health care costs is pre-eminent and, in order to be effective, such controls must apply to the industry as a whole, not just to that part which is government funded. This is especially important as we consider various forms of national health insurance because, as McClure points out, almost any plan under consideration must first come to grips with the cost control issue or expanded coverage will produce an even more rapid rise in health care expenditures.

One aspect of the rise in health care costs has been the substantial overcapitalization of health care services during the last fifteen years. The amount of capital which has been invested in health care has expanded considerably; the number of nonfederal, short-term general and other specialty hospitals increased from 5,407 in 1960 to 6,977 in 1974. The number of beds in such hospitals increased from 639,000 to 931,000, representing an increase in the bed-to-population ratio over this period from 3.6 beds per thousand population, to 4.4 beds per thousand population. Total assets in such hospitals increased from $10.9 billion in 1960 to $41.8 billion in 1974, an increase of 283 percent. Assets per bed increased from $17,000 to $45,000.[5] Similarly, the number of nursing facilities increased dramatically from 8,128 in 1963 to over 20,000 in 1974. The number of beds in nursing facilities increased from 319,000 to 1,112,000.

There is widespread evidence that many of the facilities which have already been developed were not needed and that, nonetheless, the trend for newer, bigger, better equipped hospitals and nursing facilities still persists. Thus, it is not surprising that industry-wide utilization rates and cost-effectiveness in general have not kept pace with the growth in institutional capacity. Current occupancy in short-term general and other specialty hospitals is approximately 75 percent, while a commonly accepted standard for efficient utilization is in the 80–85 percent range. In many individual communities, including large urban areas that might be expected to operate with higher occupancy rates, the situation is far worse and still deteriorating. There is also evidence that the availability of institutions such as hospitals and nursing homes and the existence of reimbursement policies which make institutional care feasible have combined to create a situation in which a large percentage of persons are placed in medical institutions when they could have been adequately cared for in less expensive facilities or on an outpatient basis.[6] There is good evidence that a significant portion of utilization is provider-induced, and that "a built bed is a filled bed."[7] Clearly, there are powerful incentives on providers to use excess space in facilities. Efforts to control this use point in two directions: on the one hand, utilization reviews which discourage physicians from overhospitalizing patients and performing unnecessary surgery and, on the other hand, limiting the availability of hospitals and nursing home beds. Many argue that the best utilization control is a tight bed supply.

The overinvestment in health care facilities as well as the overutilization of facilities cannot be understood except in relation to the expansion of third party reimbursement and the major weaknesses in the way that reimbursement rates have been established under third party systems. Currently, 65 percent of personal health care expenditures are paid with third party funds. This high and growing level of third party payment has created an unusual "market" in which the individual who receives the service (the patient) is different from the individual who makes the consumption decision (the physician) and these are most often separate from the organization which pays for the service (the third party). The result is that provider and patient decisions about health care are often made without regard to cost, and third party payers generally have not been effective proxies for a cost-conscious consumer.[b]

For the most part, third party reimbursement for institutional providers has been set on the basis of retroactive costs or institutionally set charges. For example, the original Medicare law provided that institutional providers would be reimbursed on a cost basis with a provision for both no profit and no loss for providing services to Medicare beneficiaries. The system currently operates through the establishment of an interim per diem rate of payment with a provision for final cost reporting at the end of the fiscal period. This system clearly offers no financial incentive for improved performance and reduced costs. Little, if any, discipline has been imposed either on operating costs per se or on the effects of capital budgets on operating costs since the per diem reimbursement for patient care automatically includes depreciation of capital assets and the interest costs of capital investments. The funding of depreciation on contributed

[b]Clark Havighurst, in his comments on this paper, argues that third party cost containment efforts have been hampered by legal constraints and that the opportunity now exists to remove these and allow these "purchasing agents" to recreate a market.

capital has also created cash reserves which have further improved access to capital markets. Third party payers have, thus, underwritten the risks of investment, thereby making health care institutions an attractive financial risk, increasing the availability of capital and, consequently, contributing to overcapitalization and increased health care costs. The expansion of the nursing home industry is a classic case in point where the availability of Medicaid and Medicare reimbursement has significantly contributed to the overcapitalization and overbuilding of the private nursing home industry, resulting in expensive nursing care for many people who simply need custodial room and board. The changes in health care financing in the past two decades have enabled health care providers to undertake capital expansion plans with a minimum of regulatory restraint and with little financial risk. This absence of financial risk constitutes a structural departure from classic free market practice.

It is, therefore, no surprise that every seriously contemplated form of national health insurance and other proposed legislation, such as the Talmadge Medicare-Medicaid Amendments, all include some mechanism for altering reimbursement systems, placing limitations on reimbursement and moderating capital investment decisions. The next section discusses several recent efforts to influence rising health care costs and capital allocation decisions that are currently in place or in process.

CURRENT APPROACHES

It should be clear from the preceding discussion that the question is not *whether* to influence the health care sector but *how* to do it in a manner that would accentuate the positive market incentives for efficiency through competition and other devices while ensuring a coherent and accountable health care system.

There is an extensive base of literature discussing the relative merits of expanded regulation to control the financial decisions of health care providers, as well as of efforts to develop and improve the operation of markets within the health care sector.[8] We are currently in a regulated environment from which there appears to be no real support for retreat. Few people would seriously question institutional and provider regulation with respect to health, safety, and professional credentials. Instead, the debate arises around regulation of operating expenditures, prices, and capital formation. Passage of the National Health Planning and Resource Development Act of 1974 (P.L. 93-641) represents a major federal endorsement of such regulation, particularly related to capital, and suggests that public regulation is to be a basic element in a future health care system. However, the form of that regulation and of the health care system in general remains at issue.

Traditionally, in the United States, there is a preference for reliance on free market forces over public regulation. There are three reasons. First, the notion of incentives and encouragement of appropriate behavior is preferred to dictation or coercion. Second, there remain strong doubts about the ability of regulation to achieve its goals. Regulation has not been notably successful in other areas of the economy,[9] and the limited experience in the United States as well as the experience of other countries in controlling health care expenditures through regulatory means is, at best, uneven.[10] While some studies suggest that regulation has been able to moderate the growth of health care costs and the development of unnecessary services, at least in specific locations,[11] other studies suggest that regulation has had either no effect or has actually increased the costs that are associated with health care.[12] Finally, there are the inherent limitations on what government can accomplish. These considerations notwithstanding, it must be noted that evaluations of existing regulatory efforts must be viewed with caution, since the regulations themselves are developmental, are in response to relatively recent phenomena in the health care system, and are not based on any common integrated framework. As health care costs have risen during the last decade, the response has been haphazard. On the one hand, regulation has evolved in a piecemeal, uncoordinated and, possibly, conflicting manner, creating an industry in which there appears to be overregulation with little positive effect; while, on the other hand, attempts to alter the structure of the health care system through innovative financing and delivery systems have been, with few exceptions, sporadic and, generally, small-scale efforts.

Principal among current regulatory and market development efforts are:

1. Capital Expenditure and Service Development Controls
2. Prospective Rate Controls
3. Health Planning and Resource Development Act
4. Health Maintenance Organization (HMO) Development
5. Professional Standards Review Organizations (PSROs)
6. Increased Cost Competition
7. Expanded Consumer Cost-Sharing

Over the past several years, capital expenditure and services development controls have become the principal instrument of federal and state efforts to contain the rapid rise in health costs. These controls are predicated on the belief that the supply of health capital assets and services is a critical determinant of the cost and utilization of health care. Since federal and state governments now finance a substantial portion of both the capital and operating costs of health care, controls have been established to ensure that capital investment decisions in the health industry take into account the marginal costs and benefits to the general public as well as to the individual provider institution.

There are presently two major types of these controls: state Certificates of Need (C/N) statutes and Section 1122 of the Social Security Act. In states that have adopted C/N statutes, health care institutions may not add to the existing supply of health facilities, equipment or services without prior state approval. The first C/N statute was enacted by New York State in 1965; at present, a total of thirty states have enacted some form of C/N statute.

Under Section 1122 of the Social Security Act, the federal government may deny Medicare and Medicaid reimbursement for capital costs resulting from investments that exceed $100,000 or that increase beds or services if such investments are made without prior state approval. Since Section 1122 was adopted in October 1972, thirty-nine states have contracted with the Department of Health, Education and Welfare to conduct reviews under Section 1122, including fifteen states which already had C/N programs.

At the present time, only Missouri (which recently canceled its 1122 contract) and West Virginia do not have either a C/N statute or a Section 1122 review process, though West Virginia does have a very strong C/N statute under consideration.

A comparatively new form of regulation which seems to be gaining wide acceptance is the regulation of expenditures for institutional health care through prospective rate setting. Under these systems, in which rates are set in advance and retrospective increases are either prohibited entirely or severely limited, the provider institutions are theoretically at risk to the extent that their costs exceed revenues produced by the prospective reimbursement rate. Currently, nine states have established prospective reimbursement systems applicable to at least some third party payers, and in five of these the goal is to establish a total revenue ceiling for an institution as a whole.[13] A major feature of this type of regulation is that rate-setting agencies automatically build into the rates provisions for depreciation, interest and, for proprietary institutions, a return on equity. While building these factors into the rate is an advantage for the institution, the rate-setting agency can also gain a power of review and, in most cases, of approval over both operational and capital budgets. Thus, the reimbursement process could be, theoretically, a source of considerable leverage over capital expenditure decisions.

A third major initiative has been the enactment of the National Health Planning Resources and Development Act of 1974 (P.L. 93-641) with the goal of establishing Health Systems Agencies (HSAs) covering the entire nation, each with the capacity to plan and develop integrated networks of health providers that would efficiently meet established community health needs. There are wide variations in the abilities and experience of local HSAs in moving toward this objective. Perhaps more important in the short term, P.L. 93-641 requires that all states establish C/N programs that meet federal standards or risk the loss of federal funds for health services and research. The Act also introduces officially, if only tentatively, the notion of "recertification" of the need for already existing facilities. This provision, although "toothless" at the moment, is based on the premise that patterns of need may change and existing facilities might become a burden in the future. Clearly, if this concept becomes operational, it has the potential of increasing risk for institutional providers. Since current reimburse-

ment systems provide a major cushion against failures and market exit, the introduction of recertification systems could serve as an incentive for the kind of risk
analysis that is more commonly found in market-sensitive industries.

Fourth, a policy that is currently being advocated and pursued, although on a
more limited basis, is a strategy to restructure the systems of paying for, and
delivering, health care services through Health Maintenance Organizations
(HMOs) so that a market can be made to operate more effectively without much
need for extensive, detailed regulatory review over capital expenditure decisions
or specific per service reimbursement rates. The goal of those advocating HMOs
or other prepaid group practices is to create an integrated network of services for
a specific population of subscribers. A predetermined package of services would
be available for a fixed price per year. Consumers would be free to choose the
plan which best meets their needs, based on considerations of cost, scope of service, convenience, and quality. The objective is to alter both the structure and
financial incentives of the health care system in order to improve efficiency and
service delivery. Although, to date, the experience of HMOs in acquiring start up
capital and successfully marketing their coverage has been mixed, HMOs remain
an intriguing alternative, and have been at the center of many market development strategies.

Fifth, in part to modify the relatively unlimited power which physicians
now have to order health care services, often without regard to cost/benefit considerations, the Congress has established the Professional Standards Review
Organization (PSRO) program. This effort involves establishing regional councils,
composed primarily of physicians, to set standards for appropriate care and to
review performance. The risk here, as potentially with any regulatory initiative,
is that it will operate to the benefit of the regulated (the physicians) and not to
the benefit of the consumer.

Sixth, an element often proposed in the market development strategy is for
price regulation without entry controls. The prices that third parties pay for
specific services would be fixed and based upon a uniform formula or common
price for all potential offerors of the service. Entry into, and exit from, the market would be open. Providers who felt that they could meet the price and quality
constraints imposed by the third party payer would be free to make services
available. Those who advocate this approach believe that freedom of entry is
critical to assure that inefficient providers are not protected by regulation and
that opportunities to organize services in new ways are preserved.

Seventh, another alternative that is often proposed is to increase consumer
cost-sharing in order to reduce consumer and market insensitivity to health care
costs, thereby, it is hoped, reducing demand and utilization rates. This proposal
is usually coupled with increased use of publicity, price advertising, and consumer education to increase the ability to shop for services.

Finally, some market development advocates argue that many of the government regulatory approaches—rate setting or negotiation and utilization review,

for instance—would be more energetically pursued by private third party payers competing against one another on a price basis. They advocate removing legal barriers to the private implementation of these programs. This is a plausible strategy. The operational success of existing third party efforts—Blue Cross "conformance with local planning" requirements, rate negotiation, and utilization review through reviews of bills—has not been impressive. In assessing the potential for private efforts, the reasons for their failures require further research, as does the willingness of third parties to assume these responsibilities without government regulatory leadership.

Most of the efforts which have been made, or are being contemplated, have been taken without careful consideration of their impact on access to capital. Some of these efforts, like the HMO Act, include access to federal funds to assist in development, but this cannot be considered a coordinated capital policy. The next section, therefore, explores the question of what might happen to capital availability were the regulatory strategy or market development strategy to be implemented successfully. Specifically, it focuses on whether capital funds can still be obtained as the regulation or structure of the health care system is changed, whether the sources of capital will shift, and whether the cost of capital will increase.

THE EFFECT OF POLICY ON
CAPITAL FINANCING

Capital funds for institutional health care providers currently come from a variety of sources, including standard mortgages and bank loans, to commercial loans by large private institutions such as insurance companies, and tax-exempt revenue bonds that are sold through public agencies with interest rates lower than they would be if interest were taxable. There are also a number of programs whereby private mortgages are guaranteed by the government, such as the Federal Housing Administration and the Hill-Burton programs. Direct government taxing authority may also be used to support institutional capital financing through both revenue and general obligation bonds. Finally, philanthropic donations continue to represent a major source of funds for capital expenditures.

As part of the development of a capital financing policy we need to know what can be expected to happen to the sources of capital as the environment changes, either through changes in regulation or through new efforts at market development, and we must assess the consequences of any changes for public policy. Our focus is on the private capital market and philanthropy. Government programs began as responses to limited private sources of funds, to the supplementing of these funds or to serve as seed money. Increases in government-provided funds would appear, therefore, to be a fallback position should access to private funds seriously decrease. For purposes of this analysis, the effects of regulation and market development on capital availability are considered separately.

Regulation

Analysis suggests that access to private capital need not be negatively affected by a well-conceived, integrated regulatory approach which assures some stability of health care financing on which to base investment decisions. Capital markets respond to risk associated with an investment.[c] If estimates of risk increase, funds will be less available or available only at a higher rate of return. If risks are perceived as decreasing, the costs associated with capital are likely to go down and the amount of capital available to increase.

Certificate of need, the main form of current regulations, should decrease the risks associated with a loan to an institution. A favorable certification review is a positive outside assessment that a service or bed is needed and that estimated utilization levels are sufficient to support the service. Rate review agencies have generally been bound by certificate of need judgments, so that once a project is approved, recovery of capital and operating costs will generally be built into new rates.

Certification may have a negative effect on philanthropy, however, by limiting the freedom of institutions to apply restricted funds to the capital expenditures for which they were donated. This frustration of the philanthropist's intent may, in the long run, reduce the ability of institutions to obtain such "free" capital. A recent analysis of the reasons why nonprofit institutions get into financial difficulty suggests that a key problem has been over endowment, with plants for which operating funds are not available.[14] However, if this is, in fact, the case, then the redirection or forced rechanneling of philanthropy may be warranted.

The potential impact of rate review on risk is less clear-cut. It can operate to increase risk. Indeed, one of the rationales for rate review is to place health care providers at risk with respect to their operating costs. The increased risk associated with rate review may be mitigated, however, by several factors. First, uniform rate determination can reduce the uncertainty and the special pressures imposed through the current complexities and patchwork of alternative reimbursement systems with which institutions must now deal. Furthermore, to the extent that the conditions under which an institution might gain or lose are better known, as they could be with a clearly enunciated rate review policy, investors should be able to calculate more clearly the risks that are associated with a particular investment. The influence of increases in risk is also likely to be felt more by the poor operators, and by those institutions with the weakest management, and not be felt uniformly across the entire health care system. As with

---

[c]Economic theory distinguishes between "risk" and "uncertainty." Risk is used in those cases where the probabilities of specific outcomes are known or can be estimated; i.e., in a true economic risk situation, average interest rates should be such that when they are discounted for the probability of failure, the return is equivalent to that on a risk-free investment. In cases of uncertainty, the probabilities of specific outcomes are unknown and reliable estimates cannot be made. In the discussion which follows, these two forms of hazards are both meant to be included in the term "risk." Where uncertainty is specifically meant, that term is used.

certificate of need, however, rate review is likely to have a negative effect on philanthropy if rate setting agencies follow the lead of some current programs in establishing requirements on institutions to spend unrestricted funds and other gifts on patient care in order to offset the need for patient-derived revenues.

The experience of the health care system under existing regulations would appear to bear out this theoretical view. Recent experience in the hospital and municipal bond market can be taken as a case in point.[15] Hospital bonds sell at a premium of 20 to 30 percent above other tax-free municipal bonds of comparable quality. However, bonds sold by states with extensive regulation, that is, with both certificate of need and rate review, do not appear to sell at rates different from those sold by states with only limited regulation. This is confirmed by staff in the hospital associations in Connecticut, New York, and Maryland who indicated that, in the period following the introduction of state rate review, there was no change in the ability of the institutions within those states to acquire funds. The bond market also suggests that investors are capable of distinguishing between well-managed and poorly-managed institutions.

The actual effect of future regulations on capital availability and on the costs of capital will depend on how carefully the regulators construct their policies and how carefully these policies are explained to the investment community. Regulators, particularly those involved in rate regulation, must consciously consider the potential impact of the policies which they adopt on the ability of an institution to repay debt. For example, policy may be designed to place providers at risk for both poor management and for offering unnecessary beds and services. We believe that regulation should treat each of these forms of risk separately. Managerial efficiency should be within the capacity of each provider and risks associated with it are appropriate, provided there is also an opportunity to recover deficits through improved management. On the other hand, once society has assumed a role in determining the need for facilities and services, investors should not stand alone in assuming the risk of decertification, should circumstances later make the facility unnecessary. Mechanisms can, and should be, developed for sharing the costs with government or with the payers for care. In establishing regulation, it is also important that policies among different regulatory programs (such as certificate of need, rate review, state bonds) be coordinated so that the institutions and potential investors have evidence of consistent rules, consistently applied. Only three cases were reported by individuals in the municipal bond market in which that market was, for a period, closed to hospital issues. Two of these cases reflected failures by regulators to meet these conditions.[d] Finally, regulators must explain the intent of specific policies and the

---

[d]One was during the Economic Stabilization Program, when the Cost of Living Council failed to establish a system for the consideration of long-range increases in rates to cover capital expansion plans. The other resulted from a disagreement between the Maryland Health Services Cost Review Commission and Higher Education Finance Authority over the appropriate standards for debt service ratios on new bond issues. The third case, New York, was described as a general problem with the state's bonds and not a specific reaction to regulatory policy toward hospitals.

rationale for specific controls or standards. The private capital market seems extremely sensitive to uncertainty, even more so than to known risks. Those involved with the capital markets should be pressing for explicit statements and participation in the development of regulatory policy. If these things are done, private investment capital should remain available to the health care sector under increased regulation.

Market Development

The preceding section examined the likelihood of maintaining access to private capital markets if regulation is increased, concluding that access could be preserved and that private capital could continue to be used. This section examines the likely response of private capital sources to efforts to develop a more effective market in the health care sector. Our conclusion is that market development activities are likely to reduce access to private capital.

There are two reasons for this conclusion. It is based, first, on the concept behind market development, which is to improve provider responsiveness to appropriate supply and cost cues by increasing the degree of financial risk (as well as potential for gain) that is associated with providing medical services. These efforts also seek to assure that opportunities exist for both entry into and exit from the market, exits which, at times, may be forced by financial failure. Given these policy elements, the market development strategy is likely to generate increased capital costs.

The second reason why access to private capital may decrease under a market strategy is that there is a great deal of uncertainty with respect to new forms of medical expenditures such as health maintenance organizations or ambulatory surgical centers. Questions as to their potential profitability, the extent to which a market exists for them, and the means by which to evaluate specific projects not only adds to the risks, but makes the risks unknown.

One of the dilemmas of the market development strategy is that, while investment is likely to be less attractive under this policy, the policy itself requires greater private assumption of risk. One possible source of funds is from individuals and groups looking for speculative opportunities. To attract these sources, the bases for establishing reimbursement rates, rates of return on investment, and premiums would have to be revised so that legitimate opportunities for large gains are possible. The wisdom of establishing major forms of health care delivery with a conscious intent to create an opportunity for large speculative profits can be questioned. While proprietary institutions can provide appropriate services and high quality care,[16] the experience with California's prepaid group plans under Medicaid and the situation documented by the New York State Moreland Act Commission strongly suggest that the possibility of large profits may undermine the commitment of proprietary medicine to quality service.

An alternative and more appropriate strategy would be to underwrite the costs of developing market-oriented mechanisms until a track record can be established by which the actual financial risks can be determined. This would appear to be the rationale for the federal Health Maintenance Organization Act. This type of support in a start-up period is appropriate if it is believed that the long-term benefits of an improved market should be explored.

Ultimately, under a market development strategy, financing must be shifted back to the private sector. If the risks remain too high to attract private capital, they can be eased either through more favorable reimbursement mechanisms or through tax benefits. At the same time, nonprofit organizations should be encouraged to compete in the restructured market. Financing these initiatives may represent a fruitful new role for philanthropy.

A STRATEGY FOR CHANGE

The preceding discussion examined the need for major changes in health care financing and organization to address the needs of improved access to appropriate services and cost control, and also explore the ways in which access to capital might affect the choices which can be made. In this section, we speculate on how these elements might be combined into a strategy that links planning and regulation directly to budgeting and financing and imposes external controls where necessary to assure public accountability for health care expenditures. The strategy that is presented also provides opportunities for market incentives to encourage lower costs.

Our approach is not the only scenario that might be constructed to reflect the issues facing the health care system and the likely responses of the capital market, but it does illustrate how the requirements that are imposed by each of these factors might be addressed in a coherent way.

The proposed strategy, which needs to be developed in considerably more depth and then tested, seeks to combine elements of a competitive free market approach with regulation that has both the power and flexibility to initiate and shape a coordinated health care system as well as to prevent unnecessary expenditures or overcapitalization. The strategy assumes that the government's role in the health care industry is not to be limited to that of a prudent buyer, but should include the shaping of the health care system into a network of widely accessible, efficiently run, quality services. The main elements of the strategy are:

1. The establishment of state or regional boards which have responsibility for setting regional ceilings on health care expenditures (private and public) and for establishing prospective rates of payment for institutional care. It is proposed to start initially only with hospitals, nursing facilities and inpatient physician care, since, together, they account for 55 percent of all personal health care expenditures.

2. For those services for which it is appropriate, hospitals would be reimbursed on the basis of established uniform rates rather than on budgeted costs, and their rate structures would be charges calculated from a hybrid of budgeted expendi-

tures (within the overall ceiling) and uniform rates.[e] Providers with lower costs would have the opportunity to benefit from their efficiency. The overall ceiling would help control the tendencies toward increasing volume which fixed reimbursement rates encourage. The existence of uniform rates should also create incentives for institutions to share services or contract out services (including medical services such as ambulatory surgery and laboratory work) where appropriate. Private operators, with private capital, can enter this contracting market offering services at less than the established uniform rates. The institution which contracts out can be expected to police the quality of its contractees.

3. Operating and capital costs would be subsumed under the same overall regional ceiling. Placing both operating and capital expenditures under a single regional ceiling would force consideration of the effects of capital expenditures on operating costs and require budgeting authorities to make trade-offs among projects and between existing operating expenses and the development of new services. It would also create a vested interest in health care institutions to educate physicians about the costs of overutilizing institutional services and might also encourage them to be more selective in developing arrangments with physicians. The certificate of need process would have to be adjusted to reflect the need to establish priorities for limited funds.[f] Continued use of private capital sources would introduce the additional discipline of market interest rates (whether subsidized by interest free status or not) on the rate of expansion. Debt guarantees, if they are used at all, should be the responsibility of the regional board. Philanthropy would have a clear role in this system of earning the trade-offs and allowing more to be done. The existence of an overall ceiling would discourage the shortsighted patterns of capital formation unmatched by operating resources.

4. The same board would separate out the capital expenditures, research, training, etc., from operating budgets in determining reimbursement for patient care. Reimbursement rates would be based on separate reviews of capital and operating costs. While reimbursement rates would be the same for similar services in similar institutions throughout the jurisdiction of the board, there would be flexible rates established to encourage innovative service delivery options such as HMOs and ambulatory care units, at least in an initial start-up period and to ensure that the system does not exclude competition and legitimate new entry into the market.

5. Retirement of unneeded facilities would be a part of this system, and might be accomplished in several ways. For example, a system similar to a state insurance insolvency fund might be developed. Should an unnecessary facility be

---

[e]This system presupposes the existence of a uniform accounting and cost allocation system such as that contemplated in the National Health Planning and Resources Development Act and in effect in California, Washington, Arizona, and Maryland.

[f]A variation on this approach has been used in the Rhode Island prospective reimbursement system.

closed or not be able to pay a debt, that debt would be assumed by other institutions providing comparable services in the area. While charges for these services might be increased to allow the assumption of the debt, the increases could not be so large that the overall regional ceiling is exceeded. Such a system would place the assumption of debt on the community for which the institutional closing is an advantage. It would enable each community to determine the extent to which it will commit itself to assuming existing debt, probably affecting the interest rate which institutions in that community receive in the capital market. The analysis of the costs associated with assuming the debt and shifting the services to other providers and the costs associated with maintaining the institutional service should also allow a comparison to be made of the relative advantages of each course of action.

6. Health maintenance organizations or other prepaid group practices could receive a formula apportionment of the regional ceiling based on enrollment, thereby reducing the total amount available to existing providers for non-HMO utilization. If supported by certificate of need provisions which provide special protection to HMOs in the development and marketing of their services, this apportionment would reduce impediments to organizational innovation that are otherwise implicit in the proposal. In areas where there is an adequate supply of institutional beds so that it would be preferable to transfer existing capital to HMOs through sale, lease, or service contracts rather than to develop new facilities, the allocation formulae and reimbursement rates can be constructed to create incentives for such action. The potential sources of capital funds for HMOs would be the same as those currently in use—federal funds, private venture capital, and private grants.

7. Other new organizational forms should also be encouraged. These include Health Care Alliances, which are similar to HMOs but are organized by a third party insurer who would be at risk for the covered services. Health Care Alliances would be, basically, private insurance plans which cover services provided by, or referred through, a defined set of participating providers in a community. Similar to HMOs, Health Care Alliances and other potential new organizational forms should be apportioned a piece of the regional ceiling based on enrollment.

The approach outlined above attempts to control expenditures for health care by tying them to a fixed national figure rather than by continuing the current open-ended financing which threatens to consume even greater portions of the GNP without measurable improvement in health status. The need to function wholly within the expenditure ceiling should foster reallocation of the health care dollars away from expensive high technology care and facility expansion towards better use of limited health manpower and resources. It should also produce a more thoughtful and responsible approach to capital budgeting, provide a more vigorous test of the need for new and replacement capital, and sharpen the issues regarding the cost of capital and the risks associated with private investment in health care facilities. By weakening those reimbursement practices that obscure risk, it should encourage needed and appropriate capital investment while discouraging overcapitalization.

In addition, by setting rates that are applicable to both public and privately financed care, the approach guards against the creation of a dual system of health care, one for the rich and one for the poor. Finally, by combining a coordinated approach to regulation that ties planning to budgeting with the flexibility to encourage competitive as well as innovative service delivery systems, this approach holds the promise of solving some of the structural and financial dilemmas confronting public policy on health care.

SUMMARY

In summary, it is hoped that this paper raises some appropriate questions for discussion and detailed analysis during the remainder of this conference. The paper will have served its purpose if it sets the stage for more in-depth deliberations here on many of the aspects of health care capital financing and their relation to health care policy. The dichotomies between free market and regulatory mechanisms and between public and private strategies for health care need to be examined, debated and reconciled, not as either-or propositions, but in order to implement the best of each. This conference will be successful if the sum total of our discussions can provide some relevant insights on these issues for forthcoming public policy debate on National Health Insurance.

NOTES

1. M. Mueller and R. Gibson, "National Health Expenditures," *Social Security Bulletin,* February 1976.

2. United States Congress, Committee on Ways and Means, *National Health Insurance Resource Book* (Washington, D.C.: U.S. Government Printing Office, April 11, 1974), p. 6.

3. Mueller and Gibson, "National Health Expenditures."

4. W. McClure, "The Medical Care System under National Health Insurance: Four Models that Might Work and Their Prospects," *InterStudy,* Minneapolis, Minnesota, January 23, 1976, pp. 11-20.

5. American Hospital Association, *Hospital Statistics,* 1975 Edition, Table 1.

6. For hospitals, see Walter J. McNerney, *Hospital and Medical Economics: A Study of Population Services, Costs, Methods of Payment and Controls* (Chicago: Hospital Research and Education Trust, 1962). For nursing homes, see "Health Care of the Elderly Study; Monroe County, Rochester, N.Y.," and H. Kistin and R. Morris, "Alternatives to Institutional Care for the Elderly and Disabled," paper presented at the 24th annual meeting of the Gerentological Society, Houston, Texas, October 1971.

7. Among the evidence is D. Harris, "An Elaboration of the Relationship between General Hospital Supply and General Hospital Utilization," *Journal of*

Health and Social Behavior 15, 2 (June 1975): 163. See also Robert Evans, "Beyond the Medical Marketplace: Expenditure, Utilization and Pricing of Insured Health Care in Canada," in Spyros Andreopoulos (ed.), *National Health Insurance: Can We Learn From Canada?* (New York: John Wiley & Sons, 1975).

8. Major works include Anne R. Somers, *Hospital Regulation: The Dilemma of Public Policy* (Princeton: Princeton University, Industrial Relations Section, 1969); Institute of Medicine, *Controls on Health Care* (Washington, D.C.: National Academy of Sciences, 1974); and Clark C. Havighurst (ed.), *Regulating Health Facilities Construction* (Washington, D.C.: American Enterprise Institute, 1974). Also see Clark Havighurst's comments on this paper prepared for the conference. See Irving Levenson, *Financing and Regulation of Health Services* (New York: Health Services Administration, November 1973); and Walter M. McClure, "The Medical Care System Under National Health Insurance: Four Models that Might Work and Their Prospects," *InterStudy,* Minneapolis, Minnesota, January 23, 1976, for interesting syntheses and extensions of the regulation/market literature.

9. Clark C. Havighurst, "Regulation of Health Facilities and Services by Certificate of Need," *Virginia Law Review* V 59, 7 (October 1973): 1143; Roger Noll, "The Consequences of Public Utility Regulation of Hospitals," in Institute of Medicine, *Controls on Health Care.*

10. For England, see McClure, "The Medical Care System." For Canada, see Lewin and Associates, *Government Controls on the Health Care System: The Canadian Experience* (Washington, D.C., 1975).

11. Lewin and Associates, *An Evaluation of the Effectiveness and Efficiency of the Section 1122 Review Process* (Washington, D.C., 1975).

12. Fred J. Hellinger, "The Effect of Certificate of Need Legislation on Hospital Investment," *Inquiry* 12, 2 (June 1976):187. D.S. Salkever and T. Bice, *Impact of State Certificate-of-Need Laws on Health Care Cost and Utilization.* DHEW Publication HRA 76–3163, in press.

13. Lewin and Associates, Inc., *Nationwide Survey of State and Regional Health Regulation* (Washington, D.C., 1974), pp. 1–14. Identifies four states; the Washington State system has become operational since the completion of this report.

14. Bruce C. Vladek, "Why Non-Profits Go Broke," *The Public Interest* 42 (Winter 1976):86–101.

15. The information on the bond market is drawn from conversations with several investment bankers who are knowledgeable in hospital issues, and on a state-by-state analysis of recent bond issues prepared for the authors by Kidder, Peabody & Co.

16. See the Lewin and Associates, Inc., report for the Health Services Foundation, *Investor-Owned Hospitals: An Examination of Performance* (Chicago: Health Services Foundation, September 1976), Ch. 2, which examined patient mix, services and costs in investor-owned and nonprofit hospitals.

Discussion of
Health Care Capital Financing:
Regulation, the Market, and
Public Policy

Robert G. Evans

Perceptions of "the problem" of health care capital financing have undergone a dramatic change of emphasis in the last five to ten years.

Economists in particular, a decade ago, viewed the dominance of not-for-profit institutions in the hospital industry as a significant impediment to the translation of consumer/patient "demands" for health care, through the conventional market mechanisms of prices and profits, into the expansion of existing hospital "firms" or the entry of new ones. Rosenthal, and later Stevens and Newhouse and P. Ginsburg all studied what Stevens called "the anatomy of the supply response," the problem of matching capacity to demand, in an industry where, presumptively, capital stock adjustment decisions were not profit-motivated.[1] While the general problem is, of course, symmetric in expansion or contraction, the growth of both population and income levels appeared to make the inadequacy of the supply of new capital a more pressing policy issue.

The primary focus of the Joe, Needleman, and Lewin paper illustrates how times have changed. Among the "critical questions for capital policy" which the authors identify is the control of the "existing tendency toward overcapitalization" which is one of the sources of "the most acute problem affecting health care in this country . . . [is] our inability to control health care costs." The need to formulate capital policy so as to assist in attaining such control is the central theme of the paper, and the other "critical questions," the relation between direct regulation and capital availability and the potential for development of market mechanisms, are merely issues of the evaluation and balancing of alternative strategies toward this central objective.

In this balancing of regulatory against market strategies they stress the important point that, "A functional market must be created by design and will not be achieved by merely reducing regulatory efforts." Thus, they recognize implicitly that the predominantly private arrangements for health care delivery which predated massive government intervention did not constitute a "functional" market and that any proposal for more market mechanisms and less regulation must not merely seek to turn the clock back but must include strategies for changing the organization of the delivery system of health care as well. This need is brought out clearly by Havighurst who, in a strongly argued plea for more use of market mechanisms in health care delivery, concedes that increased regulation is defensible "only if we accept as given the health care and financing systems we now have."[2] His "modest proposals" for reform imply a radical transformation of those systems, as do, indeed, the Joe, Needleman, and Lewin proposals, although in a rather different direction.[a]

The "overcapitalization" concept which is central to the authors' argument appears to be used in at least three different senses. It may imply the inefficient choice of technology for the treatment of a given patient load—too high a capital/labor ratio or wrong point on the production function—for given relative prices and marginal productivities of capital and labor. This form of overcapitalization reflects Fuchs' "technological imperative" or Lee's "conspicuous production."[3] Alternatively, overcapitalization seems sometimes to be equated with over-capacity—too many hospital beds with attendant staff and support services for a given population—as reflected in occupancy rates far below those judged either technically optimal or adequate to provide standby capacity against unexpected demand. Finally, overcapitalization can be generalized to refer to overuse of hospital facilities, relative either to less costly institutional alternatives or to no institutionalization at all. For many patients, the impact of hospitalization on health status may be zero or negative, not only *ex post* but also *ex ante;* and such unnecessary utilization based on inadequate patient or provider information can hardly be identified with "demand" in any policy-relevant (or welfare-economic) sense.[b]

Each of these alternative meanings of "overcapitalization" represents an important dimension of the health care cost-escalation problem, and each is touched upon by the authors in their background analysis of the industry. They stress, and rightly, that, "The availability of capital cannot and should not be considered apart from the related issues of health care financing, delivery, administration, and manpower." In the process, they identify many of the sources of this prob-

[a]Where the earlier view went wrong, in brief, was in assuming that a demand curve for health care could be specified independently of supplier behavior, or, empirically, that demand in the economic sense could be identified with observed utilization, and that economic rents can be drawn out of an institution only in the form of accounting profits.

[b]It is, of course, true that people may derive forms of satisfaction from the consumption of health care other than those connected with improvement in health status. Ideally, one would like to separate "health-enhancing" and "amenity" aspects and let price signals allocate resources used for the latter. In some particular cases this may be possible, but there is always danger that the distinction may become a strategic variable whereby providers can manipulate the system to their own advantage—as is asserted to be the case with pay beds in hospitals under the British N.H.S.

lem, but they do not adequately distinguish between those factors which make hospital costs too high and those which underlie the current escalation of costs. Occupancy rates of 75 percent in short-term general hospitals are pointed out as evidence of overcapacity, and so they are, but this rate is not significantly below that of a decade ago. The rapid increases in bed/population ratios referred to in the period 1960-74 seem to be matched closely by utilization, and do not, in themselves, suggest which is cause and which effect. Salkever and Bice have shown that Certificate of Need (C/N) laws tend to inhibit bed construction but not the expansion of hospital capital assets.[4] This suggests that, while existing levels of hospital utilization and occupancy may have built in an unnecessarily high *level* of costs due to unnecessary care and overcapacity, the *growth* of such costs may be traced to increasing overcapitalization in the narrower sense of too high a capital/labor ratio in the hospital—excessive gadgetry and unnecessary or low-return procedures being performed on patients. These would include, for example, extension of "heroic" medicine of the short-term life-support form which can be enormously expensive without showing up in utilization rates or health status outcomes.

Another major dynamic problem, of course, is provider incomes. In Canada, utilization rates have been reasonably stable for a number of years, drifting up in the 1960s and down somewhat since 1971. Moreover, facilities and capital equipment acquisition have been regulated with fair success by provincial government reimbursement agencies. The primary source of cost escalation appears to be the size and, particularly, the rate of earnings of the hospital workforce. Levels of utilization in Canada appear to be excessive relative to most observers' evaluation of "need," just as they are in the United States, but that is not the source of the dynamic problem.

Of course, the authors may quite validly respond that their paper focuses on capital, not labor, and one cannot do everything at once. But I think that, given the significance which they attach (I believe rightly) to the cost escalation problem, they might have identified their targets with a bit more precision before launching into the discussion of strategies for control through modifying capital-allocation decisions. Their shots are scattered rather widely, and while the availability ability of targets is such that few, if any, shots miss, the discussion could be much clearer if the sources of cost-escalation were more precisely identified. At the same time, identification of these sources would help to pinpoint the sources of decision-making authority which lead to the different types of over-capitalization problems—who's in charge here?—and, thus, enlighten the discussion of different policy responses. For example, one traditional economic (and medical) rationale for excessive hospital capacity and utilization has been the interest of private entrepreneurial physicians in access to subsidized hospital capital and labor. Scitovsky repeats an anonymous quotation that hospitals do not have patients, they only have doctors.[5] Yet, an additional, politically potent source of opposition to recent efforts in Canada to reduce the levels of hospital overcapitalization are the hospital unions, whose members have an important stake in maintaining the existing level and location of the hospital "plant."

Joe, Needleman, and Lewin identify and discuss seven different types of approach to altering the structure of the health care system, but, in fact, these appear reducible to about three and one-half, depending on where one locates the decision-making power whose exercise one proposes to influence. If the hospital itself is considered the relevant decision-making institution, prospective rate setting or other forms of price regulation may be used to create efficiency incentives for hospital management. The authors distinguish prospective rate setting as hospital-specific, and price regulation as setting fixed prices on a marketwide basis with free entry and exit. They also point out that hospital-specific prospective rate-setting might evolve into a general power of budgetary review, as it has in Canada, but this is a much more direct form of regulation.

The problems with treating the hospital as the target for efficiency-inducing incentives are several. First, it is very difficult to identify a uniform product which can be subject to rate setting or price regulation; hence, the tendency of the former to become budget review. In the absence of appropriate product definition, incentives to the hospital may well be perverse. Second, many of the key variables affecting costs may be outside the hospital's control. Decisions as to hospital use and mode of treatment are physician decisions. Wages may depend on areawide union bargaining. Price or rate regulation may, in fact, encourage further excessive hospital use in hospitals where average costs exceed marginal (as they generally do). Finally, even in hospital-targeted incentives are successful, they will tend to relate the expansion and contraction of hospitals to the relative efficiency of their managements, which may not correspond to the geographic patterns of need for hospital services.

A more broadly based strategy, involving HMOs or PSROs, targets the physician as the key decisionmaker in the health care delivery system. The HMO approach, by integrating hospital, medical, and insurance services, creates an incentive pattern which discourages "overcapitalization" in all three senses.

A paper devoted to balancing market versus regulatory mechanisms might well have given more attention to these institutions, since some authors have suggested that a world of numerous, differentiated competitive HMOs might be the proper market solution—Milton Friedman's "department stores of medicine."[6] On the other hand, the PSRO appears to be a straight regulatory device which seems at least as likely to standardize and freeze into place the existing patterns of practice as to encourage more efficient modes of delivery. As the authors point out, any regulatory initiative may operate to the benefit of the regulatee. A theme which they fail to develop, here as elsewhere, is that the central problem of cost escalation, when looked at from another perspective, is the problem of limiting the growth of provider incomes. Present patterns of capital utilization are part of the intricate mechanism whereby those incomes are maintained and increased.

The regulatory approach of C/N laws or the 1974 H.P.R.D. Act, on the other hand, is consistent with the view that the world is just too complex or the political system is too immobile. Rather than structuring incentives to modify physician or hospital behavior in socially desirable ways, one simply tightens up on the supply of capital. The rationing of access to capital becomes a political process. The difficulty here is that, as Salkever and Bice and Hellinger show, direct constraints do not seem to be working.[7] They have controlled only one dimension of capital (beds) but capital, like money, is fungible and flows into the hospital system through other channels. One might discourage this flow through the possibility of "recertification," as described in the paper, by putting investors at risk that unnecessary hospital facilities might be closed down and their bonds defaulted. As the authors note, however, this provision is currently "toothless" and its political feasibility seems dubious. Canadian experience suggests that one can get a tight grip on hospital capital spending, but only through a system of public control over the sources of both capital and operating funds. The capital control seems more successful than the operating budget control, though as British Columbia's newly announced University Hospital demonstrates, the political process is also sensitive to random shocks that are unrelated to health care needs.

The possibilities for limiting overcapitalization through increased consumer cost-sharing are dealt with in the paper in about five lines, which may somewhat overemphasize their usefulness. Within a significantly restructured health care system, such as Havighurst's world of competing HMOs, consumer responses to price signals could be an important part of a market-based allocation process. But, as long as information flows between providers and consumers remain as badly blocked as they are at present, proposals for consumer cost-sharing will tend to resemble efforts to turn back the clock. The authors rightly point out at the beginning that a functional market must be created by design; consumer cost-sharing by itself will not do so.

The section of the paper which focuses on the impact of alternative policies on sources of capital funding seems a bit obscure of purpose. The thrust of an earlier section analyzing the problems of the health care industry is the need to control and limit the flow of capital into health care, and yet, in the discussion of the effects of various policies, the concern is that regulation and increased market risk might have just this effect. It is concluded that regulation would reduce investor risk and encourage capital inflow, while increasing market type pressures would have the reverse effect. This statement seems plausible, and leads to an interesting dilemma which is not explicitly pointed out. Successful regulation which controls entry, e.g., by C/N laws, makes it easier for existing hospitals to raise private capital and, thus, defeats its purpose. On the other hand, a more competitive hospital environment, e.g., with uniform price regulation and free entry/exit, imposes much more risk on the individual hospital and its investors and may scare off the new private capital that is needed for the entry of innovating and cost-reducing types of suppliers.

The solution to this dilemma, if there is one, must lie in the care with which the regulatory or market mechanisms outlined in the paper are structured. The discussion might have been more helpful to the reader, had less attention been devoted to the hospital bond market and more been devoted to the extent to which the specific proposals relied upon current or new sources of capital or the entry of new institutions to the market. There could have been a more extensive evaluation of the policies, which tended to be reported rather than assessed. Of course, a full assessment of any one of such policies would be a major undertaking in itself, but the authors might have sketched in what they feel are the critical assumptions or variables to watch in evaluating each general strategy.

The last part of the Joe, Needleman, and Lewin paper briefly outlines an interesting and innovative proposal for the regionalization of health services delivery which they refer to as linking planning and regulation to budgeting and financing, together with external controls where necessary. It appears to me to have certain resemblances to proposals made in Canada, particularly the Report of the Health Security Program Project in British Columbia.[8] It also seems to me that it suffers from some of the same internal inconsistencies as those proposals, as well as from additional problems resulting from the absence of the necessary system infrastructure (particularly with respect to medical practice) in the United States.

The central concept of the authors' proposal is the establishment of regional ceilings, presumably on a yearly basis, on all health care expenditures, whether private or public, for hospital and nursing facility care and physician care of inpatients. These ceilings would be achieved by regional or state boards established for that purpose. But, later prospective rates are discussed, as well as the reimbursement of hospitals at uniform rates rather than budgeted costs. Reference is made to tying expenditures to a "fixed nation figure" (GNP?) which, again, implies fixed ceilings on total regional budgets. If fixed ceilings are, in fact, meant, then, since volumes cannot, in general, be controlled, the uniform rates must be subject to pro rata scaling on a year-end adjustment basis. Alternatively, one could negotiate global budgets and then use nominal prospective per diems to distribute the budget over the course of the year. In any case, fixed negotiated budgets, fixed uniform rates, and pro rata adjusted uniform rates are all very different systems, embodying different incentive patterns. The first and third are consistent with regional ceilings; the second is not.

Including inpatient physician services in this proposal and applying ceilings to public *and* private expenditure involves a revolutionary change in physician reimbursement. Again, if ceilings are to be binding, physicians must be paid on a negotiated global budget basis either as individuals (sometimes known as salary) or as an all-inclusive group like the Permanente Medical Groups with its own internal allocation rules. Alternatively, one could establish uniform fee schedules for in-patient services which would be binding (i.e., no additional payments by patients) and would be adjusted pro rata at year-end to assure that billings equal total budgeted ceiling payments. The feasibility of such a system of reimbursement only for hospital-based activities is a bit doubtful. It would obviously bear very differently on different physicians or on different activities of the same physician. Over time, it might serve to discourage in-hospital services, which may be part of what Joe, Needleman, and Lewin have in mind.

There would also be interesting regional boundary problems. Does the ceiling apply to all expenditure by people in a region, or on services of providers in a region? Do providers near a boundary get paid different amounts depending on the region of origin of the patient?

To make the ceiling constraint stick, the regional board would have to ensure that all funds passed through it, or that it had the power to review all provider budgets and tax back excesses. Either way, the usual sorts of public finance questions arise on the revenue side. If I, as a regional resident, have private insurance which reimburses my MD/hospital at a particular rate, but the ceiling requires that this rate be scaled down to stay under the ceiling, who gets the difference—I, the insurance company, or the board? Thus, it is hard to see how the board can control the reimbursement function without taking it over. If control were exercised over *rates* of reimbursement, that, in itself, would be quite complex. But global ceilings require authority greater by an order of magnitude.

Moreover, such ceilings raise very hard questions with regard to entry and exit which are highlighted in the case of physicians. Suppose that a new surgeon wishes to locate in a given region. The authors have not described how they envision handling this problem. The board might have to rule on whether the new surgeon was reimbursible, i.e., whether the ceiling would be raised sufficiently to accommodate the new entrant. If not, then, since private expenditures are included in the ceiling, the new surgeon could not practice. The national board system becomes a manpower allocator, but with no guarantee that a new physician will get in *anywhere*. If, of course, the ceiling is always raised, then it is not really a ceiling but an income policy for hospital-based physicians. Similarly, if the board sets binding fee schedules which are not prorated, then the "ceiling" floats on the locational choices of physicians. More interesting is the case of binding fee schedules in which each new surgeon entering a region increases total billings but not the total reimbursement ceiling and, thus, lowers all of his new colleagues' incomes (from hospital practice). The adjustments which would occur in access to hospitals would be fairly predictable and fun to watch— from the outside. The evolution of physicians into two classes, those with and those without hospital privileges, should follow swiftly, along with informal mechanisms for allocating access (or not) to new entrants in a region.

The same entry problems occur for institutions; the resistance to new entry would be fierce if existing institutions were to lose dollar-for-dollar. It is suggested that HMOs or HSAs (which appear to be a form of backward-linked HMO built around an insurance company with a closed panel of approved providers) could receive separate budgetary allocations. Again, this procedure would probably require "lifting the ceiling" to let new enterprises crawl under. It is suggested that the regional board would also administer the exit of unneeded facilities. Here Canadian experience is very discouraging. It is hard to discover a community which recognizes its advantage from closing facilities! The redistribution of the closed institution's revenues among others, subject to the ceiling, again raises distributional questions connected with where the revenues come from.

An additional interesting conflict of interest would be generated between hospital-based physicians and the hospitals themselves. The point that health care institutions would have an interest in educating physicians about service costs is trivial beside the physicians' realization that what is spent on hospitals is not spent on them. This realization is probably all to the good; there are signs of its emerging in Canada post-Turner. But the proposal to integrate capital and operating budgets could create new strains. Incidentally, does this proposal refer to capital *servicing*—depreciation and interest—or to actual capital *outlay* being under the ceiling? Only the former would appear to make sense. The general incentive to physicians to control overcapitalization would be acceptable, but a very powerful interest would be created to oppose any new entry—HMO or conventional—and I suspect that C/N laws would harden into stone with the whole weight of the profession behind them.

Incidentally, philanthropy is referred to as a way of easing trade-offs and allowing more to be done. First of all, as P. Ginsburg has shown, between 80 and 95 cents of every philanthropic dollar is federal money, anyway. Second, the initial point made in the Joe, Needleman, and Lewin paper is that public *and* private expenditure is subject to the ceiling. Third, if the ceiling were relaxed to permit gifts, all subsequent associated costs would fall within the ceiling, so that a recipient institution would either penalize its competitors to be unable to use the gift.

I think that the authors have not had a chance to think their proposal through; certainly they have not provided enough detail to enable one to see just what is proposed. There are, indeed, some interesting and constructive aspects to their plan, but they seem greatly to underestimate the authority which a regional or state board would require in order to administer ceilings of the sort which they propose. If the ceilings really are to bind, then the boards must have the power to manage the whole health care system—manpower and incomes, budgets, facilities and staff, entry and exit. Without this power, the ceilings would have little effect. References are made in the proposal to market-type forces, but I think that they are inconsistent with its main thrust and would tend to be subverted or controlled by the board in order to achieve its primary objective. Even so, it is doubtful that, in the United States, such a board could command the political authority that is necessary to achieve that objective.

These negative conclusions would not follow if, in fact, what is proposed were not direct budgetary allocation of shares of the global ceiling, but pro rata rate per unit reimbursement which could certainly be applied in the case of physicians' services, with significant short-run advantages. But why stop with hospital-based care? In the longer run, certain problems appear to develop as the billing and reimbursement dollars drift apart.[9] But, for institutions organized on a not-for-profit basis and under some constraint to balance budgets, the problems resulting from the uncertainty of pro rata reimbursement might well create system instability as each institution tried to ensure a given value of reimbursement by expanding output. This problem interacts, of course, with that of defining institutional output for reimbursement purposes; units of service obviously will not do.

The result is, therefore, not a balancing of market and regulatory mechanisms. Depending on the specific content which Joe, Needleman, and Lewin give to some aspects which are currently unclear it might be a first step towards a complete system of public management of health care. It might also be a move toward a world of competing HMOs by making the position of current forms of provider institution untenable and driving some into bankruptcy. In the present, rather sketchy form of the proposal, however, it is somewhat difficult to tell what such a system would look like, let alone how it might behave.

Perhaps the source of the difficulty is that the issue of regulation versus the market in capital funding of health facilities cannot be separated from that of regulatory versus market organization of the delivery system itself. The authors pointed out early in their paper that capital allocation and availability could not be considered in isolation from all of the other issues of health services delivery. Of course, there is no general solution to the regulatory/market issue at the delivery system level; the optimum policy choice depends on the characteristics of particular health services. Where a health service or product can be identified and defined with sufficient precision so that the group of such products or services is approximately internally homogenous—a dispensed prescription (but not the drug itself), a dental check-up, a well-baby visit, a refraction (but not a physician visit or a patient-day in the hospital)—then it may be possible to define uniform prices for such services. Moreover, where alternative providers of such services exist, with different costs, so that the products of each provider are roughly similar in therapeutic effect, one might very well use market mechanisms such as prices to guide consumers' decisions as to source of service. At the most general level, competition among HMOs in rate-setting does affect such decisions providing that the consumers can be assured of external quality monitoring focused on therapeutic effect (not structural characteristics).[c]

---

[c]The critical variable is that there must be grounds for believing that consumers have, or can get, information on different forms of service so that they can judge its use to them relative to its price. In particular instances, and particularly in choosing among therapeutically equivalent alternatives, this assumption may hold. In general, for health care services as a class, it does not. Hence, the universal abandonment of the market as an organizing social institution for health care by providers and patients alike—except for some economist holdouts.

Each particular type of health service will probably have to achieve a different balance between market and regulatory mechanisms, and within its own type of framework. For some services, in fact, such as immunization or children's dental care, the optimal approach is neither regulation nor market but direct public provision. A general optimal solution to the problem of mixing regulatory and market mechanisms for allocating health care resources does not appear to exist. (General schemes for consumer "participation" in health care payment, coinsurance and all that, are most completely irrelevant to this issue.)

NOTES

1. G. Rosenthal, *The Demand for General Hospital Facilities,* Hospital Monograph Series #14 (Chicago: American Hospital Association, 1964); C. Stevens, "Hospital Market Efficiency: The Anatomy of the Supply Response," in H. Klarman (ed.), *Empirical Studies in Health Economics* (Baltimore: Johns Hopkins, 1970); J. Newhouse, "An Economic Model of a Hospital," *American Economic Review,* 60, 1 (March 1970); and P. Ginsburg, *Capital in Non-Profit Hospitals,* Ph.D. dissertation, Harvard University, 1970.

2. C. Havighurst, "Speculations on the Market's Future in Health Care," in C. Havighurst (ed.), *Regulating Health Facilities Construction* (Washington: American Enterprise Institute, 1974).

3. V. Fuchs, *Who Shall Live? Health, Economics, and Social Choice* (New York: Basic Books, 1974); and M.L. Lee, "A Conspicuous Production Theory of Hospital Behavior," *Southern Economic Journal,* 38, 1 (July 1971).

4. D. Salkever and T. Bice, "The Impact of Certificate of Need Controls on Hospital Investment," *Milbank Memorial Fund Quarterly,* 54, 2 (April 1976).

5. A. Scitovsky, "Comments," in R. Rosett (ed.), *The Role of Health Insurance in the Health Services Sector,* Universities, N.B.E.R. Conference #27, (New York: N.B.E.R., 1976), p. 503.

6. See, e.g., Havighurst, "Speculations."

7. Salkever and Bice, "Impact on C/N Controls" and F. Hellinger, "The Effect of Certificate of Need Legislation on Hospital Investment," *Inquiry,* 13, 2 (June 1976).

8. British Columbia, *Report of the Health Security Program Project,* (Foulkes Report), (Victoria: The Queen's Printer, 1974).

9. See, e.g., R.G. Evans, *Price Formation in the Market for Physician Services,* monograph prepared for the Prices and Incomes Commission (Ottawa: The Queen's Printer, 1972).

Discussion of
Health Care Capital Financing:
Regulation, the Market, and
Public Policy

Clark C. Havighurst

The Joe, Needleman, and Lewin paper seems to me to fall short of fulfilling their assignment and the promise of their original outline.

Their assignment, as I understood it, included an obligation to consider using market forces as the primary allocator of capital in the health care sector, and this would seem to entail an examination of the market's possible roles in allocating resources of all kinds to health related uses. In their outline, the authors promised to contrast market-oriented and regulatory approaches and to clarify the issues which divide the proponents of each view. As a minimum, this would require stating both views to their best advantage and providing something of a scenario for the respective proposed solutions. Not only does the paper not adequately state the arguments for a market-oriented solution, but it suggests that the authors may not fully appreciate the scope of those arguments.

Because of the authors' failing, I have found it necessary to sketch the arguments myself, and I think that my statement may serve as something of a revelation not only to Joe, Needleman, and Lewin, but to others. The fact is that the market's potential, while sometimes sketched in outline form sufficient to suggest its promise, has never been fully elaborated and definitively examined by anyone, for reasons which I shall indicate later. Indeed, the market has been discussed very little except in the debate surrounding HMOs, and perhaps for this reason the authors can be excused for failing to see the true scope of the argument for a market-oriented solution.

The chief problem that I have with the paper is its excessively narrow view of the available options. Aside from a sideways glance in footnote a, the authors largely ignore the affirmative ways in which meaningful competition can be stimulated and guided and that cost conciousness can be reintroduced. Failure to show the affirmative side of the market advocates' position makes it seem that market advocates are essentially defenders of the status quo or even advocates of turning back the clock. But it is simply not true that market advocates have nothing affirmative to propose. Although it is not identified as such by Joe, Needleman, and Lewin, the HMO movement is, in large measure, attributable to the work of market advocates. HMOs remain the most interesting and potentially important policy innovation of recent years, but are treated by the authors simply as something that has been tried and found largely inadequate. Belittling it as "a promising, if limited, alternative," they do not point out that the failure of HMOs to deliver what was promised was a failure of regulation, not of the market, since the HMO Act was, at the same time—if it can be believed—both in gratification of the liberals' desire to regulate and a concession to the AMA. Market advocates criticized the law both before and after its enactment and are currently critical, not only of the recent amendments, but of such further absurdities as allowing fee-for-service doctors, who dominate PSROs, to regulate the "quality" of care in HMOs, which are their only significant competitors. While those who support market solutions would very much like to see HMOs given more room to flourish, HMOs are only one of the many innovations which the private sector would adopt, were its incentives put in order and its freedom of action restored. Later discussion supplies a positive program for affirmative market-correcting action involving much more than a reduction in the existing level of regulation and further improvements in HMO market opportunities.

A careful reading of Joe, Needleman, and Lewin suggests that they are not really so narrowly focused as to believe that government's only tools for dealing with the health sector are regulatory ones, perhaps supplemented by cash subsidies for occasional good things, such as highly regulated HMOs. Instead, it seems to be their estimate of the mood of the interest groups, Congress, and policy-makers in general—and, perhaps, of the election prospects and commitments of Mr. Carter—which leads them to skimp discussion of other, more market-oriented approaches. They say, for example, that "we are currently in a regulated environment from which there appears to be no real support for retreat." Thus, they seem to believe that market-oriented approaches are foreclosed, irrespective of their merits, by the realities of politics. I believe that this ipse dixit needs further examination.

ARE WE IRREVOCABLY COMMITTED
TO REGULATION?

One reason why I and others were originally reluctant to accept the plunge into regulation was our fear that it would commit us irrevocably to more and more restrictive regulation even if the original dose of it proved ineffective, as we feared it would. This has been the common experience in economic regulation, so common that the tendency of regulation to proliferate in an industry once it has a foothold has come to be known as the "tar baby" effect. This tendency reflects what might be called the "Vietnam mentality," since proponents of the original interventionist strategy regularly use its failures as arguments for escalating the effort. Similarly, Joe, Needleman, and Lewin are not at all dismayed by the ineffectiveness of today's regulation but use it to support their argument for total war—that is, going all the way to a regionalized system dependent on a fixed budget and on politicized decisionmaking for allocating that budget within the region. I may agree that the failures of regulation point us strongly in this direction as a practical political matter, but that is all the more reason why we should summon up the intellectual discipline at this conference to consider whether this is really the only solution left. This, I understood, was the assignment which the authors were given.

Joe, Needleman, and Lewin are not alone in refusing to engage in serious discussion of these issues. It is very common, almost obligatory, in health policy papers to assert at an early point that it is inevitable that we will have more government control. Sometimes it is observed that fundamental questions can be raised about the desirability of this trend, but the point is passed quickly over preparatory to plunging into questions about how, but not whether, to regulate. I regard the repeated assertion of regulation's inevitability as a dangerous self-fulfilling prophecy, and I believe that it is intended by many writers to be just that, since they are happy with the direction of the drift and are glad to be able to assume away the hard issues which can be raised concerning it. After all, the people who write on these subjects are experts on regulation and not on the alternatives to it, and they are anxious to write about what they know and they have no reason to object to trends which promise to expand demand for their particular talents. (I might observe that my own academic background suits me to serve in either a regulated or an unregulated environment so that whatever predispositions I may have are not a result of academic self-interest.)

I, for one, do not choose to believe in political predestination, partially because it puts such a low value on reasoned discourse and on our democratic institutions. I somehow resent being told that we have no significant control over our destiny, that we are somehow careening downhill with, perhaps, a steering mechanism but with no brakes. If so, then the only remaining questions are precisely what form the ultimate disaster will take and how bad it will be, and I do not find those issues to be very interesting. Indeed, I find the entire notion that we cannot consider health policy issues on their merits highly depressing and full of ominous portents for our society as a whole. Moreover, I do not see the country as committed irrevocably to a single course of development in health care or anywhere else, and I see many hopeful signs (even in the Carter campaign) which indicate that we still value freedom and diversity, that we would like to solve our social and economic problems without sacrificing these values (if we only knew how), and that we are still reluctant to turn everything over to government. It does worry me to find that those to whom government turns for advice on these questions are unwilling, or unable, to debate fundamental issues. I fear that they are deluding policymakers into thinking that regulation is the only way out of our dilemma and that nothing important would be sacrificed by pursuing this course as far as it leads.

WOULD MARKET FORCES FUNCTION USEFULLY UNDER THE JOE/NEEDLEMAN/ LEWIN PROPOSAL?

Although I doubt that I am required to examine, in detail, the authors proposal, sketchy as it is, I shall quickly summarize some objections to it.

The authors contend that their proposal "combines elements of a competitive free market approach with regulation that has both the power and flexibility to initiate and shape a coordinated health care system . . . ." This claim is apparently made because a role would be left to HMOs and other alternative delivery systems. It is hard to tell, from what they say, just what that role would be or whether or not the market—that is, consumers acting in their own self-interest—would have any real opportunity to balance the quality and style of care against its cost. The authors do not, for example, disclaim an intention to regulate HMOs closely, as is done under the HMO and PSRO legislation. Moreover, the fixed-budget notion, which they propound, leaves no room for private decisions about how much to spend for health services. The major allocative decisions in the system would thus be entirely political, which is to say that the market would be denied its most important role[1] and consumers would be denied significant opportunities to benefit from their economizing choices. The market can play a central allocative role only if cost-conscious consumers are offered a range of choice which permits them, rather than the providers (or regulators) to dictate the quantity, quality, and types of services that are to be provided. Regulation which helps to provide a full menu (including independent HMOs) is fine, but, so far, regulation has been resolutely directed to making everyone take potluck by imposing a single standard and allowing the medical profession the dominant voice in setting that standard. I hope that no one fails to see which approach is the more distinctly democratic in the finest sense.

The future health care system, as designed by Joe, Needleman, and Lewin, would apparently leave the door open for competition and consumer choice to this limited extent: HMOs and "health care alliances" would be able to attract enrollees not by quoting a lower price—since a fixed sum would apparently be paid by government or employers and could not be varied—but by adding benefits or other features which would be covered for the same price. This option is not the same as price competition because consumers may value the added benefits at considerably less than their cost, especially if the mandatory basic benefit package is as "comprehensive" as under the HMO Act and some NHI proposals. For example, extra dental care coverage will not appeal much to those with good teeth or with a family dentist whom they like. Perhaps the authors would consider allowing plans either to require supplemental payments for basic benefits or to pay cash rebates or experience-related dividends to subscribers. If not, or if Congress failed to see the point, the competitive features of their plan would not be worth very much. Indeed, nonprice competition is not necessarily better than no competition at all and is frequently criticized as wasteful in other regulated industries. In the airlines industry, for example, competition focuses on frills and overinvestment in expensive equipment largely because lower-price options are prohibited by law. The authors should recognize that more and better health services are not necessarily what the consumer wants or needs most. Moreover, even if this idea were a good one—and I might concede that, like cost-sharing, it is better than nothing—it is unlikely that meaningful opportunities for useful competition would be left after Congress and all of the regulatory agencies (including PSROs with their authority to keep "quality" and, therefore, cost well above market-determined levels) got through with it.

Many other problems are also raised. Health plans in the Joe/Needleman/Lewin world would compete by seeking out low-risk (or low-consuming) populations. Since price competition to enroll a specific employment group would presumably be prohibited—as it is by the community-rating requirement under the HMO Act—the best plans (in terms of service and benefits) would be those which attracted the best risks, and clinic location and marketing decisions would be made with this in mind. The suggestion that a dual system of health care would be avoided seems unfounded. The bureaucracy needed to enforce inevitable open enrollment and nondiscrimination requirements would be both costly and oppressive.

The regulatory controls over entry, as envisioned by the authors, are such that it seems unlikely that HMOs or other competitive delivery systems will bring much competitive pressure to bear on the system, since regulators charged with maintaining the financial stability and borrowing capacity of hospitals will see their job as one of stopping any development which would threaten hospital stability. Because HMOs would substitute outpatient for inpatient care, they would be seen as potentially dangerous developments to be closely controlled. Such regulatory protectionism has developed in every regulated industry, and I see no reason why the health sector will be any different. Indeed, given the widespread belief in "Roemer's law" (which says that empty hospital beds generate new demand and more inappropriate spending), the regulators in the health sector will see all the more reason for preventing developments which take patients out of the hospital. Experience with ambulatory surgery facilities has reflected precisely this approach to innovation. Regulatory controls of this kind necessarily inhibit innovation, leaving the community dependent on the regulators to initiate change, which will occur only when, and if, it can be successfully negotiated with everyone adversely affected. Even small changes become major political issues.

Conceivably, the regulators in the world of Joe, Needleman, and Lewin would recognize the value of promoting active competition and would seek to do so, but regulators have generally not done so in other settings. The tendency in the health sector has been to write statutes which are more and more inclusive, and this guarantees that the regulators will have all the opportunity they need to repress desirable market influences. The fact that Section 1122 of the Social Security Act and P.L. 93-641, the National Health Planning and Resources Development Act, contain a few clauses saying nice things about HMOs and encouraging regulators to foster their development does not convince me that meaningful competition will be tolerated. Most regulators will see their job as assuring the presence of one HMO per market, preferably one under safe and co-operative management and, therefore, not given to aggressive competition with the regulators' other clients. Moreover, the regulatory environment provides ideal conditions for negotiating issues which would otherwise be put to a consumer vote in the marketplace. For this reason, HMOs will represent less of a choice than an echo, not a lower price but more services.

The authors appear to think that regulation is good because it creates security for the regulated firm and enhances their borrowing capacity, and that markets are bad because the attendant risks make capital formation difficult, especially for innovators. The distinction which they note between risk and uncertainty is valid and important, but they do not observe the degree to which vagrant governmental policies are the main source of the latter, deterring all but speculators and quick-killing artists of the kind who exploited the Medi-Cal program. Instead of proposing the removal of this uncertainty, the reduction of other artificial barriers to change, and protection against professional retaliation so that new plans have only market risks to face, they recommend insulating innovative developments from the discipline of the capital markets by direct governmental subsidies. In thus adopting grant applications, bureaucratic reviews, and regulation as the ultimate discipline, they have chosen a course which is hardly likely to stimulate managerial competence, useful experimentation, or effective competition, since government is unlikely to foster innovations which threaten the stability of earlier investments or which depart very far from traditional medical practice. The closest model for what they propose, the HMO Act, was more an impediment than a spur to innovation, in large part because of the uncertainties that were introduced, the undue focus on subsidies, and governmental unwillingness to subsidize anything less than the "ideal" HMO or to allow consumers a lower-priced option. Of course, the authors never focus on the possibilities for making market demand once again a reasonably reliable guide to investment, both as a stimulus and as a deterrent.

It would have been helpful if Joe, Needleman, and Lewin had looked at the issues of capital investment, not as a whole, but with respect to each different type of facility. It is arguable that the case for regulating the rates and capital investments of hospitals is considerably stronger than is the case for regulating other kinds of institutions and that less comprehensive regulation would serve the public better by leaving the market more room to function. Thus, a strong case can be made for exempting HMOs and ambulatory care facilities in order that they might impose some competitive discipline on the hospital sector and its regulators. Similarly, nursing home proliferation might be desirable because it could contribute something to the quality of care by giving consumers a choice. Now, with limited entry, patients must take any nursing care bed which they can find and be glad to get it. Under these circumstances, it is not surprising that the quality of nursing home care is not all that it might be, particularly since government is unable to write a regulation guaranteeing the presence of those intangible elements which determine whether the quality of life of nursing home patients is good or bad. Obviously, effective utilization review under public financing programs would be essential if the nursing bed supply were allowed to grow, but this seems a good opportunity to blend regulation and the market to achieve what regulation alone cannot.

The authors provide us with a short statement of the problems of the health sector. Their statement of the conventional wisdom leads naturally to the conventional conclusion that more regulation is inevitable. Their treatment of the issue appears to assume that proponents of the market accept the marketplace as it is presently structured and operating. This is not the case with serious students of the problem, but the authors make no effort to consider whether the market might be improved by measures to remove the obstacles to its efficient functioning and by reshaping federal programs to restore some cost-consciousness, not by cost-sharing so much as by giving federal beneficiaries some cash benefit from their economizing in the choice of a prepayment plan. Conventional wisdom is always a handicap to any discussion, and the purpose of meetings such as this one should be to get behind it and to see if more can be learned. My belief, to be developed below, is that better understanding of the reasons why we face our present problems would point us in the direction of some constructive nonregulatory measures which the authors have not considered.

In defense of Joe, Needleman, and Lewin, it must be admitted that market-oriented solutions have not often been spelled out clearly by their proponents, who have spent most of their time in two more immediate endeavors. First, they have felt it necessary to attack regulation for its serious deficiencies in order to get people to begin thinking even a little bit about alternatives. Second, market proponents largely confined themselves to propounding the HMO strategy. This strategy was quite sound and might have worked had Congress allowed it to, but, as I shall show, the HMO is only one aspect of the market solution. Indeed, my subsequent remarks include a confession of error in concentrating too much on HMOs, thereby leading observers into thinking that HMOs were all that the market had to offer. It is regrettable that there have been so few of us working on problems from this point of view and that we were induced by expediency to emphasize HMOs to the exclusion of larger issues because the political environment seemed ready to embrace them. I plead guilty to jumping on the HMO bandwagon when I should have been doing more basic scholarly homework on the many other ways in which markets could solve not only the problem of health care costs, but other problems. To this extent, I am partly responsible for the lack of scholarship explicating the market solution so that the authors could give it the respect which it deserves and could examine its merits with greater care.

Joe, Needleman, and Lewin also promised to examine the value questions which underlie what they see as two distinct "philosophies." I think that they exaggerate the philosophical element and, thus, do a disservice to policymakers by implying that the dispute is ideological. I do not deny that there are some ultimate philosophical issues involved, but they are not, in my view, of critical importance. The important issues are pragmatic—which system will most nearly approach the correct allocation of resources and which will do it soonest and at the lowest cost? The philosophical questions revolve around the question whether the American people should be given a single health care system professing the ideal of a single standard of care for everyone. While the argument for absolute egalitarianism or, more accurately, its appearance as a symbolic ideal needs to be addressed, I doubt that this is the place to do it. Nevertheless, my subsequent remarks will touch briefly on these issues.

REDISCOVERING THE MARKET

Now let me turn to a brief statement of the case for the market-oriented solution. My basic points are that the private sector has not had the opportunity which it should have had to control the cost of medical care and that, if it were given a reasonable opportunity, it could do much of what government is failing to do. What has been lacking is any low-cost alternative which cost-conscious purchasers could select as adequate for their needs. The menu, in other words, has been too limited.

It is particularly noteworthy at this time that the private sector is now making major attempts to control health care costs. These efforts were recently documented by the Council on Wage and Price Stability in a twenty-eight-page insertion in the *Federal Register* (September 17, 1976), illustrating what management and labor are doing to bring the cost of their health plans under control. Impressive as these on-going efforts are, there is much more that might be done but which cannot be done because of certain circumstances which limit the private sector's ability to respond to the challenge. Government could, if it chose, quickly alter many of these circumstances, unleashing market forces which have long been effectively restrained. It might then be possible to see what the private sector could do while we are awaiting government's next move. It is at least possible that we would have a convincing demonstration of the private sector's capability, in time, to impress Congress that it may not be necessary to regulate our way out of our current cost problem. The following remarks are meant to underscore what the Council on Wage and Price Stability called "the heretofore unappreciated potential of the private sector to combat the problem and possibly exert substantial downward pressure on rising health care costs." (I have written a fuller statement of this argument in connection with testimony before the Council in October. Copies of that paper are available upon request.)[2]

The Problem: Third Party Payment Without Cost Controls

Health care cost problems stem from Americans' having too much of the wrong kind of financial protection against burdensome medical expenses. Contrary to the conventional wisdom, however, it is not third party payment alone which has produced our problems but the absence in third party payment programs of any significant check on the price or utilization of services. Indeed, most of the "unique" features of the health care industry that were noted by Joe, Needleman, and Lewin are merely reflections of the particular financing mechanisms which have grown up. Thus, the central decision-making role of the physician, while obvious, is of major consequence only because, when health insurance was introduced, no other accountability for the cost of care was substituted for the doctor's previous fiduciary obligation to look out for his patient's pocketbook as well as for his health. Similarly, the ability of hospitals to ignore efficiency and to invest in expensive capital equipment and in larger and more highly trained staffs flows directly from the increasing nonnecessity, due to automatic third party cost reimbursement, for keeping the cost of care within particular bounds.

These observations would normally be read to support the whole panoply of governmental controls which are being tried and further ones which are being proposed, as in the Joe, Needleman, and Lewin paper. But, for a full view of the alternatives, the analysis needs to go further—into the reasons why financing mechanisms took the form that they did. Was it inevitable that health insurance would leave providers free to spend the insurer's money without accountability? If not, why did financing mechanisms not develop in such a way as to assure that services were truly needed and that needed care was rendered in the least expensive way? Did insurance company executives simply not recognize the importance of experimenting with cost controls and different delivery arrangements in order to find acceptable low-cost alternatives? Were consumers not interested in lower-cost arrangements? Such questions make clear that our current problems stem from history, from long-established practices which have only lately been recognized for what they are—one of the most potent vehicles that we have ever seen for systematically misallocating the nation's resources.

Once third party payment patterns were established so as to free providers from controls initiated by insurers in the consumer's interest, a vicious upward spiral was set in motion, with cost increases stimulated by insurance necessitating the purchase of more insurance protection, which, in turn, stimulated further cost increases, more insurance, and so forth. Predictably, this spiral eventually reached the plane of political action. Medicare and Medicaid, designed to help particularly vulnerable groups cope with higher costs, were the first response to the emerging crisis, but, being modeled after the privately developed insurance plans which preceded them, Medicare and Medicaid simply accelerated the inflationary trend. Now, just over ten years later, still higher costs have produced pressure for a "national health insurance" program which, it is hoped, will "solve" the cost problem for everyone. The variety of direct and indirect cost controls being implemented by government are simply an attempt to supply belatedly what the private market did not.

What were the causes of the market's failure to control costs without government assistance? Excessive growth of the wrong kinds of financial protection against medical care costs can be traced to two major factors which have not been widely recognized for the pernicious influences which they are: (1) the tax law's treatment of health insurance premiums, and (2) provider dictation of the type of insurance plans that are available to consumers. An understanding of how these influences have distorted the provision of health services points towards policy proposals which could give the private sector the chance that it has never really had to control health care costs and would assure that consumers get value for money in health care.

Sources of the Problem

Tax Treatment of Insurance Premiums. As Martin Feldstein, in particular, has observed, the tax treatment of health insurance premiums has substantially weakened the consumer's incentive to self-insure, thus determining, in large measure, the character of privately purchased health insurance. Quite simply, the tax law has long encouraged employers and employees to buy group insurance with low deductibles ("shallow" coverage) in order that even routine medical bills could be paid with untaxed rather than after-tax dollars. Feldstein has estimated that a typical wage earner can purchase nearly 50 percent more health care for the same money in this manner. Such shallow coverage invites consumers to seek, and providers to give, care which would not have seemed worthwhile if paid for out of pocket. Overinsurance against routine expenses has greatly expanded the area in which normal cost constraints do not operate.

Change in the tax treatment of health insurance premiums is a prerequisite to placing significant reliance on consumer cost consciousness to discourage overinsurance and to induce the design of insurance plans (or other financing schemes) with cost-control features. Outright repeal of favorable tax treatment would, of course, be politically impossible, but an upper limit on employer-employee deductibility might be introduced without too much trouble. Better yet, in keeping with redistributive goals, a tax credit for premiums on health insurance could be substituted for the tax deductions but limited to a fixed inflation-indexed amount deemed sufficient to buy adequate financial protection (which is not to say comprehensive coverage). This would spur the purchase of insurance by those persons who are not now covered adequately, but the limit would mean that people would be spending their own money for any additional coverage and would thus be under pressure not to obtain more coverage than they really need. Shallow coverage would almost certainly be reduced as more people sought protection primarily against unpredictable expenses, and insurers would be pressed to provide optimal protection for the amount of money which people were willing to commit. They would find greater resistance to premium increases and would be led to consider greater use of cost controls as a means of giving more essential coverage for the subsidized premium.

Obviously, a fully worked out health policy would also have to address restoration of cost consciousness for beneficiaries of public programs and an expansion of those programs to cover all of those in need of subsidized care. The use of the tax system might be expanded—in keeping with "negative income tax" proposals and the "work bonus" in the recent tax bill—to permit payments to persons who had no taxes against which to apply the credit. Or a system of vouchers might be used. Price competition for the patronage of otherwise indigent citizens could be encouraged by letting plans, within some limits, pay dividends or rebates to those who spend their vouchers to enroll. (Clearly, this is preferable to requiring the poor to supplement the government subsidy, but achieves the desired result.) Though considerable, the practical problems confronted in reintroducing consumer cost consciousness while also protecting consumers against serious mistakes would seem minor when compared to those encountered in controlling costs directly under other national health insurance plans.

Provider Resistance to Cost Control. The second—and, in my view, more important—major cause of the market's failure to produce financing programs which serve consumers' interests lies in the control which medical care providers have exerted over the design and implementation of such plans. It is no accident that health insurance was, for many years, opposed by the medical profession and that it was only when the hospitals and doctors themselves came to sponsor— and control the practices of—third party payment schemes (Blue Cross and Blue Shield) that they became an accepted medium of financial protection. However, these plans were designed not so much to protect patients as to assure providers that they could easily collect payment for their services. This emphasis resulted in excessively shallow coverage on the one hand and, on the other hand, in inadequate protection against the rare but large and unpredictable costs which (but for the tax advantage) are the only risks that rational consumers would elect to insure against. State legislation, enacted largely at the behest of medical care providers, restricted the development of plans which served consumer interests, and the provider-dominated "Blues" were given unique powers to contract directly with providers. Commercial insurers, on the other hand, were barred from any role in supplying and controlling services under the prohibition against the "corporate practice of medicine." Instead, they were relegated to indemnifying patients for bills incurred, a role which greatly impaired their ability to impose controls on providers. At the same time, "ethical" standards of the medical profession and other subtle sanctions were being invoked to prevent doctors from associating with independent health care plans, primarily HMOs, which competed with the uncontrolled system.

Despite the restraints imposed, history had provided occasional glimpses into the market's potential for stimulating constructive approaches to cost problems. Prepaid group practice, the forerunner of the HMO movement, is the only mechanism which achieved any permanence, and this was achieved in only a few places and only after legendary struggles and many compromises with organized medicine. Less well recognized, because uniformity is mistaken for inevitability, is the role which organized medicine played in dictating the practices of private health insurers. The most revealing experience, which occurred in Oregon in the 1930s and 1940s, was the subject in the early 1950s of an unsuccessful antitrust suit, the record of which has recently been reexamined by two Federal Trade Commission (FTC) economists for insights into our current problems.[3] They have found that the introduction of a Blue Shield plan in Oregon, coupled with a partial boycott, by doctors, of allegedly "unethical" insurance plans, halted for all time the insurers' historic practice of requiring physicians to justify their expenditure of insurer funds. Under the pressures thus brought to bear, the insurers ceased the practices which the doctors found objectionable but which today seem to be merely rudimentary versions of precisely the kinds of cost controls which Congress hoped that PSROs would be able to impose on medical practice.

A more recent demonstration of the ability of organized medicine to maintain its freedom to spend the public's money occurred a few years ago, when the Aetna Life and Casualty Company undertook to assist its insureds in resisting in court their doctors' claims for payment of excessive charges or for unnecessary services. Medical societies the country over passed resolutions calling for boycotts of Aetna's patients, and Aetna had to negotiate a change in its policy with the AMA.

What emerges from these insights is the need to free insurers engaging in cost-control activities from the threat of retaliation by the medical profession. Fortunately, recent clarification of the applicability of the antitrust laws to the organized professions in *Goldfarb* v. *Virginia State Bar* provides a powerful legal weapon for controlling such objectionable behavior. While further legal clarification is necessary, the FTC and the Antitrust Division have recently shown interest in medical society activities and should soon declare the necessary principles, perhaps initiating litigation to make the point clearer yet.

Given only a small amount of encouragement and assistance, the market for health services could probably restructure itself in fairly quick order to allow consumers effectively to express their preferences with respect to the cost, as well as the quality, of much of the medical care which they receive. Although legislative action—specifically, tax law changes, invalidation of state legal impediments to insurer cost-control efforts, and adaptation of public financing programs—is needed to permit maximum response, market forces could begin to operate immediately if the need to defer to the preferences of organized medicine could be minimized. The HMO Act of 1973 already permits commercial health insurers to form "independent practice associations" with significant cost controls, and, once this is understood as permission for insurers to organize "closed panels" of doctors without obtaining the local medical society's permission, the process of rapid change should begin. Indeed, this provision in the HMO Act, which allows insurers to bypass restrictions in state laws, is potentially at least as important as the authorization of traditional HMOs. Although the benefit package requirements are a serious impediment, amounting to compulsory overinsurance, this law represents a significant break in the medical profession's defenses, which have long depended heavily on requiring medical "service" plans to preserve "free choice of physician," thereby preventing plans from effectively excluding physicians who failed to cooperate in cost-control endeavors. With the backing of antitrust principles, this breakthrough could be exploited, permitting consumers to opt out of the uncontrolled health care system which has dominated the scene for so long and into something more suitable.

How These Ideas Relate to the Health Policy Debate

Regulation Versus "the Market". Obviously, much of the foregoing discussion swims against the tide of the ongoing health policy debate which, like the Joe, Needleman, and Lewin paper, deals mostly with how, and how much, to regulate the system and not with the more fundamental issue of whether comprehensive regulation is really the best way to correct the industry's obviously defective performance. While there is almost a consensus that the "market" has failed, there in only poor understanding of why that market failure occurred, most people accepting as conclusive the following propositions: health care is "different" or "unique"; consumer ignorance is the source of the problem because decision-making must be delegated to noncost-conscious doctors; consumers (voters) prefer comprehensive third party coverage of as many health expenditures as possible; and, finally, third party payment is synonymous with the absence of effective controls on the cost of care. The foregoing discussion indicates that all of these propositions are too simple. To paraphrase Mark Twain, the report that the market cannot be restored to health is greatly exaggerated.

The inevitability of vastly expanded federal and state regulation of the health system is so widely accepted that many persons are now unwilling to consider any alternative. Yet, confidence in the efficacy of regulation is not high among policymakers, and recent months have seen an increasing awareness of regulation's shortcomings, in health as well as elsewhere. Although there has been no change in the direction of the drift, the pace has slowed somewhat, and long-imminent "national health insurance" is still not close to being a reality. It seems quite possible that, if a clear and persuasive alternative policy appeared, repressed doubts about regulatory approaches would rise to the surface and a fundamental reappraisal could be launched. Moreover, many of the interest groups affected, particularly those who are paying the excessive costs, might find such an alternative strategy attractive, thus improving its political prospects.

The last previous attempt to present an alternative to comprehensive regulation of the health care industry was the "HMO strategy" launched in 1970. The depressing history of that idea, culminating in its destruction at the hands of the Congress, need not be recounted here, but many people who rallied to that banner are still believers in the philosophy that it represented. HMOs are still a good idea and very much a part of the strategy that I am advocating. It should be noted, however, that the strategy which I have advanced is not just a restatement of the HMO idea. In 1971, when I first entered the debate on health policy, I made the tactical error—as others did—of seizing on HMOs as the best available vehicle for introducing privately initiated cost controls and competition in the health services industry. This proved to be a mistake because it depended on Congress to do too much, but it was an understandable mistake, since HMOs seemed, indeed, to be the "wave of the future" and the broader approach of encouraging insurer-initiated cost controls seemed too radical, too questionable under state legal restrictions, and too easily squelched by professional opposition. Indeed, it seemed that HMO competition might serve to trigger significant efforts on the part of insurers who were long accustomed to serving as a pass-through mechanism, providing only actuarial and claim payment services. But when Congress failed to embrace the opportunity which HMOs presented (the forthcoming amendments still largely miss the point), those who believe that a market-oriented response could be organized were left pretty much where they began. What seems to be needed, then, if serious attention is to be drawn to nonregulatory solutions to our problems, is a strategy which appears to be wholly new and not just a warmed-over version of the HMO idea, respectable as that was. I believe that such a new campaign can, and must be, launched.

There are at least three significant new developments in the present climate which make this an appropriate juncture for rediscovering the market's potential capacity for dealing with health care cost problems. First, employers (and the public at large) have become highly conscious of health care costs and are visibly anxious to find lower-cost alternatives; the Council on Wage and Price Stability has impressively documented this new awareness. Second, commercial insurers have begun to recognize their own responsibility for controlling costs and, under increasing pressure not only from employers and consumers to reduce costs but from government to justify their very existence, can perhaps be counted on more than ever before to compete in cost control as well as in other ways; Blue Cross and Blue Shield, while still influenced by providers, may be less likely now than in the past to serve as providers' stalking horses. Third, and perhaps most important, the applicability of the antitrust laws to the medical profession has been clarified and, due in large measure to the rediscovery of the old Oregon experience, there is new recognition in the antitrust enforcement agencies and elsewhere of the importance of preventing concerted professional resistance to insurer-initiated cost-control efforts. When these elements are combined, a new and appealing strategy begins to emerge. What it requires at this critical point, as battle lines for the next Congress are being drawn, is not further investigation and subtle elaboration in the academic literature but a solid endorsement—at least as an idea deserving serious and immediate attention—by an authoritative body such as the Council on Wage and Price Stability.

Other Values at Stake. While heavy emphasis on cost concerns is appropriate in the present climate, it is easy, in the campaign to control costs, to neglect other values which are also of great importance. For example, concern about costs has already produced far-reaching regulatory initiatives—the PSRO law, the health planning legislation, and the HMO Act—which generally confirm the medical profession's dominance and weaken the system's ability to innovate and to offer consumers a meaningful range of choice. To have any chance of success in solving problems to the public's satisfaction—and, indeed, to have any political appeal—market-oriented, cost-containment policies cannot simply exalt the market but must also be attuned to the other values which health care affects and to the special concerns which it excites. Thus, attention needs to be given not only to how costs are to be contained but also to such matters as how currently unmet health needs are to be met, how patients are to be protected against incompetent providers and dishonest operators, how geographic maldistribution of providers will be rectified, how monopolistic hospitals' rates are to be controlled, and so forth. In some respects, it will be necessary to accommodate the strong desire in the health sector to regulate things in order to protect the ignorant consumer against possible mistakes. Powerfully felt distributive-justice concerns must also certainly be addressed.

A market-oriented strategy can, in fact, be designed to address such problems and concerns. All that is essential is that the market's basic integrity not be undermined by measures dealing with specific problems. Specific emphasis must also be placed on measures to improve the market's functioning and to narrow providers' dominance over its organization, the flow of information, and the range of choices that are available to consumers. There is nothing implicit in the endorsement of a market-oriented strategy which denies the reasonable demands of social justice, and only those who demand absolute equality in this symbolic area should find reason to object to the implications of permitting reasonable diversity and relying on constrained private choice.

A market-oriented system would address itself in some ways to the public's new suspiciousness toward government. Moreover, recent repeated emphasis in health policy discussions on individual's responsibility for their own health may foreshadow a trend away from relying on government to make everyone well and toward acceptance of personal responsibility for selecting a health care plan and for deciding how much of a financial commitment to make. Perhaps most important in its implications both for cost control and for an expanded range of constrained choice is another new and increasingly dominant theme in health policy discussions—namely, the expression of serious reservations about the ability of health services to make significant contributions to human welfare in many of the cases where great expense is incurred. A corollary of this new skepticism should be a recognition that the apparent range and subjectivity of consumers' preferences in this area, as in others, does not signify irrationality, and that different people can come rationally to different conclusions about what quantity and quality of services to buy. A market system, by allowing people (many of them subsidized) to make their own decisions about how much health care is worth to them, would fit with this new awareness. On the other hand, regulatory approaches, by their very nature, narrow the range of choice, defining a single standard of care which everyone must accept.

No single standard and style of health care can, in fact, be appropriate for all Americans, given their widely varied attitudes, tastes and religious convictions, their other needs, and the necessarily limited resources at their disposal, including public funds, which might be made available to some of them. Implementing a single standard would mean either (1) "leveling down," which means denying people the right or opportunity to choose a higher, or different, standard even if they were willing to pay the added cost, or (2) "leveling up," which means bringing the entire population up to a level defined primarily by the preferences of the upper middle class professionals providing the service. At present, the rhetoric of the policy debate—e.g., "the right to health care"—seems slanted toward leveling up, though some leveling down is implicit in the expressed need to control cost and to "ration" care. A strong dose of leveling down also appears in the Kennedy-Corman Health Security bill and in the proposal of Joe, Needleman, and Lewin, both of which seek to make all Americans part of a single "insured" group, with the cost fixed politically and paid from progressive taxes and with equal, but limited, services for all.

What emerges from the new themes in the health policy debate is another new basis for reopening consideration of the value of a health care system based primarily on diversity and choice. These new awarenesses focus attention not on the value of health services in the aggregate, where there can be no real dispute, but on their highly questionable value at the margin, where benefits are frequently problematic and where preferences and alternative uses for resources are apt to be decisive. This new sophistication is at least equivalent in importance to the three new developments mentioned earlier as circumstances warranting the "rediscovery" of the market as the appropriate instrument for restoring accountability and fiscal prudence to the health sector.

THE MARKET AND CAPITAL ALLOCATION

The Joe, Needleman, and Lewin paper suggests that the market would continue to play a role in capital allocation under their fixed-budget system. This is so only in an insignificant sense, since they would leave the market no allocative function—market-registered demand would not determine supply. Perhaps the authors think that the market is at work as long as private investors supply most of the capital that is used by the health care system. But if government or the medical profession makes most of the decisions on "quality," if consumers are limited in their choices and have no opportunity to benefit themselves by economizing, and if government sets nearly all of the other conditions determining the investors' risks, the market is left no significant role to play in allocating resources. Continued dependence on private capital sources would supply some protection against the exploitation of capital invested in health facilities—just as it does in public utility regulation, where the regulators must set rates and establish policies which do not cause the cost of capital to rise out of sight or make new capital unavailable. But, to say that the capital market serves to keep the regulators fair, serving this purpose better than do judicial controls, is not to say very much for the market's role. One would not say that the British economy is under the discipline of the free market just because the pound must compete in foreign exchange markets.

In an unconstrained market in which a wide range of private sector cost-control initiatives were permitted, market demand would be a much more dependable guide to the public's true needs than it is at present. Privately sponsored controls on hospital admissions and lengths of stay and on the use of ancillary services would greatly curtail the ability of providers to create demand. If the price of services were determined by arm's length bargaining between plans and providers, excess capacity would be reflected in prices below costs. This hazard would, in turn, cause providers to be more careful in their investment decisions. Underused equipment would be a liability.

It would be claiming too much to suggest that no regulation would be required if the private sector were allowed a freer hand, but regulation could be supplemental, not dominant, as in the Joe, Needleman, and Lewin plan. The chief problems requiring regulation would be those associated with natural monopoly power that is possessed by some hospitals as a result of locational advantages and economies of scale affecting some services. Additional problems exist because of many hospitals' nonprofit status and their consequent tendency not to leave the industry even in the face of losses which would drive a for-profit firm to liquidate. Regulation might also be needed to curb the monopoly power of some private health plans, which might unfairly exploit providers. Perhaps health planning agencies would provide a useful or even the best mechanism for cost-conscious purchasers to exert their influence, but this eventuality is far from clear. On the contrary, there is a good chance that bringing these issues before public decision makers is to force consumer interests to compromise unduly with providers. Also, public decisionmakers find it hard to say "no" to more and better health services on the ground that the incremental health benefit is not worth the cost. Private decisionmakers may be better able to face such choices realistically. Judging from the British experience, even centrally managed systems which are dependent on a fixed-budget (as the authors' would be) have great difficulty in allocating resources in accordance with patients' interests rather than with providers' preferences.

There is no opportunity at this conference—as there never seems to be—to explore these interesting problems in detail. It is clear, however, that the regulatory agenda would look very different, and much more limited, if the private sector did not have its invisible hands tied. One can only plead for a more complete and imaginative review than we have yet seen of the policy alternatives and of the possibilities for blending market forces and regulatory controls. If nothing else, this paper should suggest how inadequate the policy debate on these questions has been. The fact is that there has never been a competent scholarly critique of the market-oriented approach to the health sector's problems. Joe, Needleman, and Lewin have simply added another paper to the pile of inadequate treatments of what still seems to me to be the most promising idea of them all.

NOTES

1. In this connection, I want to quote a sentence from the outline for the Joe, Needleman, and Lewin paper, which reveals to me the depth of the authors' misunderstanding of the market advocates' position. As an example of "the different focus of the two philosophies," they state that "advocates of regulation focus on inefficient uses of capital as an issue, while market-orienting individuals focus on operating inefficiencies." This is one point on which the record could not be clearer. As my subsequent remarks here will show, misallocation of resources has been my central concern from the beginning, and the central issue that I have tried to identify is whether political or market mechanisms can ultimately do the allocative job better. This entire question, including the very doubtful capacity of regulatory authorities to make hard choices, is examined exhaustively in C. Havighurst and J. Blumstein, "Coping with Quality/Cost Trade-Offs in Medical Care: The Role of PSROs," *Northwestern University Law Review* 70 (1975):6–68. This article is not cited by Joe, Needleman, and Lewin.

2. Clark Havighurst, "Controlling Health Care Costs: Strengthening the Private Sector's Hand," *Journal of Health Politics, Policy and Law* 1 (Winter 1977):471.

3. M. Goldberg and B. Greenberg, "The Effect of Physician-Controlled Health Insurance: *U.S. v. Oregon State Medical Society*," *J. Health Politics, Policy & Law* 1 (Winter 1977).

Discussion

Mr. Needleman: If we are talking about market development, we are talking about regulation which strengthens the market, and we must acknowledge the many problems of any regulatory system. The alternative to market development that has been posited is direct economic regulation of costs, supply, and utilization. In either case, we are talking about regulation.

Dr. Bice: I do not think that there is a theory of regulation that opposes itself to the market; at least that has not been the case historically in the United States. The history of regulation has been one of attempting to get the best out of the concentrations of political and economic power in terms of some ideal conception of the market. It seems to me that the real dichotomy is the market versus public ownership.

Mr. Wolkstein: To see the market-versus-regulation issue as a dichotomy is an oversimplification. The market, in the Adam Smith sense, can no longer be present in the health field. However, there can be a less idealized market with a relatively small number of sellers, where the actions of one seller can have an important effect on the market but, nevertheless, where competition of sorts among the few can be exploited. This oversimplification deals inadequately with the fact that there is a concentration of buying power in very few hands—in some places Medicare, Medicaid, and Blue Cross comprise essentially all of the purchasing of hospital care. These large buyers have the potential for exerting tremendous power over the industry and may be able to cope with the less than ideal sellers situation.

Mr. Ball: One point that I would like to see developed further is the concept of third party buyers being the proxy for individual consumers and exerting pressure on what is furnished by providers as a result of an increasingly sophisticated understanding of what they will pay for. I think that this concept applies to both private third parties and to the government. It seems to me that, increasingly, Medicare, private health insurance, the Blues, unions, and employers ought to be saying that they will pay for care only under a defined set of circumstances that require providers to adopt cost-saving approaches and quality assurance mechanisms. This is not the Adam Smith model of the market of the individual deciding what he or she will do about health care, but is, I suspect, the only version of the market that will work in the health field.

Dr. Evans: The authors are saying that capital problems cannot be disassociated from the industry as a whole, and that the problem par excellence is the problem of cost. I agree with them. The real issue, then, in regulation versus the market is what kind of handle those two different strategies give us on the problem of cost. If we are going to control cost, we have to do one of two things in this industry. We have to cut provider incomes or we have to cut the number of providers. We have to get people out of the industry or we have to make them poorer, and there is no other way.

Mr. Lewin: In discussing the question of capital investment we have to think not only about the economics, but, also, about the political dimension. The critical question, it seems to me, at the risk of stating the obvious, is the question of who decides. Who makes those decisions, who is involved in those decisions, and who, therefore, influences those decisions? The review process associated with Section 1122 and certificate of need is essentially a political process, and there is a very distinct bias on the part of those boards towards approving projects. I think that this relates to the fact that a community making a decision by itself is going to be preoccupied with notions of growth and prestige, so that even where technical and economic considerations may inveigh otherwise, we are dealing, ultimately, with a political process that is community-based. When the community has that say, its views and its concerns are going to predominate. There is a distinct lack of concern for cost containment in the 1122 and the certificate of need processes.

Mr. Havighurst: I am nervous about homogenizing our system, bureaucratizing it, and putting questions involving fundamental and highly personal values in the public sector, where I think that decision makers have a very hard time answering them in a way that is socially correct. I find government quite inept at regulating health and safety issues generally; it has the tendency always to prescribe higher standards than are realistic. I think that a lot of our inflationary problems are attributable to regulation that is not realistic.

Dr. Evans: We must accept the fact that external antitrust type measures can take us only so far in attempting to create a genuine market. In many circumstances the extent of the moral suasion that the provider is able to exercise over the patient precludes a market system and there is probably no amount of external assistance that is going to make the difference. For example, in Ontario, several unions, in negotiation with Blue Cross, whose dental insurance is still private, have contracts which do not include topical fluorides for adult patients. That makes perfectly good sense, because the marginal benefits are close to zero. What happens, apparently, is that the patients go in to see their dentists who casually look at their mouths, cluck a little, and say, "You need topical fluoride; what a pity your plan does not pay." In due course, the pressure comes back to the union, which renegotiates a plan that pays. The problem is that I am not sure of the extent to which we can establish "Truth-in-Advertising" within the doctor-patient relationship.

Mr. Havighurst: We must somehow design a system in which the doctors do not call all the shots, in which the consumers have a chance to register their own feelings and preferences. One could perhaps do that through regulation, yet, in heavily regulated health systems, one finds that the doctors still are quite influential. The British system tends to emphasize acute care excessively and to neglect services which the system is supposed to provide but which do not involve much doctor care.

Dr. Evans: I would argue that it probably is not possible to run a hospital on the basis of consumer preferences. The comment this afternoon about whether we should let a person choose $600 care or $200 care implied that it is acceptable to let people barter and receive both $200 care and potatoes, whereas the people who are already eating steak can have the $600 care. I object to that suggestion on ideological and egalitarian grounds, and I do not think that the public in Canada would support that kind of system. We may get in through the back door, because as you know, the NHS in Britain and in Canada benefits upper socioeconomic people more than lower socioeconomic people; no one has ever found a way around that in any society that I know of. But you must not build a system which makes it obvious.

✳ *Chapter 4*

Investments in Health Manpower: A Possible Alternative

Eli Ginzberg

INTRODUCTION

This essay explores whether the United States confronts a realistic option of shifting the margin of investment in health care away from facilities and equipment and in favor of increasing the number, and improving the competence, of persons engaged in providing health services. To ask the question in such gross terms invites gross answers. Consider the following:

1. Iatrogenically-induced disease accounts for a substantial number of days of hospital care. Better trained and supervised personnel would presumably be less inclined to error. But there is no basis for directly relating additional manpower investments to potential economies in the use of hospital facilities.

2. There is a widespread agreement among the leaders of the health profession that modification of the public's behavior with respect to diet, alcohol, drugs, exercise, and sleep would cut down the incidence of injury and disease, with a corresponding decline in the demand for hospital treatment. But, again, such a trade-off between health education for the public and hospital care is easier to formulate than to effectuate.

3. For a third of a century, students of health insurance have decried the fact that policies have been written which encourage the excessive use of inpatient facilities, especially for diagnostic purposes. With the exception of a small number of prepayment plans (and, possibly, for extraneous reasons such as hospital capacity constraints), neither commercial insurance companies, nor Blue Cross, nor government—the principal third party payers—has found a way to shift demand toward less costly ambulatory facilities.

The author is indebted to Karen Brudney and Miriam Ostow for assistance in developing the data.

113

4. It has been observed that many hospitals are in full operation for about four and a half days out of every seven. By Friday afternoon, preparatory to the weekend, work slackens. Except for emergencies, a great many operating rooms are in use only five mornings a week. It does not follow, however, that great efficiencies in total resource use could be achieved if hospitals were to operate routinely on a twenty-four-hour schedule, seven days a week. The issue remains moot until the personnel and related costs for night, weekend, and holiday shifts are factored into the equation, and the willingness of the medical staff and the public to accept the new schedule has been tested. Most work establishments, it must be recalled, operate one shift.

5. Many patients are forced to extend their stay in a hospital because of the delays that their physicians encounter in completing various diagnostic procedures, the results of which must be in hand before therapy can be initiated. While shortages of personnel are often responsible for these delays, they more often reflect related deficiencies in diagnostic support services including space, equipment, and organization.

6. Around 1940, American physicians began to experiment with early ambulation. They quickly concluded that extended bed rest was, with rare exceptions, counterindicated for most patients. Some time later, pediatricians changed their views about tonsilectomies. More recently, a marked reduction has occurred in the average length of stay of obstetrical patients. These developments underscore the point that substantial savings in facilities can come about without compensatory investments in personnel. The determining factor in the foregoing cases was a change in professional opinion that found acceptance among the public.

These selected observations emphasize that the issue before us cannot be treated as a simple change in what economists call the "production function," involving a different combination of facilities and manpower. The several illustrations call attention to the critical role that is played by changes in physician knowledge and preferences, reimbursement policies, and consumer flexibility in altering the input/output relationships in the production of health services. The illustrations further imply that investments in health manpower must be analyzed within the institutional framework that governs the production and distribution of health services. To ignore the institutional framework is to preclude the analysis from influencing policy.

THE INVESTMENT PROCESS: INSTITUTIONAL PERSPECTIVES

Economists operate with a simplified version of reality in which individuals or firms invest their own funds or borrowed funds in the expectation that future returns will exceed the current value of the resources that are invested. The key actors in this model are investors operating in a market economy in search of economic gains. In recent decades, under the leadership of economists at the

University of Chicago and at Columbia (Schultz, Becker, Mincer), the model has been extended to investments in human beings under the title of "human capital." The economists have pointed out that individuals are willing to undergo long periods of specialized education and training because of the higher earnings that they can later command. In developing its model, the human capital school has focused primarily on investments made by individuals (and their families) in terms of out-of-pocket expenses for tuition and living costs and an additional allowance for earnings foregone (the income that individuals could have earned had they worked rather than continued in student or trainee status). While economists are aware that society always contributes to the educational and training process through public investments—and in many parts of the world these account for the major proportion of all inputs—most of the work pursued by American economists is focused on private sector decision-making. The role of public investments and the benefits that flow therefrom are treated only incidentally.

The interested reader can obtain an up-to-date view of the status of human capital theory, its strengths and weaknesses, by reading Mark Blaug's insightful and incisive review-article in the September 1976 *Journal of Economic Literature.* The critical point in the present context is the limited help that the theory can provide in understanding the dynamics of investment in health manpower because so much of the action takes place in the public arena, not in the private one, where the principal participants pursue goals that are only distantly related to profit-maximization.

A further difficulty relates to the paucity and quality of data required for calculating rates of return. This is a problematic undertaking in view of the fact that the short-term earnings base must serve as a foundation for lifetime projections, the sensitivity of such calculations to different rates of discount, and the inability of the theory to handle the problems of uncertainty in other than an arbitrary fashion.

The present effort, which aims to illuminate the investment process in health manpower, must begin by identifying the principal investors with sufficient specification in order to facilitate differentiating among those who influence the amount of resources that are raised, those who provide the resources, and those who determine the purposes for which they are used. A preliminary system of classification would have to include the following:

Households—individuals with parental or connubial support who are pursuing a course of studies or training with the intention of entering upon a career in health.

Institutions of higher education—
a. *Undergraduate level*—junior and senior colleges which offer a range of majors, from biology to nursing, that enable some, or most, graduates to enter a health occupation.

b. *Professional and graduate level*—university or free-standing professional schools and graduate departments offering instruction from biochemistry to dentistry, whose graduates are likely to enter a health occupation.
c. *Post-graduate instruction*—a rapidly growing effort directed at the advanced training of specialists and at refresher training for professionals in active practice.

Employers—all sectors of the economy—pharmaceutical firms, teaching hospitals, the Veterans Administration—devote considerable resources to raising the competence of thier staffs through formal and informal training and educational efforts.

State governments—the principal societal organ responsible for financing higher education and a major factor in the recent expansion of investments in health manpower through a great variety of programs, including large construction and operating grants and loans to institutions of higher education and teaching hospitals to increase the number of health professionals.

Federal government—It has vastly increased its share of the nation's total investment in health manpower since World War II via the following programs:

a. *Biomedical research funding*—the source of major infusion of new funds into medical schools and major teaching hospitals.
b. *Construction and operating grants*—including capitation payments geared to the expansion of enrollments in health professional schools.
c. *Student support*—via fellowships, traineeships, teaching assistantships, etc.
d. *Reimbursement mechanisms*—a major source of new funds, under Medicare, that underpin the education-training functions of teaching hospitals.
e. *Direct educational and training programs of federal agencies*—particularly the Veterans Administration and the Armed Services.
f. *Educational and training support for paraprofessionals*—provided by the Office of Education, the Social and Rehabilitation Service, the Health Resources Administration, the National Institutes of Health, the Department of Labor, and the Veterans Administration.

Foundations—A number of foundations including Rockefeller, Kellogg, Commonwealth and, more recently, Robert Wood Johnson, as well as others, have long played a supporting role in the training of health professionals, particularly physicians. They should still be included in a listing of investors in health manpower.

Professional associations and societies—including the American Medical Association, the various specialty boards, the professional societies in the fields of dentistry, nursing, etc. Although not themselves investors, they exercise considerable influence both on the scale of public and private investments in health manpower and, more particularly, on the purposes for which the funds are used.

This listing points up the fact that private sector investments are limited to households, a few proprietary training institutions, and a limited number of employers such as pharmaceutical companies. All other investors operate in the not-for-profit sector.

The foregoing classification of the principal actors involved in the investment process in health manpower provides a basis for reviewing the dynamics of their decision-making. Many individuals who decide to pursue studies leading to a health career are, as the economists postulate, interested in the main chance, that is, in becoming high earners and entering a career that carries status and prestige. But such career decisions do not apply to all who enter the health field. From the scion of a wealthy family who decides to become a surgeon to the black woman from the South who relocates in the North or West and finds a job as a nurses' aide, the theory that every person seeks to optimize his or her future economic position, taking current costs into account, does not carry conviction.

The relative importance of proprietary training schools has been declining; the number of employers in the health industry who invest in the training and further education of their work forces is worth noting but should not be exaggerated. An important form of private investment is represented by the self-financed continuing educational efforts of members of the health professions who take time out from their practice and often incur sizable out-of-pocket costs (tuition, travel, living expenses away from home) to keep up with new developments.

The rapid expansion of undergraduate education in the United States in both four-year and two-year institutions can be best explained by rising family income, a favorable employment outlook, and such special factors as college attendance for the purposes of avoiding the draft. The vastly enlarged enrollments in training for health careers, particularly in community colleges, was tied to the rapid growth of employment opportunities in the health industry.

State governments, a major force in increasing investments in health manpower, responded to a series of pressures, including their desire to assure adequate personnel to meet the rising demands of their citizens for improvements in health care; and their effort to meet, at least partially, the desires of qualified state applicants for admission to medical school, a response to offers of federal financing that would favor the expansion of training capacity if additional state monies were allocated.

The federal government's increased investments in health manpower reflected changing goals and objectives over the years. Its first major thrust (1950s) was a concomitant of its much enlarged support for biomedical research which vastly increased the funds available to the nation's stronger medical schools. Later on, the rationale for increased federal support for health manpower reflected the widespread conviction that the nation was suffering from a physician shortage that was adversely affecting the people's health; the desire to increase, as a matter of equity and efficiency, the number of health professionals from low income families; the importance of raising professional standards of care, particularly by encouraging the preparation of larger numbers of nurses with higher educational credentials; improving the capability of federal agencies to discharge their own health functions more effectively; and encouraging the growth of paramedics in the hope and expectation both of reducing the costs of care and of providing opportunities to hard-to-employ persons for improving their position in the job market.

This summary of the principal forces underlying the actions taken by higher education, state governments, and the federal government suggests the difficulties of applying the human capital model to the investment process in health manpower where so many of the strategic decisions are made within a highly politicized environment in which profit-maximizing goals play little or no part.

SOME CONCEPTUAL NOTATIONS

The foregoing schema, concerned with illuminating the dynamics of the decision-making process, has not differentiated sharply between those who made the funds available for investment in health manpower and those who deployed the funds. But, in adding up the sums involved, one must be on the alert to avoid double counting. Certain other methodological issues should also be noted.

One difficulty, previously alluded to, arises in determining the boundary between investments in higher education in general and health professional education in particular. Consider the young woman who decides to pursue a baccalaureate degree in nursing but, for any one of a series of reasons, fails to seek employment later on as a nurse. Are the costs of her preparation, personal and institutional, either over four years or over the last two years, to be included in deriving an estimate of the nation's investment in health manpower? The answer may be in the affirmative with respect to the institutional costs, but what about her personal costs? How do the costs associated with her acquiring a baccalaureate degree differ from those of her twin sister who majored in sociology?

A related boundary problem is involved in calculating the investments to be included in the expansion of health educational facilities. Does one include the construction costs for a dormitory for nursing students, a garage at a university health science center, or an access road to a teaching hospital?

Another range of difficulties stems from investments made by students (and their families). Does one calculate "earnings foregone" at the start or conclusion of a college education? Does one differentiate between students who pursue a technical course of instruction, such as occupational therapy, from those who start—and finish—as biology majors with an intent of entering a health career? And how does one treat the "investments" made by the large numbers who, at the beginning of college, aim to enter medical school but, upon graduation, fail to be among those selected?

Another conundrum is presented by the fact that health science centers, in addition to their training mission, are heavily involved in health research and patient care while teaching hospitals, whose primary mission is to provide patient care, are also engaged in education and research. There is no easy way of breaking out the investment in health manpower from these closely related functions and outputs.

Another complicating factor grows out of accounting practices for colleges and universities which tend to exclude depreciation for plant and equipment on the assumption that the capital that is raised in the form of gifts is not directly revenue-producing. But, since the passage of Medicare in 1965, depreciation has become the rule in hospital accounting. Further complications arise from the fact that both educational institutions and hospitals have increasingly resorted to loans from public and private lending agencies, the carrying charges of which are reflected in their costs and reimbursement.

The conceptual difficulties that are involved in developing a realistic estimate of investment in health manpower have been suggested, but far from exhausted, by the issues identified above. The principal value of this brief exercise has been to alert the reader against undue reliance on the following data which represent, at best, first-order approximations suggestive of the changing levels and trends of such investment, and nothing more.

SELECTIVE DATA ON MANPOWER INVESTMENTS

One parameter for gauging the scale of investment in health manpower is to consider the growth of the total number of individuals with some type of training who were employed in the field during the past quarter century. While total employment data tell us nothing about the numbers trained but who failed to enter the field or who entered and left, they do provide the best single clue to overall growth. Again, ignoring the softness of the Census and alternative systems of counting workers employed in the health industry, the growth has been very rapid:

> 1950—1.6 million
> 1960—2.6
> 1973—4.4.

These figures[1] represent an increase of 175 percent in the twenty-four-year period, compared to a total labor force growth from 63 to 91 million or a gain of 44 percent. Restated, the increase of health professionals and paraprofessionals was at a rate four times greater than that for total employment!

The following data pinpoint the differing rates of growth in the 1960–70 period among various groups of health workers:

	1960	1970	Percent Change
Physicians, including osteopathic	233,000	282,000	21
Registered nurses	630,000	842,000	30
Health technologists & technicians	136,000	349,000	157
Nursing aides, orderlies	430,000	749,000	74

If one extends the time period from mid-century to 1971 and restricts attention to the increase in the stock of health manpower with baccalaureate or higher degrees from U.S. colleges and universities, this is what one finds:

	1950	1971	Percent Change
Medicine and osteopathy	170,000	243,000	43
Dentistry	69,000	95,000	38
Nursing, therapy and dental hygiene (all 3 degree levels)	56,000	213,000	275
Health professions, N.E.C.	57,000	164,000	188

Since the federal government's participation in expanding the supply of health manpower gained momentum only in the latter part of the 1960s and the early 1970s, attention should be focused upon the most recent changes in the number of schools, and the enrollments and graduations in medicine, dentistry and nursing.

From the mid-1960s to the mid-1970s, the number of medical schools increased from 88 to 114, with an additional 11 in development. The expansion in dental schools was more moderate but still noteworthy, from 49 to 54, with 5 additional in development.

The substantial expansion of training capacity in health professional schools was undertaken with the aim of increasing the numbers entering the health professions and, as the following data on enrollments and graduates make clear, this objective was accomplished.

In the case of students in medical school, the following decadal changes are noteworthy. In the decade after 1965, the numbers enrolled increased from about 32,400 to 54,100, or by 67 percent. Of the 21,700 new students, about 5,600 were enrolled in new schools and 16,100 in existing schools which expanded. The numbers being graduated over the ten-year span increased from about 7,400 to 12,700, or by about 72 percent. And the first year enrollment grew from about 8,900 to just below 15,000. What these last figures underscore is that, by the latter 1970s, the number of physician graduates will be twice the mid-1960 output.

The expansion in dentistry was substantial, though less than in medicine. The number of students enrolled increased from about 13,900 to 21,100 or by more than half; the number of graduates from about 3,200 to 5,000, a slightly faster increase.

The nursing scene must be differentiated in terms of program—practical, diploma, associate, baccalaureate and graduate. For all except the last the data cover 1964-65 to 1972-73, while for the last the terminal year is 1973-74. The following summarizes the changes in the number of programs:

	1964-65	*1972-73*	*Percent Change*
Practical	984	1306	33
Diploma	840	494	-41
Associate	130	574	342
Baccalaureate	188	305	62
Graduate	*1964-65*	*1973-74*	
Baccalaureate for R.N.	166	274	65
Master's	53	86	62
Doctoral	4	9	125

The succeeding table sets forth what happened to both enrollments and graduates at the several different levels of nurse preparation:

	1964-65	*1972-73*	*Percent Change*
Practical			
Enrollments	33,900	57,100	69
Graduates	24,300	46,500	91
Registered Diploma			
Enrollments	93,100	68,800	-30
Graduates	26,800	21,500	-20
Associate Degree			
Enrollments	8,500	78,700	824
Graduates	2,510	24,850	890
Baccalaureate			
Enrollments	27,700	85,200	208
Graduates	5,400	13,100	144

Programs for nurses who had acquired the RN diploma or degree increased their enrollments from 12,400 to 18,800, or by more than half. In terms of graduates, the largest gain was at the master's level, from 1,380 to 2,450, or by over three-quarters.

To expand the numbers of professionally trained personnel usually requires the inflow of new funds for the following purposes: the creation of additional facilities; the training of additional faculty; the enlargement of operating funds to support the increased student body; and the ability and willingness of applicants to assume part, or all, of the costs connected with complete or partial withdrawal from the labor market during the period of their studies.

Funding for new and expanded educational facilities comes from three principal sources: the federal government, state government, and philanthropy. Most of it is in the form of grants; some part is in loanable funds. A recent publication of the Health Resources Administration of the U.S. Department of Health, Education and Welfare provides the key data about the federal contribution to the enlargement of training capacity in the health professions.[2]

During this decade, the federal government awarded grants in the amount of $1.3 billion to 619 institutions, all but $213 million going to health professions schools and nurse training programs. The residual sum was in the form of grants to the allied health professions, medical libraries, and health research facilities.

Of the approximately $1 billion to health professions schools, over two-thirds ($670 million) was in the form of grants to medical schools. Dentistry received $210 million, with the remainder divided among veterinary medicine, public health, pharmacy, optometry, and podiatry. It is worth noting that federal funds were divided between public and private institutions in the ratio of more than 2:1. Further, of the approximately $1 billion distributed to health professions schools, about $700 million went to expanding existing schools while the remainder helped finance new institutions.

The HEW report calculates that the $217 million for new medical schools assured 1,780 new places in the first year class, resulting in a calculated average federal support of approximately $122,000 per first year student. The $430 million awarded to existing schools assured 2,080 new places while 6,545 places were maintained, representing support for a total of 8,625 first year students when the construction is completed. The federal support to existing schools for both expansion and maintenance averages about $50,000 per first year student.

About 40 percent of the above grants for construction support to medical schools represented the costs for 6,000 new beds in university teaching or affiliated hospitals, emphasizing the high cost of providing facilities for clinical instruction.

This substantial support understates the total federal contribution. For instance, facility grants from the National Institutes of Health often assisted in the launching of new medical schools or the expansion of existing ones. The substantial new construction and renovation program of the Veterans Administration contributed to the expansion of training facilities for health professionals in terms of the numbers of trainees under its own auspices, clinical support for medical schools with which VA hospitals were affiliated and, more recently, the provision of seed money and other support for selected medical schools in development. These and still additional sources of federal support are not included in the $1.3 billion total made available through the Bureau of Health Manpower (HEW).

Any comprehensive accounting of the federal contribution to the expansion of health educational facilities would also have to include the considerable sums that were made available in the form of construction loans to teaching hospitals and health science centers. These additional forms of direct and indirect assistance probably raise the federal contribution over the decade to the neighborhood of $2 billion.

Even more elusive than the federal total are data that would enable one to estimate the contribution of state governments and philanthropy to the expansion of training capacity. In the absence of reliable statistics, one is forced back upon case materials and impressions. Informed persons estimate that the federal contribution accounted for not less than a third, and possibly as much as half, of all facility expansion. That sets the total national investment in construction in the $4 to $6 billion range for the decade 1965–75. That this is a reasonable estimate is suggested by the one study in depth prepared in 1967.[3]

As noted above, the total investment cost of expanding health manpower resources must also take into account such additional factors as the training of faculty, operating costs, and the loss of student earning power. Each is briefly discussed below.

With respect to faculty, the period 1950 to 1970 saw not only a maintenance of faculty-student ratios in medical schools, but a marked improvement. In 1960, approximately 10,500 full-time faculty were responsible for instructing about 30,000 medical students or a ratio of 1:2.9. In 1970, the number of full-time faculty was about 25,000 for a medical student body of 38,000 and a total health professions student body of 93,000, resulting in ratios of 1:1.5 and 1:3.7 respectively. The ratios for 1975 show no substantial change. From the present vantage of assessing the investments in faculty development, one must take account of the 217 percent increase in total full-time faculty members during this fifteen-year period. If one assumes that each new faculty member received stipend support for an average of three years and that the total cost of his graduate training was twice his stipend, the training of new faculty represents a national investment in the $2 billion range ($80,000 salary and support over a three-year period times 26,000 new faculty).

There is no question that the federal government, through fellowships and traineeships, played the principal role in the training of faculty and research personnel. In 1970, for instance, the National Institutes of Health—the primary, but not sole, source of federal support—was funding about 3,000 pre- and postdoctoral fellows, and over 10,000 full-time trainees, a third of whom are postdoctoral; in addition, it supported some 6,000 part-time trainees, about one-third of whom were postdoctoral.

Additional support was provided by state governments and, in the case of New York, by city government. Foundations such as Markle Commonwealth, Robert Wood Johnson, various philanthropic health organizations, and interested corporations also sponsored fellowships.

There are periodic outbursts by leaders of the research community about federal cut-backs in postgraduate training support which is seen as eroding the biomedical science base. But, if federal policy swings erratically from over- to underfinancing and if conflicts among the bureaucrats, the budget-keepers, and the Congress add to the confusion, the fact remains that biomedical research is in no serious danger although the nation lacks a long-term policy of R&D investment, including investment in professional manpower. It should be noted that, at a time when federal support for postgraduate training in the health professions was at its peak, many medical schools expressed varying orders of difficulty in recruiting faculty, not because of a lack of trained personnel but because of the lure of the fleshpots. Specialists in various clinical fields saw little point in accepting a full-time academic post at one-third or less of what they could earn in private practice.

The combined impact of more students, more research activity, increases in the number of teaching beds, and the constant deepening of medical technology which resulted in ever larger expenditures on plant, equipment and staff raised considerably the operating expenses of educating health professionals. The large-scale study released by the Institute of Medicine on the *Costs of Education in the Health Professions* disclosed that in Fiscal 1972 the total expenditures of these schools exceeded $3 billion.[4] The thrust of the IOM inquiry was to determine the average *net* cost of educating a health professional in order to provide Congress with guidance for future capitation. The IOM concluded that the average annual cost of educating various health professionals was approximately $10,000 for a physician, $7,500 for a dentist, slightly above and below $5,000 for students in podiatry and veterinary medicine respectively and in the $2,000 range for nursing. With slightly under 50,000 students enrolled, medical schools were spending close to $500 million annually to discharge their basic educational mission.

In that same fiscal year, 1972, the Bureau of Health Manpower, HEW, made grants to the health professional schools of approximately $235 million, exclusive of construction, start-up monies, and loan funds for scholarships. Ten years earlier it had made no contribution to the general operating expenses of these schools.

The IOM study pointed out that, with state governments contributing $1.5 billion towards the operating expenditures of health professional schools in Fiscal 1972, their contribution exceeded that of the federal government. By inference, this level of support was at least a quarter of a billion dollars greater than it had been several years earlier. Hence, the combined increase in the annual contribution of federal and state governments toward the operating expenditures of health professional schools was in the half billion dollar range.

The final element to be considered in deriving a first approximation of the additional investments in health manpower are the losses in earnings that are experienced by students during the course of acquiring their first professional degree. In the seven academic years of the present decade the students enrolled in all health professional schools except nursing increased from about 87,000 to 124,000, or by 37,000. If one assumes that the "earnings foregone" amount to $10,000 a year for each student, and that the annual additional students average 18,000, the investment for a decade for this increased number of students total $1.8 billion.

The post-World War II period saw an increasing proportion of all medical school participants puruse their education for another three to four years, on the average, with the intent of qualifying as specialists. This investment in health manpower must also be taken into account in developing a comprehensive estimate of investment costs in health manpower.

There is no reliable study available to guide one in estimating the costs of graduate medical education because both teaching physicians and the house staff often combine education with patient care. To complicate matters further, the presence of a strong teaching program affects the selection and treatment of patients, so that the patient care in teaching and nonteaching hospitals cannot be directly compared. Additional difficulties derive from the fact that many of the teaching physicians do not receive monetary compensation for the educational functions that they perform. However, an Institute of Medicine study on Medicare and Medicaid reimbursement policies provides some suggestive data which can be used in gauging the investment involved in graduate education.[5]

In the period 1964–74 the number of American and foreign-trained residents increased from 29,000 to 49,000 or by more than two-thirds, the number of American residents from 20,000 to 30,000.

The IOM study provides some clues as to the time that residents devote to educational functions (40 percent), as well as the time that teaching physicians devote (25 percent), to instructing them. By piecing together other scraps of information about salaries and the increase in residents, and developing averages for the decade, a rough estimate has been made of the costs for graduate education to support the expanded resident pool.

To this, two additional calculations have been added. One is for the income that is foregone by American graduates only during the course of their residency training. The second is for the additional patient day costs resulting from the expansion of residency programs, predicated on one additional day's stay plus additional diagnostic procedures (15 percent of the patient day costs).

We are now in a position to summarize the order of investments that is involved in the rapid expansion of health manpower since the mid-1960s. It should be emphasized once again that the figures presented below are no more than first order approximations.

	Estimated Investments in Health Manpower Mid 1960s–1970s
Construction of additional educational facilities	$5 billion
Training of additional faculty (medical school only)	2
Additional operating expenses of health professional schools (exclusive of nursing)	5
Income foregone by additional students for a first professional degree	1.8
Graduate medical education	7.270
Additional residents	.320
Teaching staff for additional residents	.500
Patient care costs for additional residents	5.850
Income foregone—additional U.S. residents	.600
	$21.070 billion

The foregoing table helps to highlight three findings about the investment process:

1. The dominant role of the federal and state governments, which were primarily responsible for financing the $12 billion investment to expand facilities and faculty and to subsidize the higher operating costs;

2. The principal private sector effort was represented by the income foregone of the additional numbers who pursued a first professional degree or residency training. Together, this investment was estimated at $2.4 billion, or less than one-eighth of the total. (The remaining private investment consists of tuition and fees, exclusive of scholarship assistance, which may have totaled as much as $1 billion over the decade for the additional students who pursued a health professional education); and

3. The significant expenditures for graduate education of additional residents that were submerged in payments for patient care.

MANPOWER-FACILITY MIX

The extended review of the nation's investment in health manpower during the last two decades was undertaken for the purpose of exploring the potential that exists for substituting investments in manpower for investments in health facilities and equipment with an aim of economizing in the use of total resources. To this end, it is now necessary to focus on developments on the facility front, particularly short-term hospitals, which are the principal locale for major therapeutic interventions.

In the last fifteen years, that is, from the early 1960s, the level of health facility construction expenditures increased from approximately $1 billion to over $4 billion annually, the predominant part of these expenditures, particularly in the latter years, occurring in the nongovernmental sector. Short-term voluntary nonprofit hospitals report an increase in assets during this period from $8.4 billion in 1960 to $28.6 billion in 1973 or approximately 340 percent. During the same period (1960–1973) the number of beds in nonfederal short-term general and special hospitals increased from 639,000 to 903,000. Allowing for the increase in population, the ratio of beds increased from 3.6 per 1,000 to 4.3, or by about one-fifth. Clearly, these years saw an enlargement of the nation's hospital plant.

What about the utilization of the enlarged plant? In 1960, 136 persons out of every 1,000 entered a general or special care hospital. In 1973 the rate has risen to 160, or an increase of about 17.5 percent over the fourteen-year stretch. The total days that this larger number of admissions (from 230 million to 318 million) spent in the hospitals did not increase proportionately. The corresponding ratios showed an increase from 1,265 days per 1,000 to 1,414 days per 1,000, or 10.5 percent. The balancing factor was a decline in the average length of stay of approximately half a day per patient admitted, from 9.3 to 8.8 days.

Relatively little attention has been paid to the striking differences among regions in average patient stay. Between the Northeast and the West coast they are of an order of 50 percent. Any serious effort to improve efficiency in the health industry via additional investments in manpower or facilities must probe the causes for such long-standing disparities.

The much enlarged number of short-term beds, number of admissions, and days of patient care led hospitals to a substantial increase in the number of personnel to cover their much enlarged work load. In 1960, the short-term hospitals had 1,080,000 full-time equivalent personnel to take care of an average daily census of 477,000 patients. By 1973, the comparable figures were 2,149,000 for a census that had increased to only 681,000. The number of personnel per 100 patients increased between 1960 and 1973 from 226 to 315, or by about two-fifths. In dollar terms, the total expense in nonfederal short-term hospitals averaged $32 per day in 1960, of which $20 represented payroll cost. The comparison, in current dollars, for 1973 was $115 per patient day with $64 representing personnel costs.

A more detailed picture of what happened to the personnel-bed ratios in *all* hospitals in the United States between 1960 and 1970 has been built up from census data and is presented in Table 4-1. It should be emphasized that reliance on the Census facilitates comparability but the Census, like every other source of hospital reporting, suffers from serious limitations. For instance, it does not recalculate part-time into full-time personnel. It should also be noted that ratios of personnel per bed ignore the intensification of hospital use which, as noted earlier, increased over these two decades. But, for trend analysis, the Census provides the best single source.

If attention is focused solely on the 1960–1970 comparisons the following observations are noteworthy:

1. a two-thirds increase in personnel per bed;
2. a more than one-third increase in physicians per bed, with a 50 percent increase in house staff;
3. an almost three-fifths increase in nursing personnel;
4. a doubling in allied health and technical personnel;
5. and a two-third increase in all other personnel.

These data underscore the fact that, even allowing for the larger number of admissions, hospitals increased their personnel very substantially during the period.

While the trends in hospitalization hold the key to the potential trade-off between additional investments in personnel versus facilities, some attention should be paid to other locales where medical care is provided, specifically physicians' offices, outpatient departments, and nursing homes. With respect to the first, physicians' offices, a recent study disclosed that between May 1973 and

Table 4-1. Personnel Employed in All United States Hospitals

	1950	1960	1970
Number of Beds	1,456,000	1,658,000	1,616,000
Total personnel	983,820	1,691,578	2,689,722
Per bed	.676	1.02	1.66
Physicians	40,950	63,595	86,096
Per bed	.028	.038	.053
Interns & residents	24,803	37,843	51,228
Per bed	.017	.023	.032
Staff	16,147	25,752	34,868
Per bed	.011	.016	.022
Nursing personnel	476,208	790,000	1,275,900
Per bed	.327	.476	.790
Registered nurses	205,389	325,000	495,000
Per bed	.141	.196	.306
Practical nurses	49,880	105,000	221,900
Per bed	.034	.063	.137
Aides, orderlies, etc.	220,939	360,000	559,000
Per bed	.152	.217	.346
Allied health, professional and technical	79,560	166,243	338,194
Per bed	.055	.100	.209
All other	340,410	602,053	962,305
Per bed	.234	.363	.595

April 1974 an estimated 645 million patients visited a physician in his office, representing 3.1 visits per person. The total number of visits per person to all ambulatory care sources is estimated to be about 4.5 per year.

One of the noteworthy trends between 1965 and 1973 was the marked rise in outpatient visits to hospitals of all types, federal and nonfederal, but excluding psychiatric and tuberculosis. The rate increased from 640 per 1,000 to 1,084, or by about 70 percent within a seven-year span.

What this translates into is that for every person admitted to a hospital for inpatient treatment there are approximately seven persons treated in an outpatient facility. Unquestionably, part of the increase in hospital personnel per bed marks the 70 percent increase in outpatients that the hospital staff had to cope with in recent years. What remains moot is the extent to which the increased number of patients treated in outpatient facilities represents a shift from potential inpatient treatment. We know from other sources that a high proportion of patients seen in emergency rooms are not in urgent need of treatment; and we further know that many of them, especially the urban poor, use the emergency room for basic care, since they have no access to a local practitioner.

Some additional insight into the shifting locus of care between inpatient and outpatient facilities can be gained from a closer look at what has been transpiring in the arena of mental health. Here there has been both a major expansion in treatment and a major shift in treatment locale.

Between 1955 and 1973 patient care episodes per 100,000 population increased from slightly over 1,000 to about 2,300. However, the total number of inpatient services barely increased, from 799 to 807. On the other hand, the number of patients treated in outpatient settings rose from 234,000 to 1,475,000 or more than sixfold.

The magnitude of this shift (disregarding the greater use of nursing home beds for the senile aged) is suggested by the fact that inpatient treatments accounted for more than three-quarters of all patient encounters in 1955 and only slightly more than one-third in 1973. In 1960, the country had 722,000 beds used specifically for the care of mental patients; in 1973 the number had been reduced to 422,000, a decline of 40 percent.

Brief reference should also be made to the broad developments in nursing homes and extended care facilities. The cost of constructing, staffing, and operating a nursing home bed is much lower than for a general hospital bed.

The decade 1963–1973 saw more than a doubling of nursing home beds, from approximately 550,000 to about 1,280,000, with a corresponding increase in the number of patients. While total nursing home personnel increased substantially, from 242,000 to 613,000, the increase per 1,000 patients was relatively modest—from 491 to 533. The difference in costs between treating a person in a short-term hospital bed and in a nursing home is suggested by the following. In 1973, short-term hospital expense per patient day came to $115; in 1973–74, the monthly resident charge in a nursing home was $478, a difference of over 7:1. Much of this difference is accounted for by the fact that there are slightly more than three persons employed per patient in a short-term hospital while the ratio in nursing homes is about one person for two patients.

As Table 4-2 makes clear, the decade 1965–74 reveals a total expenditure of just under $30 billion on new construction for health facilities, roughly two-thirds in the nongovernmental sector and one-third by government. The substantial rise in construction expenditures by the nongovernmental sector represents, in the first instance, the opportunities that were provided to hospitals to modernize and expand once depreciation was recognized as a reimbursable expense by third party payers. Further, hospitals had access to new sources of governmental grants and loans for construction as well as to loanable funds, both private and public. Moreover, they continued to compete with considerable success for philanthropic dollars.

In addition, the private sector increased its investments to a modest degree. The number of proprietary hospital beds expanded from 46,000 in 1960 to 73,000 in 1973 and private interests dominated new investments in nursing homes, most of which are operated on a for-profit basis.

The investment process was not limited to constructing new beds in hospitals and nursing homes, but also included a substantial parallel investment in the com-

Table 4-2.   Construction (in thousands of dollars)

	Total	Private (Non-profit & Profit)	Public
Fiscal 65	1840	1170	670
66	1900	1160	740
67	1930	1210	720
68	2160	1320	840
69	2500	1560	940
70	3290	2290	1000
71	3550	2230	1320
72	4080	3030	1050
73	4150	2940	1210
74	4370	2910	1460
	$29,770	19,820	9,950

plex equipment that is required to permit physicians to take advantage of the advances in medical technology. The establishment of a neurosurgical service always involves expensive structural alterations in addition to the purchase of much new equipment. Large investments are also required when a hospital decides to open a burn unit, an organ bank, or a hyperbaric chamber.

This brief review of investments in facilities and equipment reveals that the total sums involved were substantial; that the principal sources of funds were governmental; that increasing investments in facilities did not lead to savings in manpower; and that there was little movement from the use of more costly to less costly facilities, the expansion in nursing homes and hospital-based ambulatory services representing primarily an expansion in total services rather than substitutions resulting in the more economical use of resources.

FINDINGS AND LESSONS FOR POLICY

The principal conclusion to be drawn from this review of investments in health manpower, with primary attention to the correlative investments in health facilities, is that the United States accelerated the flow of resources into the health care industry during the post-World War II period, more particularly in the last decade. Rough calculations suggest that, in the last decade alone, the manpower investment total exceeded $21 billion and that the facility total was almost half again as large.

The magnitude of these two investment streams suggests that strong forces operated to expand both manpower and facilities and that whatever substitution occurred for the purpose of economizing in the use of one resource or another was swamped by forces directed to enlarging the total health care system.

A review of the sources of funding—as well as of the principal users of the funds—disclosed that the federal and state governments played the leading role as suppliers of new funds, with the nonprofit universities, medical schools, and hospitals sharing in putting the funds to use. A closer view disclosed that the federal and state governments were not monolithic organizations but that many different agencies, both at the federal and state levels, participated actively, including those concerned with higher education, medical research, health resources, social security, manpower development, construction and lending, and still others.

Further, the goals of public policy were many and diverse and included efforts to reduce and eliminate manpower and facility shortcomings so that the public's pressure for services could be better met; enlarging the opportunities for various groups in the society to pursue a career in health; assuring the financial viability of health professional schools; enlarging the supply of paramedics in the expectation that such an increased output might help contain the sharply rising costs of health care; broadening access to the health care system for hitherto underserved populations; and still other priority objectives.

What the foregoing paragraphs underline is the limited degree to which the increased investments in the health arena, under governmental initiative, were informed by a resource economizing approach. Federal and state legislators were more concerned about speeding the accomplishment of what they viewed as priority social goals than in calculating how such goals could be achieved at least cost.

The preceding analysis called attention to the modest role of the private sector, where, presumably, economic investment criteria prevail. The principal areas where such considerations prevailed related to a modest investment in the expansion of proprietary hospitals, a more substantial growth in nursing homes and, most importantly, the willingness of large numbers of individuals to enter upon shorter or longer courses of training in the realization that the market was sending out repeated cues to the effect that they would be able to make a good career for themselves in the burgeoning health care industry.

There is scattered evidence, however, that some forces operated to bring about a more economic and efficient use of health resources. Specifically:

1. the more rapid expansion, in the pre-1965 period, of nursing and allied health personnel other than physician manpower;
2. some modest reduction in average patient stay in short-term hospitals achieved, in part, through an increased use of personnel;
3. a substantial increase in outpatient care, some small part of which represented a reduction in inpatient admissions, achieved through an enlarged hospital staff;
4. a market shift in the treatment of psychiatric patients from inpatient to outpatient facilities; and
5. a marked expansion of patients cared for in nursing homes (with their smaller and less sophisticated staff), some part of whom would have remained, in the absence of such facilities, in much more expensive short-term hospitals.

But too much encouragement should not be drawn from these examples. A closer reading of the record suggests that additional investments in health manpower were seldom the sole, or even the principal, cause of whatever modest gains in resource efficiency could be identified. Consider the following:

1. A large part of the new health workers who were trained and employed in the 1950s and 1960s were absorbed as additional members of the health team, not as substitutes for those with higher orders of training and skill.

2. There is no way to sort out whether the additional personnel per hospital bed was the critical element in shortening average patient stay. The presumption is that other factors operating at the same time, including the preferences of the medical staff, hospital administration, and patients, played the key role.

3. The substantial expansion in outpatient treatment in general hospitals was not stimulated by any radical change in insurance policies or hospital organization aimed at substituting ambulatory treatment for inpatient care. Most of the increase reflected the demands of the poor and near-poor for access to primary care.

4. Most admissions to nursing homes do not represent patients transferred from short-term hospitals but, rather, old persons whose families are no longer able or willing to care for them.

5. The striking shift from inpatient to outpatient care for large numbers of psychiatric patients cannot be adjudged a major gain in treatment and in the use of resources until more careful follow-up studies are made of the consequences of this shift for the well-being of the released patient, his family, and the community.

The foregoing analysis was directed to a single question: whether significant gains could be achieved by increasing investments in health manpower at the expense of additional investments in facilities. The following policy directions can be extracted from this exercise:

1. As long as the sources of additional funding for the health care industry remain splintered among a large number of independent federal agencies, state agencies, philanthropic and corporate enterprises, there is no practical way for substituting additional investments in manpower for additional investments in facilities. Each party at interest will make his investment decision in terms of the organizational imperatives that he confronts and few will be responding to efficiency criteria. Such considerations are not at the center of most decision-making in the health care industry. The availability principle suggests that the demand for health services, especially under third party reimbursement practices, will be determined by the level of resources.

2. The existence of gross regional differences in average patient stay, even after allowance is made for demographic and climatic factors, is presumptive evidence that many sections of the country are characterized by an excessive number of hospital beds. Federal policy affecting inpatient facilities, including reimbursement for hospital care of their beneficiaries, should aim at reducing the

presumptive oversupply of beds in regions with differentially high average patient stays.

3. Federal and state governments and the leaders of nonprofit and commercial insurance plans should explore the potentialities of modifying existing hospital insurance plans so that more diagnostic, preoperative, and postoperative care can be provided on an ambulatory basis, thereby further reducing the demand for inpatient services.

4. State planning and regulatory bodies, working in cooperation with third party reimbursement agencies and with the leadership of health services areas, should aim to close out entire hospitals or major services in adjacent hospitals when the existing capacity is clearly in excess of the present and potential demand. Unless the "excess" beds and services are eliminated, no significant savings can be achieved.

5. The studies of the General Accounting Office relating to the steep rise in the costs of Medicare and Medicaid clearly indicated that a relative shortage of nursing care beds and of home care services results in the unnecessary prolongation of patient stays in more costly short-term hospitals. The newly established HSAs should be encouraged to address these and other potential imbalances in facilities.

6. There is a serious gap between the large numbers in the health manpower pipeline and the prospective absorptive capacity of the employment market. Congress and state legislators, as well as those responsible for educating health manpower at every level, from physicians to allied health personnel, should reassess the short- and medium-term outlook with an aim of moderating the expansionary forces that have been operating since the early 1960s.

7. The period immediately ahead may provide an opportunity for tightening the rules and regulations governing the training and employment of foreign medical graduates in the United States with an aim of narrowing the gap in preparation and performance potential between them and the locally produced supply.

8. The difficulties attendant on reducing the present bed capacity through the elimination of services and the closure of hospitals will be insurmountable unless care is taken to consider the employment rights of long-term staff members in planned reductions. This adds to the urgency of improved coordination between the local institutions that train and those that employ health manpower.

CONCLUDING NOTE

In the period since the end of World War II—and more particularly since 1960—the United States has been rapidly increasing its total flow of resources into the health care industry. More investments in facilities spurred more investments in the training of health manpower and the availability of more facilities and manpower has led to increasing the flow of funds required for operating the vastly enlarged system. It should not be overlooked that if a new hospital bed costs between $50,000 and $100,000 to construct, the operation of that bed equals the investment cost before the end of the second year. If the education of a physician involves an investment in the $100,000 range, the annual salary for newly graduated physicians joining a group is in the $40,000 range. The Canadians believe that every additional physician who enters the system adds $250,000 to the total annual operating costs.

The United States, with its pluralistic structure of decision-making with respect to expenditures, education programming, and health services production, is poorly positioned to rationalize its investment outlays. The best that it can hope to accomplish at this point is to initiate, on several fronts, action that is aimed at slowing the growth of resources in the expectation that such action will slow the continuing rapid rise in total costs. If such a dampening can succeed it will create a more favorable background for the next step at rationalization which must address how changes in the delivery system can better meet consumer needs and desires at a total resource cost that is socially acceptable. This is not a counsel of despair. It is counsel for a people that has repeatedly voted with its pocketbook for consumer choice over producer efficiency.

SUMMARY

1. On the assumption that doctors drive the system, any serious effort at cost containment must aim at moderating the steep increases that are under way in enrollments and output. The FMG inflow should be brought under early control, as it is in Canada.

2. Even in the absence of potential cost containment benefits, it is desirable to encourage the broader use of nurse practitioners, especially for areas and population groups that have been repeatedly unable to attract physicians.

3. The potential expansion of the National Health Service Corps provides an opportunity for exploring new patterns of physician practice, especially in areas which previously had difficulties in attracting/retaining physicians.

4. There is practically no empirical base for assessing different combinations of manpower and facilities from the vantage of efficiency and effectiveness. The knowledge gap should be addressed.

5. Another knowledge gap relates to gross differences in total resource use among areas in the provision of patient care and the causes and consequences related thereto.

6. If hospitals are to be closed, attention must be directed to facilitating staff appointments at other institutions.

7. The potential of citizen education with respect to the uncertainties attached to many elective procedures should be more fully explored. The ability of doctors to drive the system requires consumer acquiescence.

8. Little use has been made of reimbursement mechanisms to increase the use of less costly types of health facilities and personnel.

9. There is need for the training of larger numbers of persons with expertise in health care financing and the management of large money flows.
10. It is essential that state and federal governments consider the relationships between increasing health manpower and the cost implications thereof on the delivery of health services.

NOTES

1. U.S. National Center for Health Statistics, *Health Resources Statistics,* 1974.

2. U.S. Bureau of Health Manpower, *Construction Grants for Educational Facilities, Fiscal Years 1965-75,* (December 1975).

3. Cheves Mc.C. Smythe, "Developing Medical Schools: An Interim Report," *Journal of Medical Education* 42, 11 (November 1967).

4. National Academy of Sciences, *Costs of Education in the Health Professions,* January 1974.

5. National Academy of Sciences, *Medicare-Medicaid Reimbursement Policies,* 1976.

REFERENCES

National Academy of Science. *Personnel Needs and Training for Biomedical and Behavioral Research.* The 1976 Report of the Commission on Human Resources.

Radner, Roy, et al. *Demand and Supply in U.S. Higher Education.* McGraw-Hill, 1975.

U.S. Bureau of Health Manpower. *Selected Information on Health Professions Schools.* Part I: Enrollment Data, Academic Years 1970-71 through 1976-77. Part II: Bureau of Health Manpower Support by Program, Fiscal Years 1965-75.

U.S. Bureau of Health Manpower. *The Development of a National Inventory of State Support for Health Manpower Training Programs: An Executive Summary.*

U.S. Department of Health, Education and Welfare. *The National Ambulatory Medical Care Survey: 1973 Summary.* Publication No. 76-1772.

U.S. Department of Health, Education and Welfare. *Private Foundations Supporting Health Manpower.* Publication No. 74-40, 1971.

U.S. Department of Health, Education and Welfare. *Inventory of State Appropriations Supporting Education for the Health Professions: FY 1971-72.* Publication No. 75-31.

Discussion of
Investments in Health Manpower:
A Possible Alternative

Robert J. Lampman

Professor Ginzberg's paper is an exercise in historical industry analysis. An industry is, by definition, an aggregation of firms producing a range of similar outputs. It uses inputs of land, labor, capital and, also, of intermediate products, some of which are produced by firms outside of the industry. Over time, an industry may change its level of total output and also alter the composition of its outputs. Moreover, an industry may, at the same time, change its balance among inputs. Changes in outputs and inputs may be responsive to innovations which yield either what is perceived as more effective outcomes per unit of output of more output per unit of input.

Professor Ginzberg's paper is rich with examples of recent changes in the inputs and outputs of the health care industry in the United States. All that I attempt to do here is to re-order in descriptive fashion and to review the changes to which he refers.

In 1975, the nation's output of "health services and supplies" for final use sold for $111.3 billion (see Table 4D-1). Of this, $103.2 billion was for "personal health care." This output, which could have been bought at 1950 prices for $34.1 billion, was over three times as great as the output of 1950, namely, $10.5 billion. In that twenty-five year period the real output of all industries (gross national product) "only" doubled. The high rate of growth of the personal health care industry enabled a 134 percent increase in per capita consumption of its outputs. (We should note that the data which we have do not net our purchases from other industries and, hence, do not give us a pure "value added" by the health care industry.)

It is interesting that many other nations exhibit a similar pattern of differential growth of the health care industry.[1] There appears to be no consensus on why this extraordinary expansion of output has occurred, but factors that are often

Table 4D-1. National Expenditures for Health Services and Supplies, 1950 and 1975

	(in thousands of dollars)		Ratio of 1975 expenditures to those of 1950
	1950	1975	
Total	11,181	111,250	9.9
Personal health care	10,540	103,200	9.8
Hospital care	3,698	46,600	12.6
Nursing home care	178	9,000	50.0
Physicians' services	2,689	22,100	8.2
Dentists' services	940	7,500	8.0
Other professional services	384	2,100	5.5
Other health services	534	3,000	5.7
Drugs and drug sundries	1,642	10,600	6.6
Eyeglasses and appliances	475	2,300	5.0
Other	641	8,050	12.5
Expenses for prepayment and administration	290	4,593	15.0
Government public health activities	351	3,457	9.9

Source: Adapted from Marjorie Smith Mueller and Robert M. Gibson, "National Health Expenditures, Fiscal Year 1975," *Social Security Bulletin,* February 1976.

mentioned include technological change, increased consumer and voter demand for what is simultaneously a luxury and a merit good, the shift to third party payment, and the system of rewards for suppliers.

The present mix of outputs is quite different from that produced in 1950. This is suggested by row 3 of Table 4D-1, which, based on expenditures uncorrected for relative price changes, shows a shift toward more nursing home care and less of "other" services and of "supplies." Professor Ginzberg explains some of the changes which have occurred within these broad categories, including the decline in hospital care for mental patients and the rapid rise in outpatient care.

We get another view of the change in level and composition of outputs in the top panel of Table 4D-2, which assembles information supplied by Professor Ginzberg and others. Adjusted patient-days and numbers of physician days approximately doubled, while total real output (total expenditure adjusted for price change) tripled. This apparent contradiction may be reconciled by the fact that more, and higher quality, goods and services were delivered per patient-day and per physician visit.[2]

Inputs, as distinct from outputs, appear to have increased in step with the tripling of output (see the bottom panel of Table 4D-2). Real assets of hospitals and numbers of health care workers both approximately tripled. However, Professor Ginzberg illustrates the changes within the categories of capital and labor. Workers with less training increased the most, and hospitals used increasing amounts of supplies purchased from outside the industry. These changes

Table 4D-2. Some Outputs and Inputs, Personal Health Care Industry, Selected Years 1950-75

	1950	1957	1960-61	1963	1970-71	1973	1975
Outputs							
Personal health care expenditure in 1950 prices(a)	$10.5 billion						$34.1 billion
Hospital days Outpatient visits(b)	167,530,000	227,370,000	192,600,000			297,500,000	
Adjusted patient days(c)	144,733,000		45,900,000		103,000,000	280,320,000	
Physician visits(c)		904,317,000				1,675,566	
Inputs							
Assets of short-term, voluntary, nonprofit hospitals	$3.4 billion		$8.4 billion			$28.6 billion	$35.8 billion
Beds in short-term non-federal hospitals	639,000					903,000	
Nursing home beds				550,000			
Health workers	1,600,000		2,600,000			1,280,000	
Health professionals	352,000				715,000	4,400,000	

Sources: Eli Ginzberg, "Investments in Health Manpower: A Possible Alternative," except as noted.

(a) Marjorie Smith Mueller and Robert M. Gibson, "National Health Expenditures, Fiscal Year 1975," *Social Security Bulletin*, February 1976; adjusted for price change using medical care component of consumer price index, which stood at 53.7 in 1950 and 168.0 in 1975.

(b) Julian Pettengill, "The Financial Position of Private Community Hospitals, 1961-71," *Social Security Bulletin*, November 1973.

(c) Nancy L. Worthington, "Expenditures for Hospital Care and Physicians' Services: Factors Affecting Annual Changes," *Social Security Bulletin*, November 1975.

in inputs were related to changes in outputs and, also, to technological developments in drugs, equipment, and treatment procedures.

It is not possible to tell from the fragmentary data in Table 4D-2 whether there was a change in the input mix of capital and labor. Professor Ginzberg does show an increase in the number of hospital workers per bed, but they may have been offset by a rise in capital in other forms than beds. The data do suggest relatively low ratios of capital per worker and of capital per unit of output as compared to, say, agricultural or manufacturing industries.

Professor Ginzberg looks at more than current inputs and outputs. He addresses the question of changes in the capacity to produce via investment or derived-demand outlays in research, education and training, and plant and equipment. Table 4D-3 shows that annual outlays for research have increased twenty-five times since 1950, but outlays for construction of medical facilities did not keep up with industry output. We do not have base-period information in outlay for the education of professionals, but Professor Ginzberg does provide evidence that an increase of human capital is in the pipeline. Medical school enrollments have recently doubled.

A tripling of output was achieved with what appear to have been relatively small changes in the stock of such key items as hospital beds and physicians. How different would this industry's performance be if the stock of such items had increased at twice the rate that they, in fact, did? If the mix of inputs were more capital intensive, and if the labor input were more skill-intensive, would the output be greater and less costly? The answer to those questions can presumably be found by engineering and economic analyses of physical relations in production and of relative prices of the several inputs.

Table 4D-3. National Expenditures for Health Research, Medical-Facility Construction, and Education and Training of Professionals, 1950 and 1975

	1950	*1975*	*Ratio of 1975 Expenditures to those of 1950*
Research	110	2,750	25.0
Construction	737	4,500[a]	6.1
Education and training of professionals		3,100[b]	

Sources: Marjorie Smith Mueller and Robert M. Gibson, "National Health Expenditures, Fiscal Year 1975," *Social Security Bulletin,* February 1976; except as noted.

   (a) Professor Ginzberg estimates annual average for 1965–75 at $3 billion.

   (b) NAS estimate for 1972. This covered costs for 300,000 students, in eight health professions. *Costs of Education in the Health Professions,* 1974. Professor Ginzberg estimates the annual average for 1965–75 at $2.1 billion.

Such analysis can identify least-cost combinations of inputs for a given level and pattern of outputs with a defined technology. With such information, an all-powerful industry commissar could organize the industry to achieve a static form of technical efficiency.

However, there is another level of "efficiency" that is at issue, having to do with the appropriate level and mix of outputs. Would consumers be worse off if the real output of this industry were substantially lower than it now is? (This is a little like a vegetarian asking if consumers would be better off if the output of the meat industry were lower.) Would consumers be better off if the industry produced at the same level but with an altered package of outputs? Such questions quickly take us beyond the realms of input-output analysis into that of cost-effectiveness analysis, wherein someone has to evaluate the several components of outcome from one pattern of health care as distinguished from another.

I suppose that one's opinion of the value of the historical increase in output and of possible future increases may hinge on one's view of what causes the increase. We indicated above that competing explanations of the increase involve technical change, consumers' and voters' demand increase, and financial and organizational change. One view, which Professor Ginzberg shares, is that the dynamic is supplied by a growth in the number of physicians and the number of hospital beds. In this view, increasing the stock leads to more demand, including demand for "unnecessary" services. Clues to the operational meaning of this are found in the consequences of under-utilized capital and labor of a specialized character. The logical outcome of this view is the policy judgment that an appropriate plan is to slow the growth of these key resources in order to control the rise in total costs.

I believe that Professor Ginzberg is right in his view that wisdom pushes one beyond static production functions, and that he is sound in his insight that, in our system supply and demand decisions are made at many levels and for diverse reasons. However, I am not yet pursuaded by his view that the health care industry has overinvested in physical and human capital.

NOTES

1. This pattern is documented in Brian Abel-Smith, *An International Study of Health Expenditure* (World Health Organization, 1957) and Joseph G. Simanis, "Medical Care Expenditures," *Social Security Bulletin,* March 1973.

2. This issue is explored by Nancy L. Worthington, "Expenditures for Hospital Care and Physicians' Services: Factors Affecting Annual Changes," *Social Security Bulletin,* November 1975.

Discussion of
Investments in Health Manpower:
A Possible Alternative

Richard N. Rosett

To those of you who believe, as I do, that the price system allocates resources far better than does the political system, the remarks which I am about to make may sound like treason. Still, it is worth considering the possibility that even politicians and bureaucrats reach their decisions by the rational calculation of costs and benefits. Let me begin by contrasting two possible descriptions of the growth of the health care industry over the past twenty-five years.

One possibility is that the growth of third party payment and the shift from private to public financing of investment in both human and physical capital have led to gross misallocation of resources. Third party payment tends to insulate both the patient and the provider from the influence of ordinary market forces so that the resource cost of some of the services consumed far exceeds the benefit to the consumer. Subsidized training and capital construction programs lead to investments in which the social rate of return is far below the rate at which society discounts future benefits. This is more or less the currently popular view which is shared both by those who favor a return to market allocation and by those who favor increased government intervention, regulation, and planning.

In contrast, consider the possibility that market forces are capable of overcoming many of the obstacles that have been erected in the health services industry, and that while there are effects of intervention, even important and possibly deplorable effects, they are not likely to be of the sort that are implicit in the question under discussion here. I take that question to be whether a change in the proportions of human to physical capital could produce the health care benefits which we now enjoy at far lower cost than we now bear.

If interference with market forces has led to significant misallocation, it is difficult, in the evidence which Professor Ginzberg has gathered, to detect a clue as to the direction in which improvement lies. The formation of both human and physical capital has been encouraged and large amounts of both have been formed. If nothing has balanced their growth, how do we know which way the balance has been tipped? Nothing in the data tells us, so that even if we accept that interpretation, no clear policy prescription emerges.

The alternative is that, despite the seemingly chaotic state of the health services industry, it, like the rest of our seemingly chaotic economic system, is actually surprisingly orderly, thanks to the guidance of the invisible hand. Consequently, it is likely that the present value of our investments equals the cost, that we are producing our health care efficiently, and in just about the amounts that we want to buy.

As an example of how market forces might operate in a system that seems to stifle them, consider the case of private hospitalization insurance. Few hospital patients now pay more than a trivial fraction of their hospital bills directly. For most, private insurance pays most of the bill. This has been advanced by many, including myself, as one of the principal causes of the rapid rise in hospital costs since World War II. But while we may not care what it costs to stay in the hospital, we do care what our hospital insurance costs. The insurance companies know that and are frequently influential in restraining total hospital expenditure, often by limiting the number of beds, but by other cost-restraining means as well. If there really is no restraint, why are we spending a mere $151 per day instead of $500 or $1,000? Something is obviously at work limiting what is spent, and that something is likely to be the insurance buyer's unwillingness to spend more.

Health insurance is a tax-free fringe benefit, and that tends to introduce a bias toward buying medical care. So, in fact, does the tax deductibility of medical care itself. Here we must consider the politician and his own calculation of costs and benefits. In deciding which private expenditures to exempt from taxation, he must make a calculation similar to the one that he makes in deciding which public expenditures to vote for. In the latter case, he tries to choose expenditures that will make the taxpayer willing, or at least not sorry, to part with his taxes. In the former, he exempts from taxation those private expenditures for which the exemption is most appreciated.

I do not mean to suggest here that the political allocation is identical to market allocation, only that the same consideration of costs and benefits enters the calculation.

The political process tends to allocate fewer resources to any given activity than would the market, simply because it requires a substantial consensus of the voters. Public services seldom offer frills. This allows the private sector to compensate for the failure of the public sector to spend enough. This compensation would be impossible if the public sector tended to spend too much. This assertion may seem surprising in a discussion of the one industry that seems to have been greatly overstimulated by public spending, but, in support of it, here is the one bit of empirical evidence which I have to offer. Joseph Newhouse has computed an Engel curve for medical care.[1] His data come from thirteen countries and consist of per capita medical care and per capita Gross Domestic Product. He obtains a linear regression:

$$\text{Medical care dollars per capita} = -60 + .0788 \times \text{Gross Domestic Product per capita.}$$
$$R^2 = 0.92.$$

A reproduction of his graph of the data and the function is shown in Figure 4D-1.

First, medical care, by the usual definition, seems to be a luxury. As income rises, it is a rising proportion of income, like recreation but unlike food. Second, increases in medical care expenditure seem to be explained almost entirely by increases in income. This is in contrast to empirical cross-section findings for American families which show medical care to be distributed relatively uniformly across income classes. In other words, prices seem to ration medical care across countries and over time, but not within one country among individuals at one time. Newhouse's explanation of this has no place here. I offer his data only to

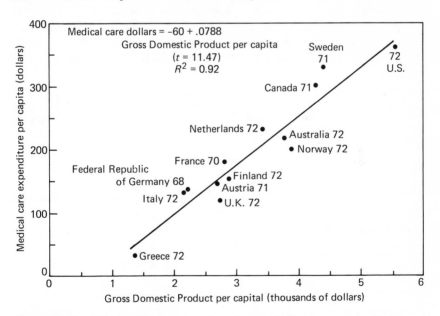

Figure 4D-1. Relationship between Gross Domestic Product and medical spending thirteen countries (recent years)

Source: Joseph Newhouse, "Income and Medical Care Expenditure Across Countries," RAND P-5608-1. Table 1. Reprinted in *Journal of Human Resources,* Vol. XII, No. 1 (Winter 1977), pp. 115–124.

support the suggestion that we are not, in fact, buying more than we want to buy. When I saw the Newhouse equation, I computed one of my own, using a United States time series from 1935 through 1970, expressed in 1970 dollars. The intercept was -41 instead of -60 and the slope was 0.0723 instead of 0.0788. The R^2 is 0.98. The similarity of the two functions is remarkable.

There is reason to believe, or at least suspect, that we are not spending too much on medical care. But are we spending badly? Could medical care be produced more efficiently? The same arguments can be advanced here: that even politicians and bureaucrats have good reason to want to give taxpayers as much value as possible for their tax dollars. The very multiplicity of programs which, to Professor Ginzberg and others, suggests inefficiency, may produce just the reverse through competition among various programs.

It might reasonably be asked why, in so perfect a world, anyone would lament the shift of privately provided services into the public sector. This is not the place to elaborate, but I will close by suggesting three reasons. First, the electoral institutions that democracy requires may tend to bias the political allocation of resources as compared with market allocations in a way that is not under discussion here. Future benefits may be more heavily discounted by politicians than by the market. We may produce efficiently in the present, but fail to provide well enough for the future. Second, political allocations tend to redistribute income, though it is unclear exactly in whose favor. As a consequence, growth may be retarded and so, again, we rob the future for the present. Finally, political allocation tends to increase governmental power at the expense of individual liberty.

These may be just part of the price that a willing electorate knowingly pays for benefits that it receives. They may well be such and still be no less cause for lament.

NOTES

1. Joseph Newhouse, "Income and Medical Care Expenditure Across Countries," RAND P-5608-1. Reprinted in *Journal of Human Resources,* Vol XII, No. 1 (Winter 1977), pp. 115-124.

Discussion

Dr. Rosett: One of the complaints that is often voiced about our medical care system is that decisions are made in many different places and that they are uncoordinated, irrational, and inefficient. Yet, I think that there is some room in such a system for the invisible hand to operate. After all, the decisionmakers face the same prices of resources, borrow at rates that are affected by the same fundamental events, face the same kinds of markets, and so on. These are the influences of the invisible hand which organize the decisions into a system. At the same time, there are enough decision-making centers to ensure competition.

Dr. Evans: I would like to comment on Dr. Rosett's interpretation of the role of the invisible hand. It is worth keeping in mind, particularly in light of Dr. Ginzberg's observations about overcapitalization of human capital, that the shadow price of the self-employed entrepreneur's time at the margin is rarely equal to the average market price. Studies of private practitioners indicate that the supply of own time is not, in fact, supply at the shadow prices that connect with the market, and that this discrepancy wipes out the invisible hand as it applies to human capital.

Dr. Blendon: Why are you so pessimistic about a capital investment policy with built in cycles which could be activated to increase or to decrease the numbers of physicians and hospital beds as needed? Why don't you think that this kind of adjustment is possible?

Dr. Ginzberg: There can be some adjustment on the supply side, but there are very long lead and lag times in any major change. Suppose we cut off the supply of foreign medical graduates, as I anticipate. There will be an effect, but not without a very serious lag. I see new pressures coming in every day for still further expansion of the schools at a time when it should be evident that we have enough physicians.

As I look at the system, the major leverage for change is the physician. I do not think that we can force physicians to change, nor do I see them wanting to change. We have very little margin in affecting their behavior at this point.

Dr. Lampman: One of the possibilities before the health care industry a few years ago was that either the insurance or the employer-union combinations which buy in wholesale lots would undertake not only to reorganize the role of the physician, but also the actual character of the output of the industry. Such a reorganization, it seems to me, would require the overriding of the vested interests and a new way of appealing to the consumer.

Dr. Ginzberg: I am hopeful that a new consumer wisdom will finally take hold and that the properly educated consumer will not feel compelled to visit the doctor all of the time. I have always felt that Spock's book on bringing up babies was the equivalent of ten or fifteen thousand pediatricians. The education of the consumer could add some new constraints to this very big system.

Dr. White: I would like to suggest that three of Professor Ginzberg's suggestions imply the need for information and that one of the reasons why we are in this troublesome state is that, for three or four decades, we have been operating in an information vacuum. The three points are related, first of all, to the examination of discrepancies in the performances of microsystems with respect to their supply and demand and the inequalities of the services that are provided. The second is the need to balance the production arm with the supply arm, which is essentially a marketing problem in sizing the capacities to the needs. Third is the notion of establishing the efficacy and the hazards that are associated with various forms of intervention.

Chapter 5

Capital Requirements and Capital Financing in a Hospital-based Group Practice Prepayment Plan

James A. Vohs
Walter K. Palmer

The delivery of health care services requires a large investment in fixed assets (land, buildings, and equipment) and a smaller, but substantial, investment in working capital. In 1975, expenditures for construction of hospitals, nursing homes, and medical clinics—excluding private physicians' offices—that were financed by public and private funds, totaled $4.5 billion, of which $2.7 billion was financed by private capital.[1] Substantial additional amounts were spent to equip the newly constructed facilities as well as to replace worn-out and obsolete equipment.

In a self-financing program, i.e., one not dependent on public funds or private donations, the money to pay for these assets must be obtained from retained earnings,[a] borrowings (short- and long-term), and/or depreciation.

To provide a base for a discussion of capital requirements and capital financing of hospital-based group practice prepayment plans, this paper describes the general characteristics of such plans. (To illustrate the operation and organization of a specific plan, the Appendix to this paper describes the Kaiser-Permanente Medical Care Program.)

The focus of attention is on the long-term capital financing requirements of health care institutions and systems, including hospital-based group practice prepayment plans, that are required to meet our health care needs. There are those who believe that, because there is an excess of hospital beds in the United States, earnings are not required by hospitals and should not be included in payments

---

[a]The term "earnings," as used in this paper, is the balance of revenue after the deduction of related costs and expenses, including interest and depreciation. In a for-profit organization, expenses would include taxes on earnings, and "retained" earnings would be reduced by payment of dividends to stockholders. Not-for-profit organizations do not pay taxes on earnings and do not pay dividends.

for services, since payment for straight-line depreciation and interest expense adequately provides for capital needs. Planning legislation is intended to correct the excess of beds. Institutions and systems that are, and will be, needed have continuing capital requirements and a need for capital financing to support those requirements. Earnings must be generated to support capital financing. Thus, the factors that determine earnings requirements in hospital-based group practice prepayment plans, as well as in other health care institutions, are analyzed. The need for appropriate earnings in the periodic rates of group practice prepayment plans, as well as in the reimbursement formulas of government health programs such as Title XVIII (Medicare), is examined in detail.

Government purchasers of health care from the Kaiser-Permanente Medical Care Program and the bases of payment are identified with particular emphasis on the Kaiser-Permanente Program's community rate as the foundation for such payment arrangements, except for Medicare.

The capital financing policy of the Kaiser-Permanente Medical Care Program is included, along with summaries of its capital requirements and capital financing covering the past fifteen years.

Consistent with the principles of capital financing presented in this paper, suggested changes in the methods of reimbursement of group practice prepayment plans and other health care providers are included in the discussion.

1. Title XVIII (Medicare) of the Social Security Act should recognize and include appropriate earnings in computing the amount of payment due to group practice prepayment plans and to other providers for services furnished to Medicare beneficiaries.
2. Retrospective cost reimbursement systems of payment should be changed to payment of fixed prospective rates.
3. Title XVIII, Section 1876, and Title XIX, Section 1903, should include payment provisions that permit health maintenance organizations[b] to be paid for Medicare and Medicaid enrollees in accord with established, fixed, prospective prepayment principles, including appropriate earnings.

Implementation of these changes would: (a) maintain and promote incentives for the effective and efficient operation of health service institutions and health maintenance organizations; (b) encourage health maintenance organizations to increase the enrollment of Medicare beneficiaries, resulting in savings to the Medicare program; (c) give recognition to earnings as a necessary financial requirement to be borne proportionately by all payers for health care services; (d) eliminate the subsidy of Medicare beneficiaries by non-Medicare beneficiaries; and (e) increase capital financing from private sources, thereby minimizing dependence on public funds of private donations.

[b]As defined in Title XVIII, Section 1876, and in the HMO Act of 1973, health maintenance organizations include hospital-based group practice prepayment plans.

DESCRIPTION OF A HOSPITAL-BASED GROUP
PRACTICE PREPAYMENT PLAN

A hospital-based group practice prepayment plan is an organized health care delivery system that serves a defined population, its members, through contractual arrangements, whether groups or individual subscribers, and provides for the furnishing of specified health services for a prospective periodic rate, usually fixed for a year in advance. Hospitals and other institutional providers, such as skilled nursing facilities and home health agencies, are related to the plan by common ownership or common control. Medical services are provided by physicians and other personnel employed by the plan or by contractual arrangements with groups of physicians or combinations of both. Contracts with physicians provide for payment on a fixed prospective capitation basis without regard to the volume of services other than that resulting from changes in the number of members. Effective delivery of health care is maximized through group practice of physicians in a system that integrates inpatient and outpatient services. The Appendix to this paper illustrates the organization of a large hospital-based group practice prepayment plan, the Kaiser-Permanente Medical Care Program.

Fundamental Principles

A number of fundamental principles guide the operation of a hospital-based group practice prepayment plan, including the group practice of physicians, the organization and integration of facilities and services, preventive health services and early detection of disease, and the significant participative role of physicians in the planning and direction of the plan.

Another fundamental principle is voluntary enrollment. Each subscriber enrolls and retains his membership on a voluntary basis. Through dual or multiple choice arrangements, group subscribers have a choice between the group practice plan and one or more other types of plans—such as Blue Cross, Blue Shield, or commercial insurance. Periodically—usually at annual intervals—subscribers have the option of transferring from one of these participating plans to another.

Fundamental to the financial stability of the plan is the principle of community rating. Periodic rates for covered services are established on a community rated basis, i.e., the rate paid by all groups and individuals for the same basic set of benefits. Community rating relates to the basic characteristics of a group practice prepayment plan, i.e., the assumption of the obligation to organize and provide comprehensive health care services on essentially a prepaid basis. A plan that is hospital based and provides direct services has substantial fixed and semi-fixed expenses of facilities as well as of staff to support a capability to serve its membership. Maximum stability of membership and financing is essential for a plan predicated on substantial fixed costs. Experience rating indemnification organizations, by contrast, do not have such fixed and semi-fixed expenses.

The principle of community rating is recognized by a variety of government agencies that purchase health care from group practice prepayment plans. The United States Civil Service Commission contracts with a number of such plans on this basis. A number of states, counties, cities, school boards, and other public agencies also recognize community rating as an appropriate basis for contracting for health care services for their employees. Further, community rating is a required element for health maintenance organizations under the HMO Act of 1973.

Incentives

Incentives for efficient delivery of health services are present in a hospital-based group practice prepayment plan. The incentive to control costs rewards early intervention by preventive and other outpatient services rather than by concentrating on costly inpatient care. Relative to the fee-for-service sector, more is spent on physicians' services in the outpatient setting and less on hospitalization.[2] The plan and the members both benefit when members are healthy and satisfied. Thus, health screening, preventive care, and health education are emphasized.

Fixed prospective periodic rates paid by subscribers and fixed prospective per capita payments to providers reverse the fee-for-service incentive to provide more service to produce more income whether or not the services are medically necessary. Within the plan, providers share financial resources determined by the number of persons served. Resources are budgeted and fixed a year in advance and within these fixed amounts decisions must be made for allocating manpower and facilities for the best matching of the needs of the persons who must be served. There is no reward for providing unnecessary services or making unnecessary expenditures. Incentive is balanced with the requirement to provide necessary services of high quality in order to retain the satisfaction of the persons served (all of whom are voluntarily enrolled). The plan receives no extra revenue for hospitalizing its members or from performing surgery. Thus, there is an incentive to avoid unnecessary surgery. On the other hand, the plan would suffer in terms of greater costs, member dissatisfaction, increased liability for malpractice, and loss of members if it failed to do necessary surgery.

The incentive to control costs promotes efficient manpower utilization, e.g., primary physicians provide primary care and refer patients to specialists, based on their medical needs. The distribution of specialists is not haphazard, as it often is in the general community; it is planned to meet the specific needs of a defined population, the membership. For example, surgical manpower is matched to the needs of members for surgical services. Surgeons are kept busy full time, thus enhancing their proficiency. In this way, quality of care is achieved as well as economy.

The incentive to control costs encourages the centralization of specialized services in order to avoid wasteful duplication of costly and sometimes scarce manpower or facilities. For example, in one region of the Kaiser-Permanente

Medical Care Program, with twelve medical centers serving 1.3 million members, neurosurgery is performed at one location; in another region serving more than 1.2 million members, open-heart surgery, radiation therapy, and treatment for renal disease are centralized in the largest medical center.

Incentives for effective planning promote efficient facility design and utilization, and emphasis on integration of inpatient and ambulatory care. The incentive to maximize ambulatory care results in substantial savings in capital as well as in operating costs for hospital beds and supporting services. Planning for a predictable, defined population improves the ability to maximize hospital occupancy rates, thus further reducing capital and operating costs. For example, over the past five years, the Kaiser-Permanente Medical Care Program has operated its hospitals at an average occupancy rate of 80.9 percent, compared with 76.1 percent[3] for the United Stated generally. The average number of days of inpatient hospital care per person served and the occupancy rate determine the number of beds required to serve a defined population. If the age and sex composition of the Kaiser-Permanente program's membership were the same as the United States' population, the program could operate with approximately two beds per 1,000 members,[4] about half the ratio for the United States generally.

In order to encourage efficient and economical health care delivery systems and to help avoid discriminatory treatment of health maintenance organizations, the National Health Planning and Resources Development Act requires that state certificate of need programs contain criteria for consideration of ". . . special needs and circumstances of health maintenance organizations. Furthermore, the author of a certificate of need bill in California has accepted amendments that would require the state to grant approval for the construction of beds or the development of special services by a hospital that is affiliated with a group practice prepayment plan if the plan can show that it cannot obtain sufficient beds or special services in a single facility that it does not control under conditions that would allow it to meet the needs of its members on a reasonable basis.

There is a discussion, beginning on page 163, of the incentives for a group practice prepayment plan, in a competitive market situation, voluntarily to plan its facility requirements for an effective use of capital.

FACTORS THAT DETERMINE EARNINGS REQUIREMENTS

There is an excess of short-term hospital beds in many metropolitan areas of the United States. The National Health Planning and Resources Development Act and state planning and certificate of need legislation are intended to correct this excess. Those health care institutions and systems, including hospital-based group practice prepayment plans, that are required to provide the health care needs of the country have continuing capital requirements and a need for capital financing. This discussion of earnings requirements is directed toward the long-term financing of the capital requirements of those institutions and systems.

Critique of Nonpayment for Earnings Requirements

Those who support payment for services on the basis of cost without any recognition of a requirement for earnings hold an erroneous view of capital financing based on the following premises:

1. Capital costs are recovered adequately through depreciation.
2. If reimbursement formulas include straight-line depreciation and interest on borrowed funds, expenditures for capital assets and the cost of capital are recovered eventually.
3. Since depreciation and interest fully reimburse capital costs, no earnings are required.

If this capital financing mechanism were to work well, or at all, the following conditions would have to be present:

1. The health care institution would have to operate without any net worth accumulated from retained earnings.
2. While having no retained earnings and, therefore, a doubtful ability to repay borrowed funds, the health care institution would have to borrow 100 percent of its capital needs (added beds, new services, new facilities, etc.) including architects' fees, equipment, landscaping, and financing fees.
3. The institution would have to negotiate with the lender for repayment terms that precisely match the straight-line depreciation on all the components of the facility. Different longevities apply to equipment, varying from three to twenty years. The building may be depreciated over forty years. With no earnings, all of these depreciation dollars must match, in point-of-time, the principal payments on the debt. Land is usually not depreciated, so the facility would have to be built on leased ground, or third party payers would have to start paying, in some form, for the use of land.
4. The institution would need to be operated so that "unallowable" costs are not incurred, since there are no earnings to absorb such costs.
5. The institution would either never need working capital or it would have to find a lender that would permanently lend it 100 percent of its working capital requirements.
6. Lenders willing to lend 100 percent of the cost of every new piece of equipment, every piece of equipment replaced, and every modernization project would have to be available when needed, even though the institution were never to expand in size or never to provide new services.

The major fallacy in this unrealistic scenario is the lack of willing lenders.

Lenders are willing to lend if they have assurance that loans will be repaid. Lenders can be attracted at reasonable interest rates if it can be demonstrated that $1.00 of retained earnings can be generated from revenues for each $1.00 of borrowing. This ratio might change from $1.00 of earnings to $1.25 or even $1.50 of borrowed funds at the cost of higher interest rates. It is doubtful that borrowed funds would be available beyond those limits. Lenders do not lend 100 percent of the value of a capital asset whether it be a personal residence, a hospital building, or an X-ray machine. Lenders have a legitimate need for security. Earnings provide the down payment essential to make borrowing possible and the assurance that the amounts which are borrowed will be repaid.

Factors Influencing Earnings Requirement

A number of factors influence the level of earnings that must be recovered from revenues after payment of operating expenses.

1. Earnings must be generated to make a "down payment" on the cost of construction or the acquisition of facilities and equipment sufficient to satisfy a lender who is willing to lend the balance of the cost at reasonable interest rates. The level of down payment can vary from one capital asset to another, such as an X-ray machine or an entire hospital structure. Down payments will vary according to the credit-worthiness of the institution. Credit-worthiness or the ability to borrow is principally measured by the ability to repay amounts borrowed from funds generated from operations, and that, in turn, is evidenced by: (a) the level of net worth (including retained earnings) compared to planned debt and (b) gross capital generation[c] from operations that are related to required repayments of principal and interest. In spite of a satisfactory credit rating, the supply of money in the hands of lenders from time to time can influence the level of borrowing that is available at reasonable interest rates and, therefore, the required down payment.

2. Inflation, both economic and technological, must be anticipated and earnings must be increased to provide for it. If an X-ray machine will cost more when it is replaced fifteen years from now, earnings must be increased now to develop the higher down payment that will be required for its replacement. A 5 percent economic inflation rate will more than double the cost in fifteen years. This higher down payment must be accumulated over a period of years as inflation affects replacement values, since the revenue structure cannot reasonably include the entire amount of the higher down payment in the year when the replacement machine is acquired.

The reality is that inflation has exceeded 5 percent for health care facilities and equipment. In the United States, during the eight years from 1968 through 1975, per capita construction expenditures for medical facilities increased from $10.64 to $20.77, an annual rate of increase of 10 percent. This percentage com-

---

[c]The total of earnings, provision for depreciation, and interest expense.

pares with the average annual increase of 11 percent in per capita expenditures for all health services and supplies during the same period.[5]

Further, the X-ray machine will not be the same machine fifteen years from now. Many technical improvements will be made and the same old machine could not be purchased even if it were acceptable medically. Therefore, technological inflation must be anticipated in the same way as is economic inflation. Because of technological inflation, plus economic inflation, replacement may cost four times as much in fifteen years instead of only twice as much.

3. Growth in volume of services can significantly increase the required level of earnings. In a group practice prepayment plan, growth in services is measured by the number of persons who are served and by the utilization rate of the services (the number of services required for 1,000 persons served per year). In the Kaiser-Permanente Medical Care Program, growth in membership has been a significant factor, averaging 9 percent per year over the past fifteen years. During the same time, the use of hospital beds per capita has decreased an average of 1-1/2 percent per year, partially offsetting the growth in persons served. Both factors are considered in planning the level of earnings to accommodate growth.

In the example of the X-ray machine, growth may require an additional machine every five years, requiring a down payment for each new machine, in addition to planning for the down payment for the replacement of the first machine. In fifteen years, earnings must be planned and generated for four machines instead of one because of growth.

4. Planning for obsolescence is difficult but necessary. In the absence of inflation or requirements for growth, even before the first X-ray machine is purchased the manufacturer begins to design an improved model. In eight years, instead of the expected fifteen years, the old machine is obsolete and must be replaced. The debt on the old machine has not been repaid, depreciation will be stopped because the machine will no longer be used and a down payment is required for a replacement seven years earlier than planned. This drama is being reenacted in the health care industry on such a regular basis that sound planning must anticipate it by increasing earnings to make sure that funds are on hand to meet the requirements of technological obsolescence which is an inherent part of continuing progress in medical science and practice.

5. In a health care institution, there are a number of required capital improvements that must be paid fully or, to a large extent, from earnings. Because of the nature of the improvement, lenders may want a very high level of down payment or may not want to lend at all. Remodeling and modernization projects may have proven economic value but lenders may not feel that they provide adequate collateral for a loan. If they do have economic value, the cost may be recovered through savings in future operating expenses but they have to be paid for at the time when they are undertaken. External sources, such as health department, fire department, or building department regulations or codes, may impose projects of a similar nature on the institution. Lenders may also be reluctant to lend

much or anything on such projects. These necessary and ongoing requirements for capital financing add to the level of earnings that must be generated from earnings.

6. New facilities and the expansion of existing facilities typically involve starting-up costs, including interest on construction loans, that must be paid before revenue is generated from the new services. Typically, such costs are deferred over a period of years. While viewed as a capital asset, they are not physical assets that can be paid for with borrowed funds. When new or expanded facilities are planned, earnings must be increased to provide the internally generated capital financing for these costs when they are incurred.

7. Most enterprises, including health care institutions, require working capital, the amount of which is affected by inflation, growth, and a variety of other factors. If it is predicted that working capital will increase, earnings must be increased accordingly to provide it. In a group practice prepayment plan, the prepayment of monthly rates can meet working capital requirements without requiring an increase in earnings.

From the foregoing, it may appear that all of the factors affecting earnings result in increases. Technology, obsolescence, modernization, and working capital needs will call for continuing increases in earnings and it is likely that economic inflation will have the same effect. An institution could, however, experience a decline in volume of services which could result in reduced levels of earnings.

Long-Range Capital Planning

How are all of these complex factors evaluated to determine the appropriate and reasonable level of earnings in a reimbursement formula or in a prepaid monthly rate in a group practice prepayment plan? In the Kaiser-Permanente Medical Care Program, long-range capital planning is based on predictions of growth of membership, changes in utilization patterns, and the hospital beds, medical offices and other facilities that are required to meet the needs of the projected members. Plans are made for five-year periods and often for longer periods when major capital expenditures are contemplated.

There is an important point to be made about long-range capital planning. It should not be associated with the rigidity and resistance to change that is characteristic of state and federal planning activities. On the contrary, all of the uncertainties, such as those cited earlier, dictate constant reevaluation and adjustment. For that reason, the Kaiser-Permanente Medical Care Program's long-range plans are reviewed every six months and revised as required.

It is a myth that one can develop a standard earnings allowance or return on invested capital that would meet the needs of all hospitals (both for-profit and not-for-profit), group practice prepayment plans and other health care institutions and providers. Such an approach would result in an unwarranted windfall for some and in gross inadequacy for others. The level of earnings is a function of needs for capital, not a vague entitlement to a "fair" return. The need must be supported by sound planning which can be effective within an organized system such as a hospital-based group practice prepayment plan.

An added view and argument of the payers who would reimburse only depreciation and interest is that including earnings in reimbursement formulas results in a duplicate payment or a current payment for a long-term capital asset that will be providing care for many years in the future. From a social standpoint, it is appropriate that the persons who are served or those who pay for their care, make sure that a capability will be available when it is required to serve future needs. Such a capability cannot be assembled and organized without an accumulation of earnings from past operations to meet future capital financing requirements. Earnings can be viewed socially and from a business viewpoint as a sound long-term investment in order to create stable and financially strong health care institutions.

GOVERNMENT PURCHASERS OF HEALTH CARE FROM THE KAISER-PERMANENTE MEDICAL CARE PROGRAM

Payments Based on Community Rates

A variety of federal, state, and local government agencies purchase health care from the Kaiser-Permanente Medical Care Program for their employees or beneficiaries. These agencies include the United States Civil Service Commission, contracting pursuant to the Federal Employees Health Benefits Act, state and county employees health benefits programs, federal and state agencies administering Title XIX (Medicaid), and the Social Security Administration (Title XVIII, Medicare). Additional large groups of personnel who are employed by cities, school boards and other local public agencies also contract with the program. Approximately 40 percent of the three million persons served by the program are public employees and their families. In addition, approximately 5 percent are Medicare and Medicaid beneficiaries. Medicare beneficiaries use substantially more services than do persons not covered by Medicare. Thus, revenue derived from the Medicare and Medicaid programs is between 12 percent and 14 percent of total revenue.

All agencies that represent public employees and beneficiaries contract with the program on the basis of payment of the program's community rate, adjusted only for differences in benefits. This rate is the one paid by all groups and individuals for the same basic set of benefits. The only exception is the Social Security Administration's payments on behalf of Medicare beneficiaries who are program members.

As a result of the separate financing that is provided by the Medicare program, the program's community rate includes the cost of providing services to all of the program's members not covered by Medicare. The community rate also includes earnings which contribute to the program's capital financing that is required to provide the hospitals, medical offices and equipment that must be constructed or acquired to meet the needs of the program's members. The principle of community rating has proven to be a sound and socially useful way of financing the health care needs of a population. It is equitable that all members should share in the capital cost of maintaining, improving and expanding the facilities and equipment that must be in place, ready to provide the services that may be needed by them. Earnings are an integral part of the cost of providing health services.

Since the implementation of the Federal Employee Health Benefits Act in 1960, the Civil Service Commission has contracted with the program on the basis of community rates which stand the test of the competitive marketplace inasmuch as they are paid by, or on behalf of, all group subscribers on the basis of voluntary enrollment in the program. The program is currently serving 338,000 federal employees and their dependents. The state of California and the University of California are contracting on this basis for 148,000 state and university employees and their dependents. As noted earlier, approximately 1.2 million (40 percent) of the program's three million members are public employees and their dependents receiving services under community rated contracts.

These contractual arrangements have been mutually satisfactory. The purchaser is assured that it is paying neither more nor less than other group purchasers in the "community" for the same benefits and that the rate has met the competitive market test. The program preserves its important incentive to operate effectively and efficiently within financial limitations that are based on fixed, prospective, prepaid monthly rates.

Payment for Medicare Beneficiaries

The payment arrangement with the Social Security Administration for Medicare beneficiaries under Title XVIII is an exception to the program's established method of contracting for services.

Under Title XVIII of the Social Security Act (effective in 1966), institutional care for Medicare beneficiaries that is provided by hospitals and skilled nursing facilities is paid for on the basis of "reasonable cost." Initially, "reasonable cost" included accelerated depreciation and a 2 percent allowance for costs "not otherwise specified." In 1969, the depreciation allowance was limited to straight-line depreciation and the 2 percent allowance was discontinued.

A legislative history of the reasonable cost reimbursement provisions of Title XVIII[6] indicates that retrospective reimbursement of cost had its origins in federal and state health programs during the thirty years prior to enactment of Title XVIII. A number of Blue Cross plans had also developed "cost-based" reimbursement formulas under arrangements with hospitals. The American Hospital Association introduced into the legislative discussions its "Principles of Payment for Hospital Care," which were first published in 1953 and revised in 1962, 1963, and 1965. The AHA principles included important criteria for a "cost-based" method of reimbursement. However, in its recommended reimbursement formula, the criteria did not clearly identify earnings as a distinct component separate from reimbursable cost. After Title XVIII was enacted and it became clear that the term "reasonable cost" was being narrowly defined and would permit no recognition of earnings, the American Hospital Association developed a new Statement on the Financial Requirements of Health Care Institutions and Services.[7] The statement has five major aims, the first of which are:

1. To set forth the obligation on the part of purchasers of health care services to collectively meet the full financial requirements of the providers of those services.
2. To establish that operating income [earnings] is an integral part of capital financing for preservation, replacement, expansion and renovation as it is in the other segments of the economy.

This new AHA Statement clearly identifies the need for an earnings requirement, over and above reasonable cost. Throughout the legislative history of Title XVIII it was not definite whether references to reimbursement of cost would recognize earnings. Despite the uncertainty as to the legislative intent, conditions have changed over the past ten years. Government financing of hospitals and sources of donated capital have declined. Inflation, progress in medical science, technological advances, and the resulting obsolescence have substantially increased the need for capital financing. The demand for services that resulted from the enactment of Title XVIII and XIX has required an expansion of capital investments that is substantially beyond the levels that were anticipated at the time when the legislation was being formulated. These and other changed conditions call for reexamination of the reimbursement provisions of Title XVIII.

With the enactment of Title XVIII, financing of health care services was provided for persons sixty-five years of age and older. Section 1861(v) of Title XVIII, as amended, reads in part:

> Such regulations shall (i) take into account both direct and indirect costs of providers of services (excluding therefrom any such costs, including standby costs, which are determined in accordance with regulations to be unnecessary in the efficient delivery of services covered by the insurance programs established under this title) in order that, under the methods of determining costs, the necessary costs of efficiently delivering covered services to individuals covered by the insurance programs established by this title will not be borne by individuals not so covered, and the costs with respect to individuals not so covered will not be borne by such insurance programs . . .

Title XVIII provided to hospitals a reimbursement of reasonable cost with no allowance for earnings except for a return on investors' equity in for-profit hospitals. Since Title XVIII does not cover the earnings that are necessary to support the services that are received by Medicare beneficiaries, the persons participating in community-rated plans who are not covered by Medicare have subsidized those who are Medicare beneficiaries. The earnings that are included in the community rate for persons not covered by Medicare included the total earnings requirement for all of the plan's members. This is contrary to the policy expressed in Section 1861(v), but such a plan cannot serve its members, including those eligible for Medicare benefits, without generating its total requirements for capital.

Section 1861(v) includes a statement which recognized that prepayment organizations operate in a substantially different way from fee-for-service hospitals and physicians.

> In prescribing the regulations referred to in the preceding sentence, the Secretary shall consider, among other things, the principles generally applied by national organizations or *established prepayment organizations* (which have developed such principles) in computing the amount of payment, to be made by persons other than the recipients of services, to providers of services on account of services furnished to such recipients by such providers. Such regulations may provide for determination of the costs of services on a per diem, per unit, *per capita,* or other basis . . . (Italics added for emphasis.)

The secretary has not given recognition to the payment and capital financing principles that were established and which proved effective by such organizations. For example, the Kaiser-Permanente Medical Care Program's hospitals in each region are not recognized as a single group sharing responsibility to provide services to a defined population but, instead, are reimbursed separately on a retrospective cost basis, like community hospitals across the country. Physicians' services also are reimbursed on a retrospective cost based payment system, whereas physicians in the community are reimbursed on a reasonable charge (fee-for-service) basis. Medicare reimbursement for physicians' services that are provided by the Program includes an "equalization" factor which can be used for capital financing related to medical offices and other physicians' services. It is probable that this "equalization" factor will be eliminated by regulations that are now being drafted.

Congress has been urged to amend Title XVIII to provide that "established prepayment organizations" be reimbursed in accord with their established principles of payment. Appropriate earnings should be recognized and included in the community rate for Medicare beneficiaries in proportion to the facilities and volume of services used by them. The subsidy of capital costs by non-Medicare beneficiaries should end.

Basic incentives to operate effectively and efficiently are eroded and destroyed by retrospective cost reimbursement systems of payment. Payment of a fixed prospective rate would maintain and support these incentives and save substantial administrative costs for both the provider and the government.

In 1972, Title XVIII was amended to add Section 1876 which provides for special payment arrangements for health maintenance organizations under either a cost reimbursement contract or a risk-sharing contract. The cost reimbursement contract essentially continues the present cost reimbursement system except to exclude the "equalization" factor related to physicians' services. The risk-sharing contract arrangement does not provide for the recognition of earnings as a financial requirement, nor does it provide for prospective fixed rates. Its sharing of risk provisions involves maximum risk for the health maintenance organization and little or no risk on the part of the government.

In comparisons of the health maintenance organization's cost with a matched Medicare cost in the community, we find unworkable provisions that cannot be fixed in advance so that the health maintenance organization will know what risk it is taking and can budget its income.

Recent Social Security Administration studies[8] have shown that hospital-based direct service group practice prepayment plans provide services to Medicare beneficiaries at substantial savings, as compared to the cost in the community outside of such plans. It is in the interest of the government and the taxpayers who support the Medicare program to encourage health maintenance organizations to maximize the enrollment of Medicare beneficiaries, thereby extending to the Medicare program the savings that result from the operation of such organized health care systems.

Title XVIII, Section 1876, and Title XIX, Section 1903, should include payment provisions that permit health maintenance organizations to be paid for Medicare and Medicaid enrollees in accord with established fixed prospective prepayment principles including appropriate earnings.

Section 1533 of the National Health Planning and Resources Development Act of 1974 provides that, "A uniform system for calculating rates to be charged to health insurers and *other health institutions payers* by health service institutions" will be established. While this provision of Section 1533 only directs the secretary to establish a system without indicating the potential uses of the system, it is possible that that system could become a standard for rate review and rate regulation programs that have been established by a number of states and that will be established by other states in the future.

The system for calculating rates that will be established under Section 1533 should include an appropriate recognition of earnings requirements supported by each institution's long-range facility and capital planning. The system should also provide for fixed prospective rates in order to maximize incentives for the effective and efficient operation of the health services institutions. Such a system cannot meet all of the conditions set forth in Section 1533 unless Title XVIII is changed to provide for the payment of fixed prospective rates that would include earnings as well as the cost of providing services.

The establishment of fixed prospective rates for all health service institutions can create positive incentives for effective and efficient operations, with the result that savings should accrue to the payers. It will also eliminate subsidies that are borne by non-Medicare beneficiaries and that result from the present payment provisions of Title XVIII which do not recognize necessary earnings requirements related to services provided for Medicare beneficiaries.

CAPITAL FINANCING POLICY AND ITS APPLICATION IN THE KAISER-PERMANENTE MEDICAL CARE PROGRAM

The Competitive Market Economy

Capital is generated in the competitive market economy by firms that can generate a profit, i.e., the market value of their output is greater than the cost of the goods and services that they use to produce it. A firm that makes a profit can build its long-term capital by saving, or by selling stock in anticipation of future profits, or by borrowing, if lenders are satisfied that the firm will be profitable enough to repay principal and interest.

This system has a number of desirable characteristics, from a social point of view, if the services that it provides are needed:

1. A firm which, by reducing cost, can widen the difference between the value of its output and the cost of the goods and services that it uses in production, can grow faster. Thus, cost reduction is rewarded.
2. Inefficient, unprofitable firms cannot grow and are choked off.
3. A firm that makes an incorrect decision and buys unneeded capacity or the wrong kind of capacity (plant, equipment and personnel) suffers a reduction in profit.

Thus, in this system, firms are rewarded for making decisions that increase the value of their products, that reduce their cost, and for matching capacity with need.

The process of capital generation for a group practice prepayment plan that owns its own facilities works in a similar manner. If the value of its services, as judged by members who have a free choice to join the plan or one or more competitors, exceeds the cost of the goods and services that it uses in production, the plan can generate capital either by retained earnings or by borrowing (based on accumulated net worth and projected net income). If the services that it offers are not needed, are not attractive to members, or are not produced efficiently, growth is shut off. If the plan invests unwisely in unneeded capacity, it must bear the cost and suffer a reduction in net income.

Thus, a group practice prepayment plan in a competitive market situation is encouraged to make socially desirable decisions. The plan's incentives to minimize capital cost result in effective voluntary planning of facilities for the defined population that it serves. Since this system is effective, a key question regarding methods of reimbursement is whether they contain appropriate incentives for the growth of such systems.

Kaiser-Permanente Medical Care Program Capital Financing Policy

The capital financing policy of the Kaiser-Permanente Medical Care Program was established to enable the program to generate enough capital to meet its goal of high quality care and membership growth, while pricing its services at competitive rates. Application of the policy should result in a sound financial position that can continue in the future.

The long-term capital financing policy of the Kaiser-Permanente Medical Care Program is as follows:

1. Program revenues and financial requirements are budgeted to include Gross Capital Generation for Health Plan and Hospitals, over and above what is required for current operating expenses, equal to the sum of the following:
   a. Depreciation based on 33-1/3 years for buildings, with shorter normal lifetimes for equipment as appropriate.
   b. Interest on debt.
   c. An additional amount (earnings) sufficient to meet long-term capital requirements.
2. Capital expenditures and capital generation for the program as a whole are planned so that all debt (short- and long-term) does not exceed the following upper limits:
   a. 70 percent of the appraised value of improved real property.
   b. The combined Net Worth (donated capital plus retained earnings) of Kaiser Foundation Health Plan and Kaiser Foundation Hospitals.

   Limiting total debt to combined net worth (also expressed as a maximum one-to-one debt to net worth ratio) is appropriate for the program. The main reason for such limitation is that, after a point, the interest rate charged by lenders increases as the debt ratio increases reflecting an increased risk. Available evidence appears to support the judgment that the incremental interest that is paid on amounts that could be borrowed as a result of increasing the debt ratio would be excessive in relation to the additional capital that would be made available. At high incremental interest rates, extra borrowing no longer reduces gross capital generation requirements.
3. Debt Service Coverage (i.e., the ratio of Gross Capital Generation to interest and scheduled principal payments) for the program as a whole will not be allowed to fall and to remain, on a continuing basis, below a two-to-one ratio.

   Another test of the adequacy of a capital financing policy is the debt service coverage ratio. This is a key to credit rating by the rating agencies, and most lenders see it as a measure of ability to repay debt. There is evidence to support the judgment that if this ratio falls much below two on a continuing basis, earnings and, therefore, gross capital generation should be adjusted to avoid paying higher interest rates for future capital financing.

4. It is appropriate to make full use of the program's borrowing power up to the limits established by the policy.

There are several reasons for a policy of full use of the borrowing capacity. Borrowing performs the valuable function of spreading a substantial portion of the capital cost of an asset over its economic life. Further, borrowing permits either a higher growth rate for a given gross capital generation rate per capita or a lower gross capital generation rate and, hence, lower prepaid charges for a given growth rate. Thus, borrowing makes it possible to even out the burden of heavy capital requirements when the growth rate is high; it permits lower prepaid charges in the early phase of rapid growth, offset by prepaid charges that are higher in the later slow growth phase when the need for new capital generation is comparatively light.

There are two significant conclusions that can be drawn from the application of the program's capital financing policy: (a) the policy results in a fair capital charge to the members for the current use of the program's facilities; and (b) adherence to the policy maintains the program in a strong financial position and results in a reasonable cost for capital that must be borrowed.

Application of the Capital Financing Policy

Tables 5-1 through 5-4 illustrate the application of the program's capital financing policy over the past fifteen years, 1961 through 1975. For convenience, the figures are summarized in five-year periods.

Table 5-1 summarizes the program's capital expenditures for property, plant and equipment and the sources of capital funds that are required to make these expenditures.

Earnings and borrowings have been the primary sources (73 percent) of capital funds. Straight-line depreciation recovered through revenues has provided only 20 percent of the total over the fifteen-year period. The program has no regular sources of donated capital. In 1970, a $3 million grant was received to assist in starting up new regions in Ohio and Colorado. In the 1971-75 period, a $2.8 million Hill-Harris grant was received to assist in the financing of one of the program's hospitals.

For the first ten years of this period, membership grew rapidly at an annual rate of 11 percent. For the last five years, annual growth has averaged 6-1/2 percent. For the six-year period, 1961 through 1966, total program revenue on a per capita basis increased at an annual rate of 3-1/2 percent. Beginning in 1967, following enactment of the Medicare and Medicaid legislation, the program followed the health care industry in experiencing sharp increases in costs that were

Table 5-1.   Expenditures for Property, Plant, Equipment and Sources of Funds ($000 omitted)

	5-Year Periods			Total 15 Years
	1961–65	*1966–70*	*1971–75*	
Expenditures for Property, Plant and Equipment	$56,000	$147,000	$315,600	$518,600
Funds Generated from:				
Earnings	$25,600	$ 54,700	$121,600	$201,900
% of total	46%	37%	39%	39%
Depreciation charges included in revenues[1]	12,000	27,900	65,000	104,900
% of total	21%	19%	20%	20%
Borrowings net of repayments	20,700	53,500	103,700	177,900
% of total	37%	36%	33%	34%
Donated capital	800	3,700	2,800	7,300
% of total	1%	3%	1%	1%
Other sources (uses)	(3,100)	7,200	22,500	26,600
% of total	(5%)	5%	7%	6%
Total	$56,000	$147,000	$315,600	$518,600

[1] Accelerated depreciation has been recorded and included in the program's financial statements since 1968. Straight-line depreciation is shown in this and succeeding tables. Retained earnings and net worth are restated accordingly, since the policy limitations on debt are related to such restated net worth.

reflected in its revenues. For the nine-year period, 1967 through 1975, per capita revenue increased at an annual rate of 11 percent.

While these increases in per capita revenue reflect general economic inflation in the health care industry, such as sharp increases in compensation of all categories of personnel and staff, the program's revenues also reflect increases in the benefits provided and significant advances in medical practice and technology. Open-heart surgery, kidney transplants, and renal dialysis have become accepted medical services. Intensive care and coronary care units have replaced special duty nurses in hospitals. These and other developments have a significant impact on both operating costs and capital costs.

Despite these significant changes in growth patterns and increases in costs, Table 5-2 shows that gross capital generation (the capital components included in revenue) maintained a stable percentage relationship to total revenue.

In spite of substantial increases in facility costs, the application of the capital financing policy resulted in a consistent and reasonable cost of capital being included in the program's prepaid monthly rates.

Table 5-3 shows the relation of increases in debt to earnings over the fifteen-year period.

Earnings add to the program's net worth and the result is a financial position

Table 5-2. Total Program Revenue and Gross Capital Generation ($000 omitted)

	5-Year Periods			Total 15 Years
	1961–65	*1966–70*	*1971–75*	
Total Program Revenue	$468,300	$1,117,400	$2,767,000	$4,352,700
Gross Capital Generation:				
Earnings	$ 25,600	$ 54,700	$ 121,600	$ 201,900
% of total Program revenue	5.5%	4.9%	4.4%	4.6%
Depreciation	12,000	27,900	65,000	104,900
% of total Program revenue	2.6%	2.5%	2.3%	2.4%
Interest included in revenues received	6,200	18,300	60,800	85,300
% of total Program revenue	1.3%	1.6%	2.2%	2.0%
Total	$ 43,800	$ 100,900	$ 247,400	$ 392,100
% of Total Program Revenue	9.4%	9.0%	8.9%	9.0%

Table 5-3. Earnings and Increases in Debt ($000 omitted)

	5-Year Periods			Total 15 Years
	1961–65	*1966–70*	*1971–75*	
Earnings	$25,600	$54,700	$121,600	$201,900
Additional Long-Term Borrowings	$31,000	$70,100	$152,500	$253,600
Less: Principal Payments	10,300	16,600	48,800	75,700
Net Increase in Debt	$20,700	$53,500	$103,700	$177,900
% Increase in Debt to Earnings	81%	98%	85%	88%

that makes private capital available at reasonable rates of interest. The 88 percent relationship of the net increase in debt to earnings compares with the policy of limiting debt to net worth (retained earnings and donated capital).

The debt service coverage ratio is also an important part of the capital financing policy since it strongly influences the credit "rating" and, thus, the interest rates charged by lenders. The program's long-term notes are currently rated "AA" by Standard & Poor's. This rating is substantially influenced by the program's maintenance of a debt service coverage ratio that is consistently in excess of the 2.0 minimum ratio which is called for by the policy. Table 5-4 shows the debt service coverage ratio that has been maintained by the Program over the past fifteen years.

Table 5–4.   Debt Service Coverage Ratio ($000 omitted)

	5-Years Periods			
	1961–65	*1966–70*	*1971–75*	*15 Years*
Gross Capital Generation (earnings, depreciation and interest)[1]	$43,800	$100,900	$247,400	$392,100
Debt Service:				
Principal payments	$10,300	$ 16,600	$ 48,800	$ 75,700
Interest	6,200	18,300	60,800	85,300
Total	$16,500	$ 34,900	$109,600	$161,000
Debt Service Coverage Ratio (ratio of Gross Capital Generation to Debt Service)	2.7	2.9	2.3	2.4

[1] Detailed in Table 5–2.

The program's long-term indebtedness is represented by the Hospitals' long-term notes which are privately placed with major insurance companies, banks, and two large government employee pension funds. Other potential sources of capital are available but have not been utilized, since the program's requirements have been readily available from present lenders.

Additional sources would include public bonds and, under certain circumstances, tax-exempt bonds. For the same credit rating, interest rates should be slightly lower for public bonds than for privately placed notes, other terms being equal. However, substantial additional legal and financing costs are required for a public bond issue which could partially, if not entirely, offset the lower interest rate. Also, some flexibility is lost in the relationship with lenders. Flexibility can prove to be of value when placing new financing at fairly frequent intervals and when it is desirable to modify the conditions of borrowing.

The program's capital financing policy, supported by satisfactory operating results, provides a financial strength that should continue to make private capital available to meet external financing requirements.

The availability of private capital depends upon maintaining a strong financial position—in other words, a strong credit worthiness. Earnings, which increase net worth, must be included in rate structures and recognized in reimbursement formulas, so that a strong credit rating can be achieved, thereby attracting adequate private capital.

The above tables show that, over the past fifteen years, the program has invested $518.6 million in facilities to serve a defined population which now exceeds three million persons. These expenditures were made pursuant to a *voluntary* planning process that matched the health needs of these persons with the hospitals, medical offices and supporting facilities that were required to meet those needs. There are no incentives to make capital expenditures beyond the needs of the program.

Earnings requirements have been included in prepaid monthly rates on a basis that has resulted in a reasonable charge for the facilities that were used to meet the members' health care needs. Because of this planned internal generation of capital, borrowed funds were available from *private* sources at reasonable interest rates.

The program has shown that a hospital-based group practice prepayment plan can redirect incentives to deliver quality health care in a cost effective manner without the need for government intervention in the planning or financing of such a system. However, continuing success of such a system requires governmental purchasers of health care to pay for services for their beneficiaries on the same basis as other payers so that all payers will share in the capital financing that is required to support the services and will also share in the operating expenses.

APPENDIX 5A
DESCRIPTION OF THE KAISER-PERMANENTE
MEDICAL CARE PROGRAM

The Kaiser Foundation Health Plan is part of the health care delivery system that is commonly referred to as the Kaiser-Permanente Medical Care Program. It is a direct service, group practice, prepayment plan whose voluntary membership includes people from most levels of our society who live in portions of six states.

In addition to its prepayment aspects, the program is the largest private provider of health care services in the United States. Several separate but closely cooperating organizations, including six independent Permanente Medical Groups, are united in a common purpose in this program. Recognizing the close and vital relationship among the Permanente Medical Groups, Kaiser Foundation Hospitals, and Kaiser Foundation Health Plan, we describe this mutual effort as the Kaiser-Permanente Medical Care Program. For several decades, the program has assumed the responsibility for organizing and delivering comprehensive health care of high quality to a defined population on an essentially prepaid basis. Membership in the plan is voluntary.

First made available to the general public in 1945, the program organizes and provides services on a self-sustaining and nonprofit basis to more than three million persons in six geographic regions: Northern California (San Francisco Bay Area and Sacramento); Southern California (Greater Los Angeles Area and San Diego); Oregon (Greater Portland Area and Vancouver, Washington); Hawaii (Oahu and Maui); Ohio (Greater Cleveland Area); and Colorado (Greater Denver Area).

Hospital and medical services are provided through the program's twenty-five hospitals, with over 5,000 licensed beds, and sixty-five medical office facilities, and by approximately 3,000 physicians in the six independent Medical Groups (one in each geographic region) which contract with the Health Plan to provide professional services to the membership.

The primary role of the program is to provide accessible, comprehensive health care of high quality on an organized, self-sustaining, prepaid basis in an efficient, cost-effective manner.

Physicians are involved in all aspects of the program. Their interest is not limited to the services that they provide directly. The physicians are intimately concerned with the services that are prescribed, ordered, or directed by them even though many of the services are provided by nonphysician personnel and by components of the program other than the Medical Group. They participate extensively in decisions regarding the allocation of resources, planning, and direction of the total program.

The regional manager and medical director in each region share a joint responsibility for the management of the program in their region. The relationship is based on mutual respect and recognition of their mutually independent roles and responsibilities. Many major policy questions are not resolved easily. This is understandable since these decisions must be carefully considered and thoroughly discussed in such an arrangement. The relationship is effective because each individual is endeavoring to achieve total program objectives related to the satisfaction of the persons served, the providers of services, and the personnel employed by the program.

Four principal organizations are united in the common effort:

1. Kaiser Foundation Health Plan, Inc., a nonprofit corporation, which contracts with individuals and groups (the members) to arrange for comprehensive health care benefits. The Health Plan contracts with Kaiser Foundation Hospitals and the Permanente Medical Groups to provide the facilities and the services that are required to provide the covered health benefits to its members.

A primary function of Health Plan in its central role as contractor under Membership Contracts is Health Plan administration. This involves member-related activities including marketing, enrollment, membership records and billing, processing claims for in-area and out-of-area emergency benefits, and general membership communications and services.

2. Kaiser Foundation Hospitals, a nonprofit, charitable corporation, which contracts with Health Plan to provide all of the covered hospital services that are required to satisfy the needs of the membership. Kaiser Foundation hospitals are community hospitals which serve nonmembers as well as Health Plan members. Staff privileges are available on the usual basis to all qualified doctors in the community.

Health Plan and Hospitals are under common management through boards of directors made up of the same persons, and through key members of management such as the president, senior vice presidents, and other managers who are officers of both Health Plan and Hospitals. This management results in an atypical financial relationship that will be discussed later.

A central staff, located in the Kaiser Center, Oakland, California, provides corporate level legal, financial, legislative, medical economics, and employee relations services and is responsible for coordinating the overall planning of Health Plan's and Hospitals' activities.

3. The Permanente Medical Groups, which are independent groups of physicians in each region, have full responsibility for providing the professional and related medical care that is necessary to meet the health needs of Health Plan's members. Physician groups are organized as partnerships or professional corporations, and each is responsible for its own physician recruitment and selection, and staffing patterns. In the California regions, the Medical Groups employ allied health professional and administrative personnel.

4. Six separate Permanente Services corporations, one in each region, whose primary purpose is to operate prescription pharmacies at nonhospital locations in all regions, and, in some regions, optical dispensing operations.

One fundamental requires emphasis. Despite legal, ethical, and historical constraints that intensify separation, even fragmentation, of the health care industry, Kaiser-Permanente has developed a way to function in a unified fashion.

The program is unified in administration. The different organizations are brought together through formal contracts and informal managerial arrangements. For example, in each region administrative functions, such as facility and financial planning, employee relations, accounting and finance, information services, purchasing and warehousing are organized to serve all of the participating organizations.

The program is unified in financing. The revenues from the various sources—prepayment, point-of-service charges, pharmacy and optical sales—are brought together within each region and allocated through unified medical and managerial judgments.

The program is unified in delivery of services. All available resources are applied to meet health care needs without regard to such traditional fragmentation as the hospital-medical office dichotomy. The various component organizations are functioning parts of a single integrated program.

The financial relationships support and reinforce the concept of joint management on which the program is based. Clearly, the program is dependent upon appropriate financial relationships. While the term "risk-sharing" in the health care field usually refers to the sharing of financial risks by prepayment organizations, physicians, and hospitals, other individuals and organizations also assume risk, e.g., those who invest in an enterprise or those who lend money to an enterprise.

In the Kaiser-Permanente Program, capital financing comes from three important sources: (a) capital generated from operations (earnings); (b) cash flow from depreciation provisions; and (c) long-term loans that are secured by mortgages on properties owned by Hospitals and Health Plan. Other sources (less than 10 percent) include donated capital and the prepayment of monthly charges. Hospitals require the major amount of capital for the construction and/or acquisition of facilities, and are, therefore, the chief borrowers of capital. Health Plan's facilities consist of outpatient medical offices at nonhospital locations and other facilities, such as warehouses and office buildings.

The Medical Groups have no legal liability with respect to external financing. They own no property or equipment; these are provided to them by Health Plan and Hospitals. They are, however, at financial risk with respect to their portion of operations and for the overall results of the operation of the program in their respective regions. The basic form of reimbursement to them is a fixed monthly capitation payment, based upon historic levels of service and staffing patterns, but not subject to adjustment for varying levels of service during the current year. By increasing the efficiency of their operation, the Medical Groups may realize additional earnings under this *basic per capita payment.* Any such gains accrue solely to the Medical Groups and may be used to increase the compensation of physicians or for other Medical Group purposes.

The Medical Service Agreements provide for additional payments to the Medical Groups: the *contingent contractual* payment, so termed because its total is contingent upon the program's financial result in each region. This payment is based upon a planned level of earnings, planned in the sense that it is included in the program's annual operating budget and, therefore, in the prepaid rates that are established for the year. The contingent contractual payment is calculated to provide a specific amount of dollars to each partner-physician in a partnership or to each principal stockholder in a professional corporation. The planned level of additional earnings for the Medical Group may be increased or decreased. Favorable or unfavorable variances from the budgeted financial results for the year are shared by Medical Group and Health Plan.

Kaiser Foundation Hospitals does not have a risk-sharing arrangement in its contract with Health Plan, because the two organizations are under common management. The contract calls for reimbursement by Health Plan of Hospitals' net financial requirements (all operating expenses and requirements for capital less revenues received directly by Hospital for services provided to nonmembers). Hospitals' debt obligations are a strong incentive to achieve financial objectives.

Because the program operates in a competitive environment, it must be attractive in terms of cost and quality to its members and to the employers and others who pay the monthly subscription charges. Thus, the program constantly seeks to improve the quality, accessibility, and attractiveness of its services to members while controlling the costs of the services that it provides. The efforts of the participating organizations are directed toward achieving these objectives.

NOTES

1. Marjorie Smith Mueller and Robert M. Gibson, "National Health Expenditures, Fiscal Year 1975," *Social Security Bulletin,* 39, 2 (February 1976):3–20.
2. Mildred Corbin and Aaron Krute, "Some Aspects of Medicare Experience

with Group Practice Prepayment Plans," *Social Security Bulletin,* 38, 3 (March 1975):3-11; and Anne R. Somers, "What Price Comprehensive Care?" *Archives of Environmental Health,* 17 (July 1968):6-20.

3. *Hospitals,* Journal of American Hospital Association.

4. Anne R. Somers (ed.), *The Kaiser-Permanente Medical Care Program, A Symposium,* March 1971, Appendix A, Table 14, p. 208, and as revised November 1975. While other demographic differences may affect comparisons between the program's membership and the United States' population, age and sex differences are considered to have the most significant impact on use of acute hospital beds.

5. Marjorie Smith Mueller and Robert M. Gibson, "National Health Expenditures, Fiscal Year 1975," *Social Security Bulletin,* 39, 2 (February 1976):3-20.

6. Irwin Wolkstein, *The Legislative History of Hospital Cost Reimbursement,* U.S. Department of Health, Education and Welfare, Social Security Administration, Office of Research and Statistics, Research Report No. 26, (1968), pp. 1-15.

7. American Hospital Association, "Statement on the Financial Requirements of Health Care Institutions and Services," approved by House of Delegates, February 12, 1969.

8. Mildred Corbin and Aaron Krute, "Some Aspects of Medicare Experience with Group Practice Prepayment Plans," *Social Security Bulletin,* 38, 3 (March 1975):3-11.

Discussion of
Capital Requirements and Capital
Financing in a Hospital-based Group
Practice Prepayment Plan

James Brindle

In my experience with two prepaid group practice programs—in Detroit and New York—one of the most serious and persistent problems was obtaining capital financing for facilities and equipment. It was a constant scramble to develop capital resources, and there was little opportunity to indulge in the kind of orderly allocation of income for this purpose that the Kaiser-Permanente Medical Care Program pursues. So, my first reaction on reading the Vohs-Palmer paper was one of green-eyed envy!

The Kaiser Program is an integrated plan that makes it possible to provide the regular allocation of funds in a self-financing program for capital formation. With forward planning and in an expanding operation, the system is ideal. To those of us in a prepaid group setting who have been involved in scratching for such money from outside of the plan, and without the ability to adjust premium income on a regular basis, there is only admiration for the systematic and continuing capital financing arrangements of the Kaiser Program.

Capital Financing
Representing, as it does, the rationale and long experience of the largest and most successful hospital-based group practice prepayment plan in the United States, the Vohs-Palmer paper gives an excellent blueprint for capital financing and forward planning. It stands in sharp contrast to the fragmentary and largely unplanned processes common to most health insurance and health care delivery systems.

The Kaiser Plan
Especially useful is the Appendix 5A analysis of the internal forces and counterforces in the Kaiser-Permanente system which provide incentives for efficient,

effective, available and acceptable health delivery operations. This Appendix also describes clearly the reasons for the long-continued progress of the plan and its success in withstanding the competition of more conventional health care and health insurance schemes.

Other Programs

It is evident that there is great strength in a comprehensive, well-integrated plan and that, in such a framework, it is possible to have systematic capital financing, which is much more difficult in many other prepaid group practice programs. The Kaiser system does not seem to be in prospect for newer developing HMOs. While Kaiser's capital financing plan is probably crucial to the long-term survival of HMOs, in most instances it is not applicable to newly developing programs which cannot, or will not, be organized on an integrated hospital-based framework. And, most other HMOs are not, or are not likely to become, hospital based. Newly strengthened governmental controls on the further proliferation of hospital beds and equipment, as well as growing constraints on both governmental and private insurance reimbursement, militate against the development of new inpatient facilities for the principal use of group practice prepaid programs. Widely publicized declarations of community general bed surpluses and concern over escalating publicly financed health service costs assure the continuation of limits on hospital construction, enlargement, and reimbursement.

Most new HMOs are likely to provide in-hospital care in community institutions which devote only a portion (usually a small one) of their services to the enrolled population of a prepaid group practice. Few programs will be able to integrate hospital and ambulatory activities. It can be very difficult to secure properly the allocation of the demonstrated lower hospital utilizations for inpatient care to the effectiveness and cost of an HMO. Rather, the inflationary forces of cost-plus hospital reimbursement are likely to persist in new prepaid group practice systems. In the Kaiser framework, the substitution of less expensive outpatient care for more expensive inpatient care is crucial to the plan's effectiveness. In community hospitals that are related to new group practice HMOs, Kaiser's incentives, which benefit the medical groups financially for holding down unneeded inpatient hospital utilizations, are absent or are only partially effective. The community hospital's doctrine of "keep the beds filled" and the incentives to hospitalize patients who do not have adequate ambulatory insurance coverage operate to inflate institutional costs rather than to provide incentives for economy. Of course, if hospitalization insurance is integrated coverage for medical services, there is an advantage to cutting hospitalization, but the full benefits that accrue in the Kaiser system are not likely to be realized in non-hospital based plans. The total system needs to be tied together; fragmented, it is not sufficiently effective.

THE IMPORTANCE OF CAPITAL FINANCING

There is need for some perspective in evaluating the importance of the capital cost component of health care. As cited in the Vohs-Palmer paper, construction costs, nationally, in 1975, constituted only 3.8 percent of total national health expenditures. Kaiser Plan's capital generation for fifteen years amounted to about 9 percent of program revenues. But this relatively small percentage is often a controlling factor when it is involved in the development of a new HMO.

Being self-contained, with integrated hospital and medical systems, and largely self-controlled, and with capital costs representing a modest portion of a three-quarter billion dollar annual income at this point, capital expenditures in the Kaiser-Permanente system are well-balanced and under control. Kaiser's "track record" is excellent—a key factor for borrowing. Not so in many other programs. Here are a few examples:

The Community Health Association of Detriot (CHA)

This program is now a Blue Cross-Blue Shield program titled "Metro Plan."

Backed by the United Auto Workers in the mid–50s, after an attempt to get Detroit hospitals to incorporate the plan, a base hospital (Metropolitan) was purchased at a bargain price from the Tuberculosis Association, with mortgage money on very favorable terms from Nationwide Insurance. The loan was backed by UAW, but before the plan got well under way, the union had advanced or guaranteed about $6 million for planning, start-up and initial operating costs, and for the construction of three branch centers and alterations to the hospital. The risks involved would not have been undertaken by conventional commercial lenders. And, of course, there was no "track record" to furnish support for loans.

Health Insurance Plan of Greater New York

Now approaching its thirtieth anniversary, the plan initially had practically no funds for capital expenditures. This lack has left a legacy of serious problems. Originally funded for about $850,000 from local foundation loans and grants, the money went mostly to setting up a central HIP staff, organizing medical groups and promotion of the plan. There was no provision for capital financing of hospitals, medical centers, or equipment. In the post-World War II period, with a good number of New York physicians having had some experience with group practice in the military services and with serious problems of renewing or starting solo practice, HIP offered capitation payments for enrolled New York City employees to almost any group of doctors who would band together to provide medical care to HIP members. The medical groups (eventually there were more than thirty) were required to set up centers, finance their development, and equip them, but with no help from the plan. A heavy initial caseload of city employees made haste necessary; a slower, early development would have been advantageous. If Central HIP had been able initially to provide and equip centers, the plan could have encouraged and required a more logical geographical distribution of the medical groups, as well as of adequately equipped attractive facilities, and have been able to influence the size and composition of the medical groups. Most of the physicians were in the plan only part time, with separate fee-for-service patients, and often practiced from their solo practice offices. As it was, there were great diversities in size, illogical geographic distribution, many unsatisfactory facilities, and other weaknesses which have been very hard to correct.

There was no opportunity to develop a hospital integral to the plan. There was certainly no shortage of hospitals in the city, but it was not possible to get medical group physicians concentrated in any one institution. There was considerable discrimination against HIP doctors. The physicians in any one group often had staff privileges in a number of different institutions, so that, in effect, group practice ceased at the hospital door.

Initial capital funding by the plan would have encouraged full-time practice. When, in the 50s, HIP built a medical center and set up a new group on Long Island, physicians were required to be full time in the center and most of them practiced in one hospital. Attempts to buy this institution and tie it more closely to the group's operations were unsuccessful, largely due to inadequate capital fund availability. Finally, HIP did secure a hospital in the Borough of Queens and effected the consolidation of three medical groups related to the institution. Physicians in these groups are coming into the program on a full-time basis and the operation is being substantially improved.

The initial weak design of the program in the area of capital financing has been responsible for a whole string of related problems which might well have been avoided by a better initial design.

There have also been continuing external forces affecting the development of a sound capital formation program. The State Insurance Department and the principal contractor (New York City, whose employees constitute about one-half the caseload) would not agree to premiums incorporating a reasonable allocation for capital development.

Hospital Insurance

A most serious added problem is the fact that hospital insurance is not included in the HIP premium. Thus, the advantage to the plan and to the medical groups of lower-than-community-hospital utilization escapes plan control. In effect, lower hospital use constitutes a subsidy to the hospitalization carrier—mostly Blue Cross.

The Scramble for Funds

The absence of readily available capital funds forces serious compromises in developing group practice programs. It affects the adequacy of facilities, site selection, adequacy of equipment, and other characteristics. In both HIP and CHA this weakness has led to attempts to combine the plans with other organizations. In New York, we had extensive discussions with Blue Cross with a view to either integrating or merging the two agencies, using Blue Cross money for extensive capital improvements. We also discussed the possibility of combining with a large insurance company, with the prospect of a very large long-term loan for a radical reform of HIP into a framework like the Kaiser Plan. The possibility of having Kaiser take over HIP and CHA was also discussed. None of these combination possibilities could be worked out.

Kaiser Principles

The description of "The Competitive Market Economy" on page 163 is a greatly oversimplified outline of the way our country's economy works. There are many other forces at work. The forces and counterforces in the Kaiser system provide incentives and disincentives which are much more clear-cut and uncomplicated and have a validity that hardly applies to the market economy generally. Here is a summary of these forces:

1. The need to maintain enrollment by the provision of attractive facilities and good service to patients is of primary concern to the plan, the hospitals and the Permanente groups. This objective gets prime attention from all of these agencies.

2. Economy in operations that is encouraged for all components of the program. Physician group income is maximized by holding down hospitalization, by not overelaborating facilities and equipment and by the provision of attractive services.

3. Centralized large scale planning and hospital administration improves economy—an objective very infrequently realized for community hospitals.

4. A mature and continuing relationship among the agencies and components of the system. In the face of interests that are sometimes in conflict, decisions get made through a series of meetings and encounters that set the whole direction of the program. This is not a trouble-free device, but it seems to work out in the Kaiser system.

Described in the Appendix 5A, these principles of operation are most important and long experience was needed to develop them. It was not easy, but a pattern has been set for future change and continuing development. In Kaiser, it works.

Controlled and Planned Capital Financing

The paper gives a detailed description of the expanding and increasing costs of capital construction and equipment, and how these needs are projected. In too many hospital and equipment cost projections, changing cost levels and the proliferation of new apparatus and new techniques are ignored—or worse, overestimated. Kaiser's techniques in this regard are rational and flexible. They take account of steady growth, but they can be adjusted to possibly static operations, which is the condition that many group practice plans have already reached and which all will arrive at eventually.

In particular, the technique of borrowing from private sources as a means of shifting later higher demands to future populations and increasing costs is one that is well brought out. In too many other situations, borrowings are a reflection of current need and opportunity rather than of careful forward planning. At any point, Kaiser's decisions to borrow or not to borrow and to be selective about its sources are under much more rational control than are similar decisions in plans which need to scramble continually for capital financing from a great variety of sources and where departure from optimal planning and control is common.

SOME SUGGESTIONS

The Vohs-Palmer paper indicates the sources for capital financing funds that Kaiser utilizes. Notably, they have avoided the utilization of governmental subsidies to any significant extent, although they do serve government programs. They are practically 100 percent self-supporting at competitive rates and with a high level of benefits, even though their conventional competitors often have direct or indirect government support and lower benefits than does Kaiser.

Many other group practice prepayment plans have been aided by federal, state and local government help in various forms, and, probably, more such help is needed. Here are several suggestions for helping group practice prepayment with capital financing:

1. Liberalization of HMO support provisions from government at national, state, and local levels and, particularly, in the form of capital investments, guarantees and grants. Added help should be a very good long-range investment.

2. Further encouragement of the development of HMOs by insurance companies and Blue Cross-Blue Shield, where some good starts have been made. Typically, such agencies have the ability to furnish capital support.

3. Development of a comprehensive catalog for capital financing in HMOs. Perhaps elements of such a catalog can be developed at least partially from the discussions at this Conference.

4. Adjustment of Medicare and other governmental payments for service so that, as Kaiser recommends, payments to group practice plans follow their regular payment practices—a single capitation amount for all services—and so that there is no longer a subsidy by insured patients for Medicare services.

5. Encouragement of existing plans—and, especially, Kaiser—to expand their programs and to move into new areas. On the basis of performance, such extensions would be worthy of outside subsidy.

6. Classification of nonprofit prepayment group agencies under 501.c.3. rather than 501.c.4. for tax purposes. Some are now so classified. Lately, founda-

tions, organizations and individuals have been reluctant to support such programs because of this tax problem.

THE FUTURE

Assuming that we will not move to extensive government operation of the health care delivery system and that any national health insurance program will accommodate to present diversified health delivery, then there are good grounds for substantial expansion of group practice prepayment. Such programs have demonstrated their value and acceptability potential for improving health care and for limiting costs. They can serve as real and healthy competition with traditional systems—competition that can be most useful. Therefore, more support and encouragement for this form of program is merited. I believe that such help can be provided without undue control—certainly with much less effort than is involved in the growing control programs that are attempting to regulate health care and health insurance generally.

Finally, I repeat the hope that the Kaiser Plan and other similar programs will make substantial further moves into new territory and expansion.

Discussion of
Capital Requirements and Capital
Financing in a Hospital-based Group
Practice Prepayment Plan

D. Eugene Sibery
Presented by
Howard J. Berman

In responding to somebody else's presentation, there are two principal ways that one can proceed. The first is to go through the other presentation, more or less line by line, either praising or criticizing it. That would be, in effect, a book review of the original paper. The second is to take the same subject—by using the original paper as a foundation and a launching point—to build new ideas and explore new concepts. My choice is to take elements of both of those alternatives. I will comment on certain portions of the Kaiser-Permanente paper, and will also share with you some of our thoughts—the thoughts of the Blue Cross Association—on the overall subject of health care financing.

I am glad to be able to begin by saying that I think that, overall, James Vohs and Walter Palmer have developed an excellent paper on capital financing in a self-contained, hospital-based group practice prepayment plan. The fact that I shall take issue with some of their points does not in any way detract from that level of excellence. As a matter of fact, the Kaiser program—and I shall abbreviate its title as a matter of convenience to myself and to you—brings to its presentation more ingredients to support its point of view than almost any other organization could bring.

Whenever the subject of discussion is prepaid group practice, Kaiser must be prominently included. It is both the prototype and a unique operating example of the prepaid group practice model. Its record is well established and its results are there for anyone to see. With its emphasis on primary care, early detection, patient education, and preventive medicine, it provides a type of care that, while still requiring significant amounts of capital, is capital balanced—as opposed to capital intensive. As a result of this and other features it obtains efficiencies that other health delivery models are still striving to learn. I am optimistic that these other models will achieve similar operating results.

Other group practices, of course, have achieved those same efficiencies—including many affiliated with Blue Cross plans across the country. As an aside—call it pausing for a commercial, if you will—I would like to inform this group that thirty-one Blue Cross plans are now involved with 107 operational HMO programs, of which fifty-seven are delivery points of five HMO network programs. Enrollment in our affiliated HMOs now stands at 1,400,000, which represents a 23 percent increase in enrollment in the last year. Forty-nine of our plans are involved in all phases of alternative delivery system activity, including planning, development, and operational programs. Perhaps more important—and more pertinent for today's discussion—than these statistics is the fact that these Blue Cross plans (in the period 1970 to 1975) invested $35 million of risk capital in group practice development and expect, over the second half of the decade, to invest another $35 million.

First, we believe, it is important to understand that Kaiser is not representative of the general health care delivery/financing model. The fact that I use the term "delivery - slash - financing" is indicative of the special character of the Kaiser model. Obviously, as I have said, there is much which can be learned from the Kaiser experience. However, we cannot pick up the Kaiser "system and experience" whole, and apply it to the more general problems of health care capital formation.

Kaiser is a more integrated health system than is typically the case. Moreover, it is a system which, in its totality, is closer to the market and the functioning of the market mechanism than is the typical institutional health provider. Now, these features may have much to commend them—and from a personal perspective I think that they do have much that is beneficial. However, unless we have a mystical catalyst which will convert the current delivery and financing system structures—the Kaiser model is an inappropriate operational standard.

Second, we believe that the issue has to be placed within the proper context. On the one hand, we are dealing with a larger general issue than just group practice capital financing. The issue of concern is really the matter of total health care institutional capital formation. The roots of this issue—as I will discuss in a moment—go all the way back to the basic core of the health care financing system. On the other hand, the problem is not a new issue. While it has recently assumed greater visibility, the matter of capital formation has always been a principal concern of the health care system. In fact, it was, in part, capital formation considerations which led to the initial establishment of the health delivery and financing systems as nonprofit enterprises. Of late, though, the traditional capital formation processes have begun to show themselves to be inadequate. Philanthropy—in absolute terms—has continued to grow. However, when laid against the capital demands of inflation and technological development, philanthropy has not been able to keep pace with capital demands. Similarly, in many institutions, retained earnings have also been unable to cover necessary capital investment.

Other factors, such as unprecedented rates of inflation in the health sector and an acceleration in the obsolescence of capital intensive technology, have combined with this set of circumstances and been labeled a "capital crisis." I would also argue—and again I believe that it is important for all of us to recognize—that we do have a capital formation problem and that the old solutions are no longer going to suffice. What is needed is a rethinking—in terms of the unique economics of a nonprofit, private sector industry—of our capital formation policies, and the development of some innovative solutions. If the accountants and commercial industry can talk about price level accounting—as a reasonable alternative to the objectivity of acquisition cost—then we should be able to begin to show similar flexibility and imagination.

In this vein, let me dispose of two notions which often clutter the capital formation discussion—so that we can move on to explore some pragmatic alternatives. The matters of depreciation, and the possibilities of accelerated payments and/or payments based on replacement cost, are often injected into the capital formation issue. Depreciation acts to provide a "real" economic brake on the "continued existence" notion which underlies all corporate operations. Admittedly, it is important that the proper corporations not only be allowed to continue, but, also, be encouraged to do so. However, recognition of this point also forces recognition of its corollary and the fact that all institutions do not need a return on capital or some other form of additional funds for either growth and/or continued operational purposes. If we—or any other major payer—were to apply a blanket capital growth factor in the payment formula, then what we would in effect be doing is sanctifying all of our present problems and errors. Certainly, depreciation is a legitimate cost and must be paid to all those who have expended capital. A capital growth factor, whether paid prospectively or retrospectively—is also, for the appropriate institutions, a legitimate cost. The real issues, then, are how do you identify the appropriate institutions—and what type of mechanism do you use to provide the necessary capital financing?

With respect to the first point, the solution is rather clear—we must rely on the health planning process. Our reliance, however, must be more than passive. We must actively involve ourselves in health planning and make the process work. There are no acceptable alternatives other than all of us being actively and knowledgeably involved in the local health planning process.

The solution to the second point is a bit more complex, for it is unrealistic to discuss mechanisms for providing capital financing outside of the context of the basic health care financing system. Certainly, a return on capital factor—whether in the form of an earnings rate or prepaid depreciation—could be laid on top of the existing payment system. Such an approach—when combined with health planning—might even solve, at least for the near term, the present capital formation problems. Such an approach, however, unconscionably side steps the fundamental financing issues which we face now—and which will not go away by our simply ignoring them.

The Kaiser report appears to make no distinction among various classes of health care financers or purchasers regarding who should pay what amount of the capital financing element—whatever it might be. We feel strongly that any method of rate calculation for a hospital or other facility should neither demand nor assume a single rate of payment for all purchasers. Rather, we believe that the method should require only that contracting agencies pay their appropriate share, that is, that each class of purchaser pays its own unique economic cost.

Economic cost per class of purchaser can be defined as the total present and future tangible and intangible costs which an institution incurs in providing care to that particular class of purchaser. For example, Blue Cross Plan subscribers generate significantly smaller amounts of certain costs than do other classes of purchasers. Some of the reasons are the plan's contract with providers which reduces business risks—the plan's prompt payment—and, in some cases, the plan's provision of working capital advances. To be fair to both payers and providers, rates must be calculated to reflect not only the elements of cost, but, also, the impact of each class of purchasers on each element of that cost.

In practical terms, that means:

1. Cost elements, such as working capital financing, credit and collection expenses, and nursing care expenses, which vary because of the business practices or other characteristics of a class of purchaser, should be reflected in payment rates on the basis of actual cost, not on the basis of uniform distribution.
2. Approved (by the planning process) capital expenditures should be reflected among payers on a proportionate basis. For existing approved capital, historical cost should represent the basis of payment. Whether straight line or an accelerated payment formula is used, it should be a negotiated decision reflecting the institution's financial position and its plan for usage of the funds.
3. Funding for approved future capital should be provided through a variety of alternatives, with the specific mechanism that is used being tailored to the financial needs of the institution. Thus, in one setting, loan guarantees may be appropriate, while in another, prepaid depreciation or capital advances may be best.
4. Financing free services for patients unable to pay should be reflected in payment rates on a negotiated basis. The economic cost concept demands that government and other programs that have traditionally paid less than their full economic share should close the gap as rapidly as possible.
5. In calculating a Blue Cross Plan's obligation, its open enrollment, extensive conversion and transfer privileges and its service benefits must be taken into account. Those factors set Blue Cross plans apart from other carriers and also cut down the amount of both free services and reductions of hospital income by making coverage available to persons who otherwise might not be able to

afford it. That economic fact should be recognized in determining a plan's economic cost.

6. The cost of community services, such as research and education, should be borne primarily by the community, with payment by purchasers only on a negotiated basis.

7. Reductions of hospital or organizational income because of such things as bad debts should be reflected in payment rates on the basis of actual experience and performance—and not on a proportionate basis.

Research by the American Hospital Association has demonstrated that economic cost can differ significantly by class of purchasers. Similar research by Blue Cross of Massachusetts has not only demonstrated the same result, but has shown that the potential size of cost differential between classes can be as much as 12 percent. Overall, rates of payment should be established on the basis of each class of purchasers' economic costs and should vary—if economically justified and only to the extent of that justification—to reflect differences in cost. We believe that it is essential for all parties in the delivery system to recognize that principle, because it is only by determining rates for all purchasers on the basis of economic reality that an adequately and fairly financed health care system can be achieved.

The fact of continuously rising health care costs and the potential of national health insurance have combined with several other factors to create a climate which demands improvement in the present system of financing health care. The Blue Cross organization not only recognizes the need for reform, but, also, the equally critical need to develop working models to help guide future decisions. If real reform is to be achieved, it has to be grounded in solutions whose practicality and workability have been proved.

In the view of many persons, the issue centers on the relative merits of government regulation of carrier rates and contracts, combined with rigorous negotiation between carriers and providers, versus all-out government regulation of both carrier rates and contracts and provider rates. I am sure that few of us want to see that, including most people in government who recognize the complexities and difficulties of health care financing and delivery.

For the last part of my remarks, I would like to lift three statements from the Kaiser report and comment on them at some length. I realize that it is often unfair to take isolated statements out of context, but I believe that the statements that I want to quote, plus their surrounding material, make a clear enough point so that it is not unfair of me to use them. I do not mean to be terribly critical of them, I am simply using them as the basis for some points that I want to make.

Early in the report, Kaiser points out that "Incentives for effective planning promote efficient facility design and utilization, and emphasis on integration of inpatient and ambulatory care." One assumes from that statement that Kaiser embraces the concept of community, regional and, perhaps, statewide health care planning. However, at another point, the report says that "Long-range planning should not be associated with the rigidity and resistance to change characterized by state and federal planning activities. To the contrary," the report continues, "all of the uncertainties . . . dictate constant re-evaluation and adjustment. For that reason, the Kaiser–Permanente Medical Care Program's long-range plans are reviewed every six months and revised as required." These remarks are followed, near the end of the report, with the statement that, "A firm that can widen the difference between the value of its output and the cost of the goods and services it uses in production by reducing cost can grow faster. Thus, cost reduction is rewarded."

Those last two statements are the key to the point I want to make. They say that a given organization's planning should not be restricted by state or federal planning rules, and that the firm or organization that can reduce cost can grow faster. That is, naturally enough, a narrow view of the aspirations of the Kaiser program. I would expect a Kaiser report to concentrate on the needs and potential future of the Kaiser plan. A report on a Blue Cross Plan would be equally restricted, just as a report on physician participation would pretty well limit itself to the needs and desires of physicians.

That, as I see it, is much of the problem that we have today. All of us in the health field tend to take a parochial view of our own situation. But, to solve the problems that face us, all of us are going to have to look at the overall view from the standpoint of the community or the region. Our goal must not be the success or growth of an institution or organization. Our goal must be access to appropriate health care services for the people of the whole community. And that means that decisions about what is needed, what will grow, what should be created, what should be eliminated, what should be altered, must be made by, and for, the community as a whole. It will do little good for each institution and organization to plan for its own good and its own future unless that planning is a part of overall planning for the community as a whole. Knowledgeable people representing every element of the community, inside of the health care field and outside of it, must determine how much money the community has to spend on health care, and what kinds of services are needed by the population of that community. Then they must set about making those services available.

Within that overall community budget, and within that overall plan for community services, each individual institution and organization will do its own planning and determine the part that it will play. For some, that role may be smaller than it now sees for itself because of differing needs of the people of that community. For others, the role may grow—again because of community need. For still others, the role may change and their future might lie in an entirely new direction. The key to the future is not what each institution and organization needs—whether in terms of capital financing, personnel or anything else—but what the community as a whole needs, balanced against what the community can pay for.

We have long supported such an approach to health care services and financing, and we are now undertaking a program to see, to a large extent, just how well it can work. Beginning December 1, 1976, the Blue Cross Association in Rochester, New York, will begin a development program among its twenty-three hospitals. Others directly involved are the Hospital Association of New York State, the Rochester Regional Hospital Association, the Finger Lakes Health Systems Agency, and the Blue Cross Plans of Rochester and Syracuse. The Social Security Administration is putting up $6 million, the other participants will provide more than $100,000, and the Blue Cross Association will donate $80,000 in time and services of its research and development division to supervise the program.

Through committees representing the hospitals, the rest of the health care industry of Rochester, the business community and the public, the goal is to spend two years setting up a program that will determine what types of hospital care the people of Rochester need and use, how many community dollars should be budgeted to cover those needs, and what inpatient and outpatient services the area hospitals can offer while keeping their operating cost within the predetermined budget and without reducing quality of care. Following the two-year developmental phase, there is to be a three-year demonstration to see how well the program works and where adjustments have to be made. After that, the hope is to go statewide and cover all of New York's 324 hospitals and 85,000 beds.

I sincerely believe that such programs as that—and there are others in other locations—will ultimately draw the design for health care services in the future, for the financing of the organizations and institutions that are part of it, and for the role that each element of the health care field will play in the overall community program.

Those are my comments on the Kaiser report, both those based specifically on it, and those which departed from it. If there are any questions, I would be glad to try to answer them.

Discussion

Mr. Brindle: My hopes are that we can develop more HMOs like prepaid group plans. I think that they have a greater potential for development and have greater validity than do the individual practice types of HMOs which have a very hard time with enrollment and high cost, much higher, typically, than does the prepaid group practice. But, on the other hand, the individual practice HMO can get acceptance by organized medicine and, perhaps, get some development there.

Dr. MacLeod: In 1971, the AMA published a survey in the *American Medical News* on the attitudes of physicians toward working in prepaid plans, whether independent practice associations or group practices. They found among the AMA membership some 30 percent who prefer prepaid plans over the fee-for-service practice. Close to 50 percent of the non-AMA members—about one-half of the physicians in the country—prefer prepaid practice plans.

It took about forty years for thirty HMOs to get going in our country, sometimes under the most adverse conditions. We have heard about some of the scars at this meeting. In the last six years, some 140 additional HMOs have been started. The great innovation in health care delivery that occurred as a result of Kaiser-Permanente, the Ross-Loos Medical Group, the group health cooperative of Puget Sound, and other early prepaid plans should continue along with the multiple and diverse activities that are just now getting going, if given half a chance.

Mr. Berman: Palmer and Vohs point out that there is an excess of hospital beds in many metropolitan areas. However, they rather quickly sidestep that problem by saying that planning legislation will correct these excesses. The track record of planning, at least to date, does not support that kind of conclusion. It is important to recognize that the issue is multifaceted, and that the real problem is to develop a mechanism which gets the right amount of capital to the right place.

Talking about the addition of an earnings factor is a quick and easy answer. The paper itself notes that you cannot just have a simple standard of earnings but that the level of earnings should be a function of need, not a vague entitlement to a fair return. This statement again brings out the fact that the key point is not really earnings, but how you provide capital. Let me point out once more that we cannot look at the issue in a relative vacuum. The problem has to be solved, but it has to be solved within the context of solving the larger problem of health care financing.

Mr. Vohs: We do not propose any kind of blanket formula for our recommendations for earnings or a recognition of the cost of capital. We are not proposing any kind of rate of return on investment. I think that what we say is that where there is a need for capital, and where that need can be demonstrated and justified, then it ought to be recognized. We certainly do not feel that there ought to be some kind of overall formula that would apply to every institution or every kind of health system.

Mr. Havighurst: I think that the debate about the scope of planning legislation was so mild that the importance of the issue may have escaped some people. I would not like to see what I would call a total protectionist kind of regulation of the sort that the ICC and the CAB have established. It would lead to results like this: a shipper finds that a certain trucker can provide the cheapest, fastest, and best service. They both go to the ICC and ask for a Certificate of Public Need and Necessities so that they can strike up an arrangement that will satisfy both of them. The ICC might say that there is another trucker who is also providing service to this shipper and, though his service might not be as good, it would be too bad to deprive an existing trucker of the business and the revenue. In view of the interests of the total national transportation system, therefore, the application is denied. The same thing could happen in the health sector. It has happened already; the surgi-centers have run into it and the HMOs will run into it in time. The argument is that anything that could possibly adversely affect the existing institution should not be allowed to happen because its capital might be jeopardized, its ability to cross-subsidize services and existing programs might be jeopardized, and so forth.

Mr. Berman: Let's take the surgi-centers for an example because the Blue Cross position there is rather interesting. Blue Cross has said that if you add to the system without changing the rest of the community's capital configuration and capital structure, all you have done is to increase total community health costs. We do not want to see this kind of suboptimization. We also do not want to see the distortions that the Havighurst argument implicitly requires as you go to a new optimization through all these suboptimizations. We cannot afford to see total community costs go up and this is how we are electing to contend with it, by trying to drive those decisions back into the community.

Mr. Brindle: You cannot use reimbursement alone to effect radical, aggressive, or even significant change in the operation of a typical community health program, but you can use it in combination with other items. I was involved in the planning agency in Detroit some fifteen years ago. Blue Cross worked with the planning agency and, through holding back reimbursement payments, they were able to drive some unneeded facilities out of business. A hospital-oriented planning organization, coupled with the Blue Cross muscle, was able to accomplish something. In addition, they had strong backing from industry and from labor, which are not inconsequential forces in Detroit.

Mr. Vohs: It is our view that alternative systems are necessary. Cost-effective organized systems ought to be encouraged; we must be careful not to discriminate against innovation. In seeking solutions to the overbedding and the over-capitalization in some areas, we should not overlook the need for capital in other areas. Finally, we think that all government purchasers, such as the Civil Service Commission, ought to recognize the need for adequate capital reimbursement based on demonstrated need.

✳ *Chapter 6*

Inducements and Impediments for Private Corporate Investment in the Delivery of Health Services

John A. Hill

THE MARKET FOR HEALTH CARE

A Changing Market

In a recent report on the health care industry by a New York consulting firm, the following statistics were presented:

Medical care per person has gone up 122% since 1950, with nearly 20% of the growth in the past four years. A 40% growth in population combined with the increase in care per person has ballooned the output of medical care since 1950 over 200% or three times the 1950 rate; and a 179% increase in medical costs combined with the increased output makes the dollar growth of medical care nearly 800% in less than 25 years.[1]

Tables 6–1 and 6–2 illustrate the changes which have taken place in the health care industry over the past twenty years, and particularly since enactment of the 1965 amendments to the Social Security Act. Due to these changes, the health care industry is currently the nation's third largest industry and, possibly, its fastest growing one.[2]

The nonprofit form of hospital organization is the traditionally favored and dominant form for the delivery of health services, particularly hospital care. Nonprofit hospitals pay no taxes; receive substantial government loans, grants, and subsidies; and, due to the charitable contribution deduction on personal income taxes, are able to attract substantial philanthropic contributions. However, nonprofit hospitals do make a profit and, frequently, a substantial one. As shown in Table 6–3, net income in nonprofit hospitals has been consistently high and increasing over time, although the recent rate of increase in total revenue has leveled off somewhat because of increased regulation (e.g., the Nixon wage-price controls). Furthermore, Davis found that, while average nonprofit hospital net income in 1969 ranged from 0.0 percent of plant assets in Rhode Island to 9.62 percent in Mississippi, it was positive in forty-nine of the fifty states.

It is traditionally assumed that nonprofits attempt to maximize output or patient services. However, as Davis and Ogur point out, accumulation of substantial surpluses is inconsistent with long-run output maximization.[3] Nonprofits apparently maximize the same thing as investor-owned facilities: cash flow.

As in the arts and private higher education, philanthropy plays a unique role in the nonprofit sector of the health industry. Bruce Vladeck discussed "the pitfalls of philanthropy" and pointed out how philanthropy can lead to overinvestment by nonprofits.

> If an influential member of the board of trustees desires to memorialize himself (and diminish his estate tax liability) by putting up half the cost of a new and essentially useless auditorium, the institution has precious little incentive to say no. Indeed, administrators of non-profits have little incentive to say no to anyone desiring increased capital expenditures, so long as they remain relatively confident that someone can be found to pay for them. The way in which non-profits set their prices, and the low price elasticity of consumer demand, permit administrators to hide from themselves the true implications of such spending. Investment projects come before the administrator as sources of "free money" . . .[4]

Vladeck also points out the preference of philanthropy for capital expansion projects and observes that "as with Morgan's yacht, it's not the price but the upkeep that dooms many institutions. . . ."[5] As shown in Table 6-3, nonprofits "plow back" their profits into plant assets, and the annual rate of increase in plant assets over the past years is greater than 9 percent.

Role of Investor-Owned Groups

Recent changes in the health care industry (see Tables 6-1, 6-2, and 6-3) challenged certain groups to organize alternative delivery systems and a "new generation" of proprietary hospitals emerged. The most important aspect in "the comeback" of proprietary hospitals is the emergence of large investor-owned hospital groups. As shown in Table 6-4, the number of proprietary hospitals declined from 1946 to 1972.

However, Table 6-5 shows the dramatic increase in the growth of major investor-owned groups which began in 1970.

In 1964, the investor-owned groups provided only $20 million worth of services or just 3 percent of the total for-profit segment of the hospital industry. By 1974, the investor-owned groups were doing $1.05 billion in business annually or 57 percent of the $2.8 billion for-profit segment. In just ten years, investor-owned groups increased revenues fiftyfold, their market share twentyfold, and

Table 6-1. National Health Expenditures

Year	Health Spending ($ billions)	% GNP	% Change	Per Capita Health Spending
1950	$ 12.0	4.6	–	$ 18
1960	$ 25.9	5.2	+13.0	$142
1965	$ 38.9	5.9	+13.4	$198
1970	$ 69.2	7.2	+20	$334
1974	$104.2	7.7	+ 5	$485
1975	$118.6 est.	8.3	+10 est.	$547 est.

Source: Statistical Abstract of the U.S., 1975.

Table 6-2. Medical Economic Summary

Year	Medical Price Index	Billions Output 1974 ($ billions)	% Change	Output Per Person ($ 1974)	% Change
1950	100	$ 34	–	$224	–
1955	120	$ 40	17	$241	8
1960	149	$ 49	22	$271	12
1965	168	$ 66	34	$340	25
1970	227	$ 80	39	$390	15
1974	280	$104	30	$488	25

Source: Proprietary Hospitals and Associated Products (New York: Frost and Sullivan, Inc., 1974), p. 121.

they currently constitute approximately 35 percent of the nation's nongovernment hospitals.

Several inducements to private corporate investment (debt and equity) spurred the development of investor-owned group hospitals.

1. Competition within the hospital industry is limited. Despite the recent clamor over physician assistants, LPNs, etc., medical care in the United States is almost unequivocally rendered by a licensed physician, either in his office or within a hospital facility. All but simple diagnostic procedures and the majority of all surgical ones are performed in the hospital setting. In short, there are currently few available substitutes for acute inpatient hospital care.
2. There is a low percentage of hospital financial failures, and the problem has been centered among nonprofit hospitals which, for reasons previously discussed, are increasingly subject to financial peril.
3. In addition to limited competition, recently enacted Certificate of Need legislation in the National Health Planning and Resource Development Act (P.L. 93-641) may strengthen and "protect" the market position of already established health facilities. However, it may also "protect" inefficient hospi-

Table 6-3.   Revenue, Expenses, and Net Income for Nongovernmental, Nonprofit Hospitals, 1961-1975

Year	Total Revenue (in millions)	Expenses (in millions)	Net Income (in millions)	Plant Assets (in millions)	Net Income Ratio		Annual Rate of Change		
					Total Revenue	Plant Assets	Total Revenue	Expenses	Plant Assets
1961	$4,675	$4,584	$91	$6,541	1.94	1.39	9.86	10.74	5.99
1962	4,995	4,999	--3	7,010	-.06	-.04	6.87	9.04	7.17
1963	5,622	5,491	132	7,592	2.34	1.74	12.54	9.84	8.29
1964	6,154	6,039	115	8,217	1.87	1.40	9.46	9.99	8.23
1965	6,870	6,643	227	9,078	3.31	2.50	11.63	10.00	10.19
1966	7,674	7,435	239	9,752	3.11	2.45	11.70	11.93	7.42
1967	9,146	8,806	339	10,457	3.71	3.24	19.18	18.44	7.23
1968	10,655	10,317	337	11,490	3.16	2.93	16.48	17.15	9.87
1969	12,537	12,137	400	12,523	3.19	3.19	17.68	17.64	9.00
1970	14,552	14,163	389	13,783	2.67	2.82	16.07	16.69	10.06
1971	N.A.	16,344	—	15,529	—	—	—	15.40	12.67
1972	18,742	18,384	358	17,007	1.91	2.11	—	12.48	9.52
1973	20,751	20,418	333	18,945	1.61	1.76	10.72	11.06	11.40
1974	23,927	23,494	433	20,963	1.81	2.07	15.31	15.07	10.65
1975	28,501	27,965	536	24,005	1.88	2.23	19.12	19.30	14.51

Sources: Statistics for 1961-1969 are from Karen Davis, "Economic Theories of Behavior in Nonprofit, Private Hospitals," *Economic Business Bulletin,* 2, 2 (1972): 6.
Statistics for 1970-1974 are from *Hospital Statistics,* 1975 Edition.
Statistics for 1975 are from *Hospital Statistics,* 1976 Edition.

Table 6-4. Investor-Owned Hospitals

Year	Hospitals	Beds (thou-sands)
1946	1,076	39
1950	1,218	42
1955	1,020	37
1960	896	37
1965	857	47
1966	852	48
1967	821	47
1968	769	48
1969	759	48
1970	769	53
1971	750	54
1972	738	57
1973	757	63
1974	775	70

Source: Hospital Statistics, 1975 Edition, Guide Issues (Chicago: American Hospital Association, 1975), p. 5.

Table 6-5. Growth of Major Hospital Investor-Owned Groups

Year	Hospitals	Beds	Revenues ($ millions)
1964	—	—	$ 20
1965	—	—	32
1966	—	—	—
1967	—	—	59
1968	—	—	81
1969	—	—	264
1970	135	16.4	409
1971	169	20.9	561
1972	236	28.2	735
1973	253	31.8	891
1974	280	26.9	1,050

Source: Proprietary Hospitals and Associated Products (New York: Frost and Sullivan, Inc., 1974), p. 9.

tals and, therefore, make it more difficult for new facilities to obtain a certificate of need.

The large percentage of the health care industry business that is underwritten by financially strong third party payers boosts credit standing, imparts financial integrity, and diminishes the threat of bad debts. It also allows for the predictability of revenues. As shown in Table 6-6, the per capita percentage of hospital expenditures paid by third parties, by persons covered by hospitalization insurance, and by hospital insurance benefits has risen dramatically. Further, coverage is skewed in favor of inpatient hospital co-payment.

With the advent of the investor-owned groups came the infusion of modern management and progressive corporate financial practices into the health care field. The groups grew without the subsidies of Hill-Burton and other such government programs, used both creditor and equity financing, and engaged in "judicious acquisition" of existing facilities.[6] Currently, they provide a wide range of services that are not found in the traditional range of hospital service. The major groups engage in management contracts, consulting services, hospital financing, construction, and operation. Many provide EDP and lab services and inhalation therapy to other hospitals. Furthermore, because of significant economies of scale (bulk purchases, standardization, access to professional personnel,

Table 6-6. Third Party Payments

Year	% Total Hosp. Exp. Pd. Third Party	Persons Covered Hosp. Insurance (% Total Pop.)	Hosp. Insurance Benefits Paid Per Capita	% Change
1965	81	71.9	27.90	—
1966	82	73.2	29.60	+ 6
1967	88	74.4	30.13	+ 2
1968	90	76.4	33.10	+10
1969	90	77.2	38.19	+16
1970	88	78.2	44.26	+16
1971	90	78.8	50.80	+15
1972	89	79.2	55.62	+ 9
1973	91	80.0	61.12	+10
1974	90	81.6	68.72	+12
1975	92	82.5	76.99	+14

	Medicare-Medicaid Government/Per Capita	
Year	Benefits	% Change
1965	25.08	—
1966	27.17	+ 8
1967	41.93	+54
1968	50.67	+21
1969	57.72	+14
1970	63.40	+10
1971	72.19	+14
1972	83.34	+15
1973	89.30	+ 7
1974	99.28	+11
1975	118.38	+19

Source: Robinson-Humphreys, *Special Report on Hospital Management* (Atlanta: Robinson-Humphreys Co., Inc., May 1976), p. 7.

etc.), the investor-owned groups were constructing hospitals in 1974 at a cost of approximately $35,000 per bed while the average cost for Hill-Burton hospitals was $50,000 per bed.[7]

The investor-owned group has been able to provide care in areas where rapid population growth occurred and where limited primary and/or secondary care existed. Many investor-owned hospitals have located in communities which were too poor to finance tax-exempt facilities. The large corporate group form of organization facilitates mobilization of private capital and quickens responses to changes in the need for health care faster than do individual hospitals. As of 1975, there were 346 communities in which four to five million people resided, and the only hospitals were investor-owned. In fact, in 103 counties in thirty-four states, there is only one hospital, and it is an investor-owned facility.[8]

With respect to quality and quantity of care, the existence of the investor-owned groups enhances the reputation of the for-profit segment as a whole and enables it to attract equity investment. As shown in Table 6-7, investor-owned groups have expanded their market share in certain key areas vis-à-vis nongovernment, nonprofit hospitals. At the present time, 96 percent of investor-owned hospitals are Blue Cross certified, 83 percent are Medicare certified, 77 percent provide emergency service, and 75 percent are accredited by the Joint Commission on Accreditation of Hospitals.[9]

Currently, investor-owned facilities provide high quality care in an efficient private enterprise setting. They are a dynamic segment of the dynamic health care industry and, potentially, have an even more effective role in the delivery of health care. As of February 1976, it would require $6 billion in public funds to replace the beds built by investor-owned groups.[10] Their future participation will be determined, of course, by their ability to attract private capital. The remainder of this discussion will focus on several key policy areas in which existing intra- and interindustry inequities impinge on the viability of the investor-owned sector.

POLICY AREA ONE: THE PROBLEM OF REGULATION

At the present time, a complicated administrative bureaucracy exists, with myriad reporting requirements for all phases of a health facility's operations. This has direct impact on costs and may reduce efficiency since resources are diverted from alternative uses. The key areas of regulation at the present time include Medicare-Medicaid reimbursement, professional standards review under P.L. 92-603, and certificate of need legislation that is contained in the recently passed National Health Planning and Resource Development Act (P.L. 93-641). Regulation of Medicare and Medicaid reimbursement is particularly important since approximately 37 percent of all revenue in investor-owned hospitals is derived from these sources.

Table 6–7. Percentage of Investor-Owned and Nonprofit Hospitals Offering Same Services: 1968, 1974

Service	Percentage Total Investor-owned Hospitals Offering Service			Percentage Total Nongovernment, Nonprofit Hospitals Offering Service		
	1968	*1974*	*% Change*	*1968*	*1974*	*% Change*
Pharmacy	55.1	65.5	+10.4	79.0	72.0	– 7.0
Premature Nursery	29.1	16.5	– 8.6	56.8	43.8	–13.0
Outpatient Department	40.8	10.8	– 3.0	48.7	31.5	–17.2
Emergency Room	77.2	72.8	– 3.4	91.7	89.7	– 2.0
Postoperative Recovery	62.0	80.5	+22.5	86.7	86.0	+ 7.6
Organ Bank	.5	.2	– .3	3.6	2.1	+ 1.5
Renal Dialysis	14.3	9.6	+ 4.7	28.5	32.5	– 4.0
Inhalation Therapy	40.8	75.6	+34.8	81.3	54.8	–32.5
Intensive Care Unit	27.1	56.6	+29.5	74.1	50.9	+23.2

Sources: Hospitals, 43, Part 2 (1969): 492–493; and *Hospital Statistics,* 1975 Edition, Guide Issues (Chicago: American Hospital Association, 1975), pp. 188–192.

Table 6–8. Sources of Revenue[1]

Year	Cost Basis			Private Insurance
	Medicare	*Medicaid*	*Blue Cross*	
1970	29%	4%	11%	56%
1971	30	4	8	58
1972	30	5	7	58
1973	30	5	7	58
1974	32	5	6	57
1975	32	5	6	57

Source: Robinson-Humphreys, *Special Report on Hospital Management* (Atlanta: Robinson-Humphreys Co., Inc., May 1976), p. 10.

[1]Figures are computed for the three largest investor-owned companies.

Until the present, the government has imposed significant administrative costs, but investor-owned health facilities have withstood the demands of increased regulation and are meeting well the regulatory requirements of P.L.'s 92–603 and 93–611. Since P.L. 93–641 does provide for consumer and health care industry representation in state health systems agencies, the investor-owned segment of the health care industry will be able to gain representation and have an input into the policy process. The enactment of P.L. 92–603 (1972) is correlated with a decline in length of hospital stay and an increase in outpatient utilization rates and revenue (See Table 6–9); and, while P.L. 93–641 has not been in effect long enough truly to have an impact, estimates are that certificate of need will not reduce total dollar investment, but, rather, alter its composition—i.e., cause a substitution of new services and equipment for additional beds.[11]

Table 6-9. Changes in Outpatient Service

Year	Length of Stay	Outpatient Revenue	% Change
1973	6.8 days	$31.3	+17.2
1974	6.7	40.0	+27.8
1975	6.6	55.9	+39.8

Source: Robinson-Humphreys, *Special Report on Hospital Management* (Atlanta: Robinson-Humphreys Co., Inc., May 1976), p. 10.

Due to the significant rate of inflation in the health care industry, there is a trend toward modification of cost reimbursement. The government (both state and federal) is concerned with its apparent inability to control health care costs and attributes the problem to a lack of efficiency and cost control incentives under current reimbursement programs. Within this framework, Senator Herman Talmadge (D-Ga.) introduced the Medicare-Medicaid Administrative and Reimbursement Reform Act (S3205). The bill calls for a Medicare-Medicaid incentive cost reimbursement system, consolidation of Medicare and Medicaid into one agency, reimbursement for closing down or converting underutilized facilities, regulation of contractual agreements between hospitals and hospital-based medical service providers—i.e., pharmacies—and increasing the rate of return on equity for Medicare reimbursement to twice the average return of the Hospital Trust Fund.[12]

In addition to the Talmadge bill, other pricing control legislation is currently under consideration by Congress. President Ford proposed a 7 percent cost increase ceiling on government reimbursed hospital costs, and such legislation could virtually halt private capital formation. Another bill proposes that, between now and 1980, Medicare reimbursement be limited to 133 percent of the Consumer Price Index (CPI) in a particular region. Finally, the approved Senate-House Conference budget included a general $800 million cutback in Medicare-Medicaid funding, and the House sponsored a "catastrophic coverage" proposal for Medicare reimbursement which included limiting hospital cost increases for Medicare to 9 1/2 percent. Of particular concern is the impending passage of the Clinical Laboratories Improvement Act, which will have a significant impact on administrative costs for hospitals, particularly those in rural areas. Many laboratories are currently unable to comply with the standards set in the proposed act, and its passage may increase the cost of clinical laboratory services.

One continuing dilemma is the future of national health insurance in the United States. While the proposed Health Security Act, Long-Ribicoff bill, and the National Health Care Services Reorganization and Financing Act (Ulman bill) differ in their specific concepts, financing, administration, and reimbursement mechanism, any type of national health insurance will enormously increase the demand for health care. However, the private sector will most likely be an integral provider in any national health care program. Support for the legislation is diminished by ever-increasing federal expenditures, and continuing disputes in the House of Representatives between the Ways and Means Subcommittee on Health and the Commerce Health Subcommittee probably preclude passage of any of the pending bills in their present form. Several years of implementation would be required subsequent to passage of such a bill, and, therefore, the concept is probably not a threatening one to investor-owned groups in the short run.

Additional regulatory concerns are the extent to which state governments will participate in price regulation. In March of 1976, the New York State Legislature passed an amended version of Governor Carey's Medicaid cutback proposal. This new law gives the state budget director the right to reject "reasonable costs" rates for Medicaid patients and to have the state's Medicaid rates revised according to his findings.[13]

Given the recent health care cost explosion, increasing regulation, and control of hospital revenues, many supposedly cost-effective substitutes for inpatient hospital care have "grown like Topsy."

As shown in Table 6-9, the ambulatory care market is one area that will probably benefit. Proponents of ambulatory care contend that this type of delivery of health services is useful since patient care can be provided at reduced charges, while existing hospitals can increase total revenue per bed, and patient day and can improve profit margins and cash flow. Currently, government support of ambulatory care is favorable. P.L. 93–641 requires that, in any fiscal year, 25 percent of a state's allotment of Hill-Burton funds be allocated to outpatient facilities.[14]

One particular area of interest in the ambulatory care market is outpatient surgery. Developments in medical knowledge and technology in the last decade precipitated the use of outpatient settings for surgical procedures in which the total time for preoperative workup, surgery, and recovery is less than one working day. The first freestanding surgical unit (FSSU) was opened in 1970, and today there are approximately twenty FSSUs, mainly in the Western United States. In the East, hospital adjunct units are favored.

Potential advantages of outpatient surgery may accrue to both the patient and the provider:

1. Outpatient surgical procedures are routine operations, all inputs (labor inputs by the doctor and other staff, and goods or supply inputs) are highly predictable, and the procedures can be efficiently scheduled throughout a working day to obtain maximum facility utilization.
2. Performing surgical procedures in outpatient facilities may be cost-saving to the patient and, sometimes, to the hospital. In minor surgery cases it eliminates the cost of at least two days' room and board and of twenty-four hour nursing care.
3. In addition to reduced dollar costs, outpatient surgery involves minimal disruption of normal activity and reduces patients' opportunity (time) cost.

4. Utilization of outpatient surgical facilities allows hospitals to allocate hospital beds more efficiently to patients who really need them.

Perhaps the largest impediments to investment in outpatient surgical facilities (particularly by existing hospitals) are related to existing utilization patterns and organizational difficulties. First, typical surgical facility utilization rates are far less than 100 percent and vary tremendously according to time of day. Generally, there are three operating schedules:

Prime Time I   =   7:00 a.m.– 3:00 p.m.
Prime Time II   =   3:00 p.m.–11:00 p.m.
Prime Time III = 11:00 p.m.– 7:00 a.m.

Prime Time I is the schedule most demanded by doctors, patients, and surgical staffs. When there is an apparent overload of surgical cases, it is usually the result of "crowding" elective cases into *one* of three operating schedules rather than any absolute shortage of surgical facilities. Prime Time II and Prime Time III "slots" are generally used for emergencies. Utilization of Prime Time I ranges from 60 to 80 percent while utilization of Prime Times II and III is only approximately 20 to 30 percent. Given such utilization patterns, most hospitals simply cannot afford to reallocate patients away from existing facilities. Furthermore, one must not confuse patient charges with hospital cost. As long as total utilization rates of existing inpatient surgery facilities remain at the current low level, most hospitals will not find it profitable to invest in outpatient units. The charge to the outpatient might be less, but, given excess inpatient capacity, the overall cost to the hospital would not be reduced. If hospitals were to charge outpatients less, they would have to charge inpatients more just to break even. Such cross-subsidization is inequitable and self-defeating. It would also appear that health systems agencies would hesitate to issue certificate of need, given such patterns of excess capacity. One alternative to creating a separate outpatient unit would be for hospitals to reorganize and offer outpatient surgery during Prime Times II and III. However, this creates substantial additional staff demands, particularly in the admitting and discharge offices.

The decision to invest in ambulatory care facilities is not, however, a simple, straightforward one. Analysis by the Blue Cross Association saliently summarizes the problem.

The transfer of appropriate services from an inpatient to an outpatient basis can serve to reduce total community costs if accompanied by commensurate adjustments in capital structure and operating behavior. However, it must be recognized that inappropriate utilization of the existing capital structure or unnecessary additions can nullify some or all of the cost savings incurred through the increased utilization of ambulatory services . . . . In the health field, where the goals of the system are complex and the methods of best attaining them uncertain, it is easy to make decisions that will maximize the production of one type of care without optimizing the operation of the entire system. This kind of decision must be avoided.[15]

In addition to these financing aspects of outpatient surgical facilities, there are significant impediments to current corporate investment in these ventures. Insurance carriers, particularly those in the Eastern United States, have been slow to provide reimbursement for outpatient surgery. Medicare did not reimburse for operating room charges for outpatient surgery until after litigation was won against them. Each outpatient surgery facility must be individually approved by the Social Security Administration, and Medicare payment still is often uncertain. Although few surgery outpatients are over sixty-two years of age, the continuing lack of Medicare payment is a problem because of the precedent effect which emanates to other third party payers. The lack of third party payment creates disincentives on both the demand and the supply sides. Patients will not demand the service since it would increase their out-of-pocket medical expenses. Providers of care will be unwilling to finance freestanding surgical units because of the risk of uncollectable bills.

Medical societies and physicians in many states have opposed the concept, and the opposition has been particularly damaging to attempts in Virginia and Rhode Island. While the specific reasons vary, the most common objection is that physicians are reluctant to jeopardize their relationships with hospitals where they perform inpatient surgery and which oppose FSSUs. Also, some contend that outpatient surgery is potentially hazardous, and they are unwilling to accept the increased liability, particularly in FSSUs.

Outpatient surgery facilities are subject to the provisions of P.L. 93–641. Therefore, one can expect the success of FSSUs to vary regionally according to the attitudes of individual health agencies. While the attitude of the federal government is increasingly oriented toward cost-saving mechanisms in the health field, unless the demand for surgical procedures increases significantly, any federal "push" for outpatient surgery would result in unused and unneeded hospital beds and surgical theaters, which could eventually lead to the closing of some hospitals or hospital wings entirely. The reimbursement mechanism of the Talmadge bill would mitigate this problem.

The malpractice problem is also a problem in the development of outpatient surgical facilities. In the East, where the general attitude toward the service is unfavorable, carriers charge higher premiums or even refuse to write coverage.

Due to potential cost-savings, the concept of outpatient surgery is likely to be important in the future. Most outpatient surgery units are relatively small; the largest freestanding facility in the country is only 17,000 square feet. However, substantial equipment requirements can result in $1 million to $2 million expenditures for these facilities. Feasibility of such investment will be influenced by government fiscal policy toward the investment tax credit, the attitudes of health systems agencies, and the willingness of third party payers to reimburse for outpatient services. The doctor-owned FSSU could be particularly profitable since the doctor who owned an FSSU and also worked there could accumulate total earnings greater than his fee-for-service income. (Anesthesiologists were among the first to open FSSUs. Gynecologists, who are the most frequent users of typical outpatient surgery facilities, could particularly benefit from the ownership of FSSUs which provide pregnancy terminations and sterilizations). However, doctor ownership of the facilities may be expected to expose FSSUs to additional contentions of overutilization of facilities. Furthermore, at this time, many feel that peer review under PSRO legislation can occur only in a hospital setting and, therefore, that some investor-owned FSSUs might have to hire physician consultants to conduct peer review.

Policy Intervention Area

As was written in a recent issue of *Hospitals,* "The issue is no longer whether there will be controls; it is now a question of whether these controls will be effective in achieving social goals."[16]

The Talmadge bill is the first true attempt by policymakers to modify health care costs. It contains proposals which are both favorable and unfavorable for the investor-owned segment of the industry. Consolidation of Medicare-Medicaid offices is desirable if it would reduce administrative reporting procedures. The cost control incentive is useful, and few investor-owned hospitals, particularly the large groups, would be unable to meet the cost targets. An increase in return on equity is desperately needed and warranted and is viewed as a past-due necessity (see Policy Area Two for a discussion of this point).

Recent legislation by the State of New York directly contravenes federal law as specified in Title XIX of the Social Security Act. Such arbitrary action by other states would seriously restrict the ability of investor-owned hospitals to service Medicaid patients and would create substantial cash flow problems for hospitals. This type of state regulation is an area of growing concern and certainly diminishes the feasibility of investment in the health care industry, particularly hospitals.

Another type of price regulation could result from additional pressure that might be exerted by third party payers who have previously acted as "pass-through" organizations. If premium costs continue to increase, policyholders may protest and cause third party payers to exert pressure to control hospital pricing.

The short-run aspects of the regulation problem seem manageable. While any government regulation diminishes investor enthusiasm, investor-owned facilities are likely to survive since economies of scale and efficient management enable them to operate with considerably more price flexibility than many nonprofit organizations. However, in the long run, additional price regulation or the advent of a radical form of national health insurance would seriously damage the viability of the investor-owned market.

POLICY AREA TWO: RATE OF RETURN FOR INVESTOR-OWNED HOSPITALS

Title XVIII of the Social Security Act provides for reimbursement of all "reasonable costs" that are incurred by hospitals in the treatment of Medicare patients plus a "reasonable return on equity capital" which is currently equal to 1 1/2 times the yield of the hospital trust fund. This yield is approximately equal to 11 percent. However, HEW regulations issued pursuant to Title XVIII do not allow reimbursement for such costs as "stock maintenance" and the payment of federal income tax even though these activities and costs are required by law. This 11 percent return is, therefore, a *pretax* yield, and the effective *aftertax* yield is 4.4 percent! Therefore, the investor-owned sector is put at a serious interindustry competitive disadvantage in attracting scarce investment dollars. In 1973, the average aftertax return for all United States industry was 14 percent. For the service industry it was 14.1 percent and for public utilities the aftertax return was 12 percent.[17] The situation creates a definite bias for investors who compare alternate rates of return, and it creates inequity for private patients who must bear higher charges as a result of the government's unwillingness to provide appropriate reimbursement. While Title XVIII and P.L. 93-641 expressly forbid cross-subsidization in the form of higher charges to private patients, hospitals cannot absorb these unmet costs and will make rational economic responses to the situation.

Medicare Reimbursement for Federal Income Taxes

In every other industry which performs a public service and operates on a cost reimbursement basis, the payment of income taxes is considered to be a legitimate reimbursement item. The logic is simple—income taxes must be paid before one can determine how much is left as the return on common equity—and based on well-established judicial precedent. Corporations cannot be required to use their property for the benefit of the public without receiving compensation at "rates which acknowledge financial interests of investors."[18] In 1967, it was determined that federal income taxes are a reasonable element of the cost of service in establishing just and reasonable rates of return for public utilities.[19]

This theory is generally accepted in public utility law and, at the present time, the Federal Power Commission, the Civil Aeronautics Board, the Federal Interstate Communications Commission, the Interstate Commerce Commission, and the Federal Maritime Commission all recognize that payment of federal income taxes is a cost of service in calculating reasonable rates of return.

That hospitals fulfill a necessary public function and that their property is used for public benefit is undisputed. As shown in Table 6-8, 37 percent of investor-owned group revenue is derived from "public patients." Payment of income taxes is a cost of providing a public service for the government; like public utility companies, facilities are entitled to inclusion of payment of federal income taxes as a reimbursement item. Failure of Medicare to reimburse for payment of federal income taxes reduces the real level of a corporation's equity and, essentially, allows the government to use that equity without providing fair compensation.

Medicare Reimbursement and the Costs of Raising Capital—Debt vs. Equity

It is often argued that present federal income tax laws make it more "expensive" for a corporation to use equity financing because dividend payments are not allowable income tax deductions and mortgage payments are allowable. Therefore, corporations can maximize income and protect cash flow by favoring debt financing. Also, since dividend payments are taxed as additional personal income to shareholders, double taxation is said to exist.

However, differences in reimbursement for the costs incurred in the raising of debt and equity capital result in additional discrimination against equity capital, and this is of significant concern for investor-owned groups. Under HEW's present interpretation of Title XVIII, costs incurred in arranging, servicing, and repaying debt financing are classified as "reasonable costs" of providing patient service and are Medicare reimbursable. However, while virtually identical costs are incurred in a stock issue, none is classified as a reimbursable cost. These so-called "stock maintenance" costs generally amount to at least 5 percent of the total value of stock issue, and nonreimbursement creates several financing problems for investor-owned hospitals.

1. Omission of "stock maintenance fees" is essentially an additional tax on corporate equity. For investor-owned groups, debt capital represents approximately 60 percent and equity capital about 40 percent of total capital. The lack of reimbursement for the costs associated with 40 percent of their total capital is an impediment to overall investment in the industry and fosters a capital formation process which is biased toward the use of debt financing.
2. Voluntary, religious, and other nonprofit health facilities raise approximately 40 percent of their total capital through philanthropy, and *all* costs of raising and maintaining philanthropic contributions are considered to be "reasonable costs" of providing patient service and are Medicare reimbursable. Therefore, the investor-owned sector is put at a significant and unjustified intra-industry disadvantage.

Policy Intervention Areas

The original Medicare legislation does not specify that "stock maintenance" and payment of income taxes are not "reasonable costs." The Act only requires the Secretary of Health, Education and Welfare to determine the "reasonable costs" of providing service and to reimburse these costs to facilities providing

Medicare service. The determination that "stock maintenance" costs not be re-imbursable was apparently made on the perception that equity would be reim-bursed in other ways—i.e., through provision of a return on equity capital and through the profits which normally accrue to investor-owned facilities. However, clear justification for the exclusion of "stock maintenance" as a reimbursable item is not made.

HEW apparently determined that income taxes were nonallowable "costs," based on the accounting concept of "costs." Specifically, all "costs" of doing business are deducted from earnings before a corporation's tax liability is com-puted and, therefore, income taxes are *not* "costs." However, payment of income taxes *does* reduce a corporation's equity, and income taxes must be paid *before* one can determine the amount of any equity. As previously mentioned, approxi-mately 37 percent of all investor-owned hospital revenue comes from Medicare-Medicaid reimbursement, and the current aftertax yield of 4.4 percent results in next to zero profitability in this 37 percent of total revenue. Unless HEW can provide a more competitive rate of return, investor-owned facilities—and particu-larly hospitals—will find it difficult to offer potential investors a return commen-surate with risk. An aftertax yield of 4.4 percent is totally inadequate to attract sufficient capital for maintenance, expansion, and new construction.

On June 2, 1976, the United States District Court of the District of Columbia ruled in *Humana of South Carolina* v. *Matthews* that, while Title XVIII expressly provides for a rate of return on equity capital in extended care facilities of not more than 1 1/2 times the yield on the Federal Hospital Insurance Fund, the original legislation was silent as to the treatment of proprietary hospitals. The court ruled that the Secretary of Health, Education and Welfare had not made any formal subsequent determination that such a yield was adequate for propri-etary hospitals, set aside the current HEW regulation, and remanded the matter to the secretary for appropriate economic study and decision making. Litigation may also be necessary to secure reimbursement for costs of "stock maintenance" and the payment of income taxes.

The Talmadge bill increases the current formula to provide for a return equal to twice the yield on Social Security investments. However, providing twice the yield on the Federal Hospital Trust Fund and not including income taxes and "stock maintenance" as reimbursement items will not be sufficient to provide adequate rates of return on private investment in hospitals.

Similar and dramatic changes in utilization and financing patterns have oc-curred in other areas of the health care industry, and Medicare-Medicaid reim-bursement policies will directly affect the developmental pattern of investment in these areas. Two examples will be discussed.

The Nursing Home Industry

The nursing home industry had its true genesis with the 1966 passage of Medicare-Medicaid provisions and, currently, 50 percent of all nursing home residents receive Medicare and/or Medicaid.[20] Medicare provides limited reimbursement for nursing home care in licensed extended care facilities which provide skilled nursing care and related services; Medicaid provides for care in licensed skilled care and intermediate care facilities. While the federal government lends some support to the construction of nursing homes under the Hill-Burton program and the Community Health Services and Facilities Act of 1961, few states provide funds for nursing home construction, and the level of support varies tremendously. For example, Massachusetts and New Jersey provide no financial support for any long-term care facility while New York offers mortgage loan guarantees and subsidies for up to 90 percent of a project's costs to voluntary nursing homes and long-term care hospitals. At the present time, the bulk of capital required for nursing home construction and renovation is raised commercially by proprietary firms. While the proprietary sector amounts to only approximately 13 percent of the acute and chronic disease hospital market, 75 percent of all nursing homes are proprietary.[21] Proprietary facilities may receive mortgage insurance under the Housing Act of 1959 from HEW and loans from the Small Business Administration.

Because of several factors—the decline of the extended family, increased mobility of siblings, smaller homes, increased labor force participation of females, an increased proportion of the population with Social Security benefits and/or private pension funds, as well as the existence of Medicare and Medicaid—the demand for institutional long-term care has increased. Also, if the present birthrate continues, an estimated 17 percent of the population will be over sixty-five by the year 2050. Today, the over-sixty-five population is approximately 10.5 percent of the total population.[22] In addition to this demographic problem, recent developments in medical science have succeeded in prolonging the life of the sick and/or aged. Fuchs has noted that "successes" in some areas of medical technology frequently impose significant costs on the other segments of the health care delivery system.[23] The drawing in Figure 6-1 is particularly useful to demonstrate the changing nature of health care in the United States.

It is estimated that, due to these changes in demography and medical science, there will be an approximate 8 to 9 percent growth in nursing home revenues in the next three to five years. While this enhances the feasibility of investment in nursing homes, the bulk of investment has been by small partnerships or private entrepreneurs. One principle reason for this ownership pattern is low reimbursement patterns and low profit levels. Medicare-Medicaid reimbursement rates vary by state, but the average is less than $20 per patient day and facilities may not charge a recipient more than the per diem Medicare-Medicaid rate. Currently, 77 percent of all proprietary nursing homes are Medicare-Medicaid certified.[24] There are basically three types of reimbursement: flat rate systems, reasonable cost reimbursement, and multiple rate structure differentiated by levels of care. The more profitable nursing home facilities have located in areas with flat rate reimbursement, have engaged in vigorous cost control, and have attained a favorable patient mix of relatively "well" patients requiring minimum care.

"Front end" capital requirements for the nursing home industry are relatively

In the previous layer of the onion were TB and other infectious diseases and many causes of death in children.

In the next layer will be the problems of old age, the chronic degenerative diseases and mental illness.

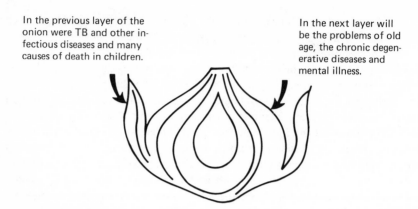

Figure 6-1. A New Generation of Medical Problems Has to Be Tackled

Source: Robert Maxwell, "The Case for Intervention," in David Ehrlich (ed.), *The Health Care Cost Explosion: Which Way Now?* (Bern: Hans Huber, 1975) p. 28.

low. The average cost of construction of proprietary facilities is approximately $12,500 per bed, compared to $35,000 to $50,000 per proprietary hospital bed, and the percentage of total area available for patient care utilization is greater than in hospitals. Labor costs in nursing homes are significantly less than similar costs in hospitals, as the ratio of professional staff to total staff is low, employees are relatively low paid, and turnover is high.

While profit margins in most nursing home facilities are low, positive cash flow can be generated. For this reason, nursing homes have been favored tax shelters for entrepreneurs who could take advantage of the depreciation allowances on personal income taxes and enjoy the benefits of positive cash flow. However, the current low profit margins are not sufficient inducements for dynamic participation by investor-owned groups.

The Market for Home Health Care

Another interesting and newly developed facet of long-term care in this country is the home health care agency. Medicare and Medicaid provide reimbursement for home health care and, between 1966 and 1974, the number of home health agencies doubled, while the number of hospital based programs increased by 300 percent.[25]

There is little current regulation of home health care agencies, and they are not subject to certificate of need legislation. In order to obtain Medicare certification, an agency must simply provide skilled nursing services in addition to at least one of the following five services: physical therapy, occupational therapy, speech therapy, medical social service, and home health aides. (Firms currently in the market generally are quite small.) In 1969, only 4.4 percent of all agencies provided all six services, and over half provided only two of the services.[26] Also,

Medicaid certification of home health care varies by state, and distribution of home health agencies among states is, therefore, skewed.

There is currently no reliable income and expense data for home health agencies. However, given the "boom" in their development, they may become interesting ancillary investments for proprietary health facilities in the future. In 1974, 2.2 percent of all investor-owned hospitals offered some home health services.[27] Regulation is apt to be favorable since this type of noninstitutional care is a potentially cost-effective method of providing some types of long-term care. Increased Medicare, Medicaid, and other third party payment would certainly precipitate greater participation by the investor-owned sector.

POLICY AREA THREE: INEQUITY UNDER
PRESENT TAX LAWS

Under existing tax policy, proprietary hospitals pay or accrue taxes which are not levied on nonprofit hospitals or "charitable" hospitals. And yet, as previously demonstrated, both exhibit the same or similar services and similar accumulation and utilization of funds for replacement purposes. Teaching hospitals are, of course, notable exceptions, and ample justification exists for their nonprofit status.

The history of federal taxation of charitable or nonprofit hospitals indicates that the government granted "tax-exemption" status as a corollary with "nonprofit" status and in a reciprocal agreement with these hospitals for their providing free care to indigents. However, it is possible that the basis for this tax-exempt status has eroded, since federal and state payment for personal health care—which includes indigents—has risen nearly 177 percent since the inception of Medicare and Medicaid and since their payments currently account for almost 58 percent of all health care expenditures. Total third party payments account for 92 percent of all hospital expenditures (see Table 6-6), and direct out-of-pocket expenditures have been cut almost in half since 1950.[28]

While these existing tax provisions create intra-industry bias in favor of nonprofit or charitable health care facilities, other inequities in the current tax law create interindustry biases and impair the ability of the proprietary sector to compete in the investment market.

The 1962 Investment Tax Credit

The 1962 Investment Tax Credit (ITC) enables hospitals to receive a tax credit against their federal income taxes equal to a percentage of the total cost that is incurred for certain categories of assets. Primarily, this category of assets involves items which are essentially equipment. The present rate is 10 percent. The ITC had the much needed effect of reducing the cost of these assets or increasing the rate of aftertax return.

The 1962 law specifically allowed certain types of companies to claim a larger portion of their assets as being eligible for the investment tax credit. A good example of this is a textile manufacturing plant which can obtain the ITC on approximately 90 percent of its total construction costs, which include the central air-conditioning systems and other special construction components necessary for the processing of textile fibers. The for-profit hospital industry firmly believes that hospitals and health care facilities should be able to obtain the ITC on a much larger percentage of their total construction costs. Hospitals have many unique construction attributes, stricter building code requirements, and more specialized output than does a textile manufacturing plant. Thus, the industry should be able to avail itself of an increased amount of ITC. The very necessity of asepsis in virtually all areas of hospitals should automatically render the associated construction costs of these areas eligible for the ITC just as are other special purpose facilities, such as textile manufacturing plants. For example, laminar flow suites used in operating rooms provide 100 percent continuous air filtration during surgical procedures, turning the air over approximately forty to fifty times per hour and costing approximately $50,000 per suite. Notwithstanding the foregoing, the present inclination of the Internal Revenue Service is to deny the ITC on this type of very specialized equipment on the rationale that it is attached to the building. The for-profit hospital industry strongly believes that the original intent of Congress would allow the ITC for the above described types of equipment. However, litigation will probably be necessary to resolve the matter.

Fiscal policy must constantly be updated to accommodate the changing character of the economy. The hospital industry is an essential part of the delivery of health care, and, as in other industries, needed and necessary investment should be encouraged via the ITC. Federal law exists to prevent overexpansion and construction of unneeded facilities or additions of unneeded services.

POLICY AREA FOUR: FINANCING HIGH TECHNOLOGY EQUIPMENT

Since 1965, the health care industry has experienced tremendous acceleration in the cost of medical equipment. The costs of equipment for a hospital currently amount to at least 20 percent of the total cost of a hospital project. For example, in 1966, the cost of a standard radiographic and fluoroscopic (X-ray) room was approximately $75,000. In 1976 the cost of the same radiographic and fluoroscopic facility is nearly $135,000—an 80 percent cost increase in just ten years. With similar cost increases in general construction costs over the same time span, many prospective hospital endeavors are made prohibitively expensive because of the large initial investment and/or excessive debt service requirements. As a result, a combination of additional equity participation, equipment financing, or leasing is required to equip a modern health care facility adequately.

Medical equipment cost increases are due to both increases in the general price level during the past decade and technological advances which have rendered obsolete much existing equipment and provided a new and improved supply. All areas within a hospital have seen changes in technique and instrumentation, but the most significant improvements during the past decade have been made in the laboratory, surgical, and radiology departments. To illustrate this point, Table 6-10 indicates certain items of equipment which have been developed or dramatically improved in these areas.

In addition to the above-mentioned supply factors, certain demand factors dictate that health facilities offer a certain amount of "high technology equipment" to be competitive:

1. Consumer demand for health care is almost entirely dependent on the decisions of physicians. Since clear-cut measures of "output" and "quality of care" are not available, problems arise associated with "Cadillac tastes" for medical services. Frequently, doctors and patients "demand" the newest, most modern medical equipment. Doctors expect the best which medical technology can offer and utilize facilities which offer the "best" in equipment. To the extent that patients must go to facilities where their physicians practice, consumers also "demand" this equipment. Perhaps the most recent example of such

Table 6-10. Schedule of Major Hospital Equipment Developments

| | | Life | | Additional |
Item Description	*Current Cost*	*Eco-nomic*	*Financial*	*Personnel Required*
Laboratory				
Blood Gas Analyzer	$18,000	5 years	10 years	1
Electrolyte Automation	15,000	5	10	0
Automated Chemistry Analyzer	100,000	5	10	3
Automated Cell Counters	58,000	5	10	2
Automated Differential Counter	100,000	5	10	0
Surgery				
Surgical Monitoring	1,400	5–10	10	0
Image Intensification	55,000	10	10	1
Hypo-Thermia Units	3,000	5–10	10	0
Advanced Orthopaedic Power Unit	1,000	7–10	10	0
Laminar Flow Suites	50,000	N/A	N/A	2
Phaco-Emulsifier	25,500	7–10	10	1
Surgical Microscopes	15,000	10	10	1
Radiology				
Mammography Unit	57,000	5–7	10	1
Cardiac Catheterization Laboratory	250,000	7–10	10	–
Computerized Axial Tomography (Head)	360,000	5–7	10	3
Portable X-Ray Unit	23,000	7–10	10	–
Ultra Sound Unit	70,000	5–7	10	1

Source: Hospital Corporation of America.

"demand" for high technology equipment is the new, computerized axial tomography (CAT) scanner. This scanner sometimes provides additional diagnostic information and with less discomfort and secondary hazards to the patient. However, that the diagnostic information will lead to a better outcome of a patient's illness is quite unclear at this time.

2. To the extent that the ominous threat of malpractice suits persists, physicians and hospitals will insist that all available technology and equipment be used as a "defense" against potential malpractice litigation. Patients will demand that they be treated with all available technology and equipment, or they will allege malpractice and poor quality of care.

However, financing this "high technology equipment" can be extremely troublesome:

1. One notable characteristic of today's medical equipment is its very rapid rate of obsolescence. As shown in Table 6-10, the economic life of much of this equipment is approximately five years. A health facility must constantly engage in a planning and financing process to obtain the latest in equipment. And, since equipment manufacturers are among the more aggressive in their research and development activities, one can expect an ever-increasing rate of obsolescence in many areas of medical equipment.

2. Due to this extremely limited economic life, neither major nor minor movable equipment is mortgageable. Most of this equipment has little resale value and, while mortgages are sometimes available, they are rare. Innovative financing arrangements are required. Health facilities must find additional equity or make substantial debt financing commitments and suffer the debt service requirements. For many small investor-owned hospitals, these capital requirements are unmanageable, and, while investor-owned groups enjoy a comparative advantage, they are still faced with an absolute financial hardship.

3. As shown in Table 6-10, the economic life of much of this equipment is only one-half of its financial life, and a serious cash flow problem arises. Health facilities are forced to "carry" a piece of equipment on their books long after the equipment has become obsolete and been replaced.

4. Traditional economic theory regarding substitution between inputs (labor and capital) does not often apply in the health care industry. Invariably, when a health care facility adds a new piece of capital equipment, several additional workers are required (see Table 6-10). As the technical aspects of equipment increase, these workers are increasingly more skilled *and* more expensive. The inelasticity of substitution of capital for labor was recently discussed by Vladeck.

When General Motors buys an automated welding machine, it engages in classic substitution of capital for labor. More cars can be produced by fewer employees. But when a teaching hospital buys a new blood analyzing machine or equips a new cardiac surgery unit, it is expanding the range or improving the quality of services that can at best be provided with the same personnel and that may, more likely, require the time and effort of still more expensive professionals.[29]

Costs associated with the additional labor demand weigh heavily on institutions' operating budgets. For example, while the purchase price of the CAT scanner is $360,000, its operation requires three additional skilled personnel and its estimated yearly operating cost is closer to $500,000.

Policy Intervention Area

At the current time, there is no answer to just how much technology is enough. Quality of care depends on continuing research and the development of appropriate technology for diagnosis and treatment. Through certificate of need legislation, health systems agencies are able to control the proliferation of equipment with costs greater than $100,000 in the delivery of health care services. Physicians, however, are not subject to certificate of need legislation and, therefore, danger of some perverse "equipmentation" persists. PSRO legislation and third party payer cost containment pressure could reduce superfluous utilization.

Several policy areas are amenable to change to facilitate equipment financing where it is deemed necessary and is approved by the appropriate health systems agency.

1. Because of rapid rates of obsolescence, shorter depreciation schedules should be enacted to equate more evenly the financial and economic life of equipment and to allow for more reasonable recovery of costs.
2. Due to the risky nature of equipment financing and the substantial capital sums that are required, government loan guarantees to health facilities would lessen the risk of such ventures and mitigate the risk to equity and/or debt financing.
3. The 1962 investment tax credit provisions could be altered to provide additional tax credits in certain high technology equipment approved in the certificate of need process.

While the "easing" of fiscal policy financing provisions for equipment will be interpreted by some to be analogous to "adding fuel to the fire," one must remember that there are many areas of the country where health care facilities, particularly acute-care hospitals, are nonexistent. Given the equipment requirements of hospitals and the unique attributes of today's high technology equipment, equipment financing is currently a significant impediment to private corporate investment in health care facilities.

The government should address the financing problems attendant on equipping health care facilities to insure adequate quantity and quality of health services in all areas of the country.

POLICY AREA FIVE: INDUSTRIAL REVENUE
BOND FINANCING

On April 1, 1976, Senator Lloyd Bentsen introduced S-3241, a bill to amend the Internal Revenue Code of 1954, to provide an exclusion from gross income for the interest on certain government obligations, the proceeds of which are used to provide hospital facilities. Since 1968, the Internal Revenue Code has allowed government agencies to issue industrial revenue bonds in six categories with all interest being tax exempt. These categories include:

1. air or water pollution control facilities;
2. convention or trade show facilities;
3. sewage or solid waste disposal facilities and facilities used to furnish electricity, gas, or water to communities;
4. airports, docks, wharfs and other mass commuting facilities and any packing, storage, and training facilities directly used by mass commuting facilities;
5. sports facilities;
6. residential real estate used for family units (urban renewal bonds).[30]

Normally, there is a $5 million ceiling per issue on tax exemption for industrial revenue bonds. This ceiling applies to total capital expenditures made on a project during the first three years preceding, and for three years following, the issuance of bonds. The interest exemption was allowed because of the high cost of constructing facilities in these six categories and because the facilities were deemed to be needed by the public and to serve a public interest. Senator Bentsen's bill simply added "hospital facilities" to the above list of six categories that are not subject to any ceiling.

When Senator Bentsen introduced S-3241, he said, "Hospitals serve a vital public need. There is no justification to give priority to convention halls and sports facilities as compared to health facilities."[31] Indeed, the exclusion of hospital facilities places the entire health care industry at a competitive disadvantage vis-à-vis the six exempt categories in the sale of industrial revenue bonds. However, Senator Bentsen went on to point out that the legislation was uniquely needed in another way. He noted: "This legislation is needed to assure an adequate supply of health services in rural and inner-city sections of the United States. Historically, investor-owned hospitals have located in rural areas with inadequate health facilities."[32] Unfortunately, the Bentsen bill was defeated in September, 1976.

Policy Intervention Areas
Industrial revenue bonds are dominant financial instruments in underwriting the costs of hospital construction. When the 1968 amendment to the 1954 Internal Revenue code was made, the $5 million ceiling sufficiently covered the

cost of constructing a 200-bed hospital facility. However, the 1976 construction cost of the same 200-bed facility is over $11 million. With current construction costs, the $5 million ceiling permits construction of only an 80-bed hospital, and such a small facility is often uneconomical.[33]

There has been much recent debate on the problem of surplus unnecessary hospital beds. However, certificate of need provisions in P.L. 93–641 should prevent perverse building of hospital facilities. Furthermore, extensive feasibility studies are typically required by bond underwriters to document the needs of a community before any bonds are marketed. Because of these two "checks," more lenient bond financing by investor-owned hospitals simply would not result in the creation of unneeded facilities.

Nonprofit hospitals finance approximately 40 percent of all new construction and/or modernization through industrial revenue bonds and, in 1975, financed over $4.3 billion of hospital projects with this instrument.[34] In addition to being tax-exempt, nonprofit hospitals are also subject to unlimited use of industrial revenue bonds and this imparts an additional bias against investor-owned hospitals, which are subject to the current $5 million ceiling.

POLICY AREA SIX: THE MALPRACTICE QUESTION

Problems related to malpractice insurance have been thrust into prominence recently because of dramatic increases in malpractice awards by juries and the concomitant increases in costs for physicians and hospitals. Since 1974, the annual cost of investor-owned hospitals' malpractice insurance premiums has risen from $4 billion to $15 billion,[35] and the cost of the premiums alone currently amounts to approximately $5.00 per patient day.

Given this scenario, managers of hospitals carefully assess the impact of the malpractice problem. Insurance premiums are significant cost items, and expenses ancillary to any litigation are generally exorbitant. Contingency fee financing creates an incentive for attorneys to encourage malpractice litigation. Furthermore, involvement in malpractice litigation may result in surplus requirements and unfavorable ratings by insurance companies which impinge on the medium- and long-run financial flexibility of a corporation. While few hospitals or other health facilities cannot now obtain malpractice insurance coverage, in some areas the policies are available from only one company and rates are almost prohibitively high. In seven states in the United States there is only one malpractice carrier, and in eleven other states there are only two. Investors are, therefore, uneasy about the ability of health care facilities to prevent large future increases in the cost of malpractice insurance coverage even if they have group buying power leverage, good claims experience, and adequate quality control. One of the larger proprietary hospital groups has resorted to self-insurance with the purchase of excess liability in the marketplace.

Policy Intervention Areas

Gradually, people are realizing that the profits and assets of insurance companies and the incomes of physicians are derived from policyholders and patients, who suffer the cost of health care as a result of malpractice and often still receive less than one-third of the settlement, if any damages are ever awarded.[36] The federal government is beginning to engage in additional control and regulation. During 1976, thirty-seven states plan to take specific action toward mitigating the increasing costs and resolving other problems associated with malpractice litigation. Potential investors view the limitation of recoverable damages, the scheduling of attorney fees, and reasonable statutes of limitations to be potential tools for reducing the financial risks from malpractice litigation. However, such actions are frequently being challenged for constitutional reasons. Insurance pools jointly underwritten by many carriers and the state or federal government would guarantee malpractice coverage to all care providers at reasonable rates. Action by other states and an expanded role of PSROs may mitigate the future negative impact of malpractice litigation on private investment in health care facilities. Without policy changes, the malpractice dilemma looms as one deterrent to private corporate investment in the health field, since prudent investors will consider the alternative investment value of the huge sums currently devoted to the area of malpractice.

POLICY AREA SEVEN: THE COST-EFFECTIVENESS OF BUILDING CODES AND THEIR IMPACT ON CONSTRUCTION COSTS OF HEALTH FACILITIES

In 1971, the Comptroller General of the United States completed a comprehensive study of the construction costs of health facilities. With respect to the impact of building code requirements on construction costs, he reported:

> The problem of multiple regulatory and code requirements, often conflicting and duplicative, has plagued the construction industry for years. The full effect in terms of construction costs, delays in construction, and suppression of innovation can probably never by precisely measured; but . . . it is certainly significant.[37]

The basic problem is the great degree of duplication and fragmentation of building codes. For facilities receiving Medicare or Medicaid reimbursement, compliance with the Hill-Burton regulations (General Standards of Construction and Equipment for Hospital and Medical Facilities) is required. In addition to this set of regulations, three other "model codes" provide the basis for most state and local building codes. These codes are used randomly across the country:

West — Uniform Building Code (1927) of the International Conference of Building Officials, Inc.

South — Southern Standard Building Code (1946) of the Southern Building Code Congress, Inc.

North — Basic Building Code (1950) of the Building Officials and Administrators, Inc.

In addition to these codes, the National Fire Protection Association (an open membership organization) publishes the Life and Safety Code and National Electric Code which set standards regarding fire safety.

The multiplicity, duplication, and fragmentation which result from these several codes imposes significant administrative costs on health facilities. The following situation was cited in the Comptroller General's report. Medicare required automatic sprinkler protection in all hospital areas, while the state and local codes required sprinkler protection only in nonoccupied areas and smoke detectors in patient rooms. Hospitals, however, had to comply with both sets of codes and install *both* smoke detectors and sprinklers in patient rooms. It should also be pointed out that the Comptroller General found that the different code requirements were based largely on "the subjective views of the groups' members" and that, generally, specific requirements were "proposed by members or other interested parties, such as suppliers of materials . . . ."[38]

In addition to numerous codes, there are numerous federal, state, and local agencies which are involved in their interpretation and enforcement. Tables 6-11 and 6-12 dramatically illustrate the great duplication and fragmentation of codes and code enforcement agencies.

Table 6-11. State and Local Codes and Regulatory Agencies Applicable to Health Facilities in California

State
California Public Health Code
California Public Safety Code
California Building Standards Code
California Professional and Vocational Standards Code
California Institutions Code
California Industrial Relations Code

Local
Building Department
Fire Department
Planning Department
Public Health Department
Sanitation Department
Air Pollution Control Agency
Flood Control Agency
Industrial Waste Control Agency

Source: The Comptroller General of the United States, *Study of Health Facility Construction Costs* (Washington, D.C.: U.S. Government Printing Office, 1971), p. 202.

Table 6–12. Non-Federal Agencies Affecting Hospital Projects in New York City

---

State
Department of Mental Hygiene
Department of Education
Department of Health, Division of Hospital Review and Planning
Department of Health, Bureau of Maternal and Child Health
Department of Health, Division of Environmental Health
New York State Hospital Review and Planning Council

Municipal
Planning and Zoning Commission
Building Department
Fire Department
Department of Water Supply, Gas and Electricity
Department of Hospitals
Board of Standards and Appeals
Department of Health

Non-Governmental
Regional Planning Councils
Joint Commission on Accreditation
Insurance Companies

Source: The Comptroller General of the United States, *Study of Health Facility Construction Costs* (Washington, D.C.: U.S. Government Printing Office, 1971), p. 202.

Policy Intervention Areas

At the present time, there is no reliable knowledge as to the cost effectiveness of health facility building code requirements. Furthermore, the incidence of serious high-loss fires in health care facilities is very low, though these few fires receive substantial unfavorable publicity. For example, in a survey of 938 fire situations in seventy-five hospitals, the National Fire Protection Agency found that only 11 percent were large-loss fires (property damage greater than $1,000 or loss of life) and only 0.7 percent resulted in bodily injury. Furthermore, only 6 percent occurred in patient-occupied areas.[39]

Duplication and fragmentation of existing codes and a lack of knowledge as to the cost-effectiveness of building codes result in substantial construction cost increases for health care facilities. Time delays are inherent, and in one state the total time required for inspection and approval of health care facilities is six months while construction costs increase approximately 1 percent per month.

While the Comptroller General found that the model code groups were able to act as a "clearing ground for suggested code requirements," he concluded that these groups lacked technical expertise and financial resources to conduct appropriate comprehensive analysis. The Comptroller recommended that HEW adopt a common code for Hill-Burton, Medicare, and Medicaid inspections and direct the Facilities Engineering and Construction Agency (FECA) and the National Bureau of Standards (NBS) to pursue scientific research in the area of fire prevention and to make the data available to the model code groups for appropriate utilization.[40]

Such recommendations are useful. However, more direct coordination of the model code groups and other codes is necessary. The three model code groups recently formed an "umbrella" organization, the Council of American Building Officials, which has indicated interest in cooperation with the FECA and NBS research.

If the health care industry is to obtain optimal allocation of the health care dollar, careful future attention should be focused on building code requirements in order to insure cost effective construction of health care facilities. More cost effective codes would also certainly facilitate private financing of health care facilities.

SUMMARY

The investor-owned hospital industry is currently a $3.8 billion business and is the fastest growing segment of the health care industry.[41] As shown in Table 6-13, traditional contributed sources of capital construction funds are diminishing and there is increased dependence on debt financing.

The 1977 Bill-Burton funding provides for no construction funds for hospitals. Given the dynamic increase in third party payment (particularly federal and state) for health services, strong participation by the investor-owned sector is needed if a capital shortage similar to that currently experienced by Great Britain is to be avoided. As one observer wrote: "The new generation of proprietary hospitals began with the firm conviction that socially responsible, creative capitalism, with reasonable profit as an incentive, can place the operation of the health care system on the same efficient basis as that of other industries."[42]

The various policy areas discussed in this paper will exert substantive impact on the future role of the investor-owned sector. In most cases, the problems result from inequitable treatment under dated legislation and the persistence of

Table 6-13. Sources of Capital for Construction Projects: Nonfederal Short-term Hospitals

	Year	
Source	*1969*	*1973*
Private Grant	15.1%	10.4%
Government Grant	26.1	15.7
Retained Funds	23.8	16.4
Borrowing	35.0	57.5

Source: Paul Ginsburg, "Inflation and Hospital Capital Investment," in M. Zubkoff (ed.), *Health: A Victim or Cause of Inflation?* (New York: Prodist, 1976), p. 167.

the health industry to favor "unchanging organizational concepts that have existed for years."[43]

The matrix in Figure 6-2 summarizes the impact of existing inequities, in each of the key policy areas that are discussed in this paper, on investment behavior in the investor-owned segment of the health care industry.

NOTES

1. *Proprietary Hospitals and Associated Products* (New York: Frost and Sullivan, Inc., 1974), pp 1–2.

2. Stuart Altman and J.P. Eichenholz, "Inflation in the Health Industry: Causes and Cures," in M. Zubkoff (ed.), *Health: A Victim or Cause of Inflation* (New York: Prodist, 1976), p. 7.

3. Karen Davis, "Economic Theories of Behavior in Nonprofit, Private Hospitals," *Economics Business Bulletin* 22, 2 (1972), and Jonathan Ogur, "The Nonprofit Firm: A Test of the Theory for the Hospital Industry," *Economic Business Bulletin* 26, 2, (Winter 1974).

4. Bruce C. Vladeck, "Why Nonprofits Go Broke," *The Public Interest* 42, 1 (Winter 1976):93.

5. Ibid., p. 91.

6. Frost and Sullivan, *Proprietary Hospitals,* p. 102.

7. Daniel J. Edelman, "Fact Sheet on Investor-Owned Hospitals," (Washington, Federation of American Hospitals, 1975).

8. Ibid.

9. Ibid.

10. Michael D. Bromberg, "Rates of Return for Investor-Owned Hospitals," (Washington, Federation of American Hospitals, Feb. 9, 1976), mimeographed, p. 5.

11. D. Salkever and T. Bice, "The Impact of Certificate of Need Controls on Investment," *Health and Society* 59, 3 (Summer 1976):209.

12. Robinson-Humphreys, *Special Report on Hospital Management* (Atlanta: Robinson-Humphreys Co., Inc., May 1976), pp. 17–18.

13. State of New York Budget Bills S–7287–A and A–9257–A, January 1976.

14. Joseph G. Sprague, "The Need for Ambulatory Care Facilities," *Hospitals* 50, 3 (1976):57.

15. *Hospitals* 49, 20 (October 16, 1975):61.

16. *Hospitals* 50, 12 (June 16, 1976):13.

17. Bromberg, "Rates of Return," pp. 1–2.

18. *Smith v. Ames,* 169 U.S. 466, 1898.

19. *FPC v. Memphis Light, Gas and Water Division,* 411 U.S. 458, 1973.

20. George Washington University, *The Evolution of Long-Term Care in the United States,* School of Government and Business Administration, monograph, September 1969, p. 41.

21. National Center for Health Statistics, *Selected Operating and Financial Characteristics of Nursing Homes,* Division of Health Resources Utilization Statistics, 1974, p. 3.

Figure 6-2. Impact Matrix

Key Policy Areas	Capital Formation — Fixed Capital: Debt	Equity	Depreciation	Replacement Obsolescence	Working Capital	Capital Allocation: Inter-Industry	Intra-Industry	Intra-Firm	Service Areas: Acute Care	Long-Term Care	Ambulatory	Equipment	Intervention: Legislative	Judicial	Regulatory Agency
1. Regulation:															
a) Certificate of Need	±	±	±	±	0	±	±	±	±	±	±	±	X		Health Systems Agencies
b) NHI	?	?	?	?	?	?	?	?	?	?	?	+	X		
c) PSRO	0	0	0	0	0	+	0	±	-	+	+	+	X		PSROs
d) Price Regulation	-	-	0	-	-	-	-	±	-	+	-	-	X		States Fed. Govt.
e) Incentive Cost Control	+	+	+	+	+	+	+	±	+	+	+	-	X		3rd Party Pyrs/HEW
2. Medicare-Medicaid Reimbursement:															
a) Return on Equity	+	-	0	-	-	-	-	0	-	-	0	0	X	X	HEW
b) Stock Maintenance	0	-	0	-	-	-	-	0	-	N	-	0	X	X	HEW
c) Income Taxes	0	-	0	-	-	-	-	0	-	-	-	0	X	X	HEW
3. Investment Tax Credit	-	+	-	-	0	-	-	±	-	-	0	-	X		IRS
4. Financing High Technology Equipment	-	-	-	-	-	0	0	-	-	N	+	-	X		IRS
5. Industrial Revenue Bond Financing	-	0	0	-	-	-	-	0	-	-	-	-	X		IRS / HEW
6. Malpractice	-	-	0	0	-	-	0	0	-	-	-	-	X	X	
7. Building Codes	-	-	0	0	-	-	0	-	-	-	+	0			Various Code GRPS

+ = Positive Impact
- = Negative Impact

N = Only Minimal Negative Impact
± = Net Uncertain

? = Policy Outcome Uncertain

22. *The New York Times,* June 1, 1976.

23. Victor L. Fuchs, *Who Shall Live?* (New York: Basic Books, 1974).

24. National Health Center for Statistics, *Selected Financial and Operating Characteristics,* p. 3.

25. Social Security Administration, Office of Research and Statistics.

26. Ibid.

27. *Hospital Statistics,* 1975 Edition, p. 194.

28. Altman and Eichenholz, "Inflation in the Health Industry," p. 10.

29. Vladeck, "Why Noprofits Go Broke," p. 95.

30. Bromberg, "Rates of Return."

31. U.S. Senate, *Congressional Record,* S. 3241, April 1, 1976.

32. Ibid.

33. Ibid.

34. Bromberg, "Rates of Return."

35. Federation of American Hospitals, *Review* 8, 3 (June-July 1975).

36. Ibid.

37. The Comptroller General of the United States, *Study of Health Facility Construction Costs* (Washington, D.C.: U.S. Government Printing Office, 1971), p. 207.

38. Ibid., pp. 31–32.

39. Charles C. Spalding, "The Frequency, Cause, and Prevention of Hospital Fires," *Fire Journal* 69, 2 (March 1975):36–37.

40. Comptroller General, *Study of Health Facility Construction Costs,* pp. 23–24.

41. Federation of American Hospitals, *Review,* p. 8.

42. Mark S. Levitan, "The Impact of the 'New Generation' of Proprietary Hospitals on Health Care," *Hospital Progress* 51, 7 (July 1970):65.

43. Ibid., p. 62.

Discussion of
Inducements and Impediments for
Private Corporate Investment in the
Delivery of Health Services

Martin Feldstein

Mr. Hill has emphasized the specific impediments that currently exist to corporate investment in hospital care. He has also discussed in some detail the types of tax incentives, reimbursement rules, and loan programs that he believes would stimulate each investment. I want to deal with a more basic question: What is the reason (if any) for society to encourage *corporate* investment in hospitals instead of relying exclusively on the currently dominant nonprofit form of hospital ownership? I believe that our current approach to financing hospital care leaves little social justification for corporate investment. Moreover, if we continue the current comprehensive insurance financing, corporations and investors will be understandably deterred from entering the hospital care field. I believe that only if we change our financing method to stimulate more diversity of care will there be a legitimate role for corporate hospitals. Let me now explain these remarks more fully.

I would preface this explanation by saying something more general about the desirability of relying on the market and on profit-seeking companies:

I believe that one of the most important things that we teach in economics is that the competitive market and the profit motive are generally the best way to allocate resources.

At least since Adam Smith, economists have understood that individuals who act out of self-interest can thereby achieve the allocation of resources that is *socially* most desirable.

The social virtue of the profit-seeking company is easy to understand. In their search for profits, companies are forced by competition to produce the goods and services that consumers want (and are willing to pay for) and to produce them at the lowest possible cost. Since we generally assume that individuals are the best judges of their own best interest, firms that seek profits are induced to provide the goods that consumers should have.

I believe that even when the conditions required to make this argument fully valid are satisfied only approximately, it is generally the best policy to leave the allocation of goods and services to the market and to rely on profit-seeking firms rather than on public bureaucracies or voluntary organizations.

Despite my general preference for the market and the profit-seeking firms, I believe that the conditions in the hospital care industry today do not imply that for-profit hospitals are a socially efficient or desirable way to produce hospital care.

A crucial step in the argument for relying on profit-seeking firms in general is that that is the best way of making the provision of goods and services correspond to the *preference of consumers* as indicated by their willingness to pay. However, because of extensive insurance, consumers' demand for hospital care is greatly distorted. The use of profit-seeking firms may be the best way to make providers sensitive to consumers' demands but, when those demands themselves are distorted by insurance, there is no social virtue in encouraging such a responsiveness of providers.

I think that the most important thing about hospital care today is that insurance (both private and public) pays 92 percent of all hospital costs. At the time that they receive care, patients pay only 8 percent of the cost of that care. The decisions that patients and doctors make about the use of hospital care is overwhelmingly influenced by the fact that the patient pays such a small share of the costs. We should not be surprised by the explosive increase in spending on expensive tests or other services when an extra $100 of spending will cost the patient only an extra $8. With this financing situation, hospitals compete primarily in terms of the quality and style of care. There is little *diversity* in the styles of hospital care because our heavily insured patients are essentially unconcerned with cost at the time that they consume care. Moreover, the doctors who advise patients and make the detailed choices on their behalf are aware of their patients' thorough insurance coverage. The result of this extensive insurance has been to extend the provision of hospital care far beyond the point where an extra dollar's worth of cost is justified by the benefits that it produces. It would not be much of an exaggeration to say that our current insurance provides a strong incentive to expand spending on hospital care until the last dollar's cost is worth only 8¢, as perceived by patients and their doctors. Much of the increase in hospital cost that has become such a subject of public concern is really a reflection of the growth of insurance.

This problem of a *demand for care that is distorted by excessive and almost complete insurance* has three implications for corporate investment in hospital care:

1. *It would be wrong at the present time to encourage more investment in hospital care.* Since insurance has already led to an overextension of investment

in hospital services, there is little reason to encourage corporations to do more investing in hospital care. While there may be particular locations in which more hospital building would be desirable, in general we should be interested (at least for the next decade) in less building and fewer additions of equipment.

2. If there is a further case for private corporate investment in hospital care, the case must be that private corporations respond better to market incentives to provide efficiently the products that consumers really want. *Since the current hospital market incentives are so grossly distorted by insurance, there is no reason to believe that the profit motive will encourage provision of the socially correct level of hospital care or the provision of care in an efficient way.* If our financing system were reformed to place more emphasis on extensive coinsurance for middle and upper income households,[1] the market incentives would improve and there would be a clearer case for the private hospital corporation. Moreover, substantial coinsurance rates would encourage the provision of a diverse mix of different styles of hospital care. Private corporations and the competitive process might respond best to this new opportunity.

I might summarize my first and second points by saying that what we need is not more investment in hospital care of the current kind, but the creation of greater diversity of hospital care. The market incentives to provide such diversity will be present only if we reform the financing of care by replacing our current comprehensive "first-dollar" insurance by an insurance system that places more emphasis on out-of-pocket payments by individual patients. Only then will there be an extensive role for private corporate investment.

3. With 92 percent of hospital costs paid by insurance, hospitals cannot be left for long to decide their own standards of care and charges. The federal and the state governments have responded to the explosion of hospital costs by proposing and introducing detailed controls on hospitals. This provides a very insecure framework for corporate investment. As long as the vast majority of hospitals are nonprofit institutions, the regulatory agencies are unlikely to be responsive to the concerns of the for-profit hospital corporations. While short-term profit opportunities may now be considerable, the potential growth of adverse regulation makes long-term commitments to hospital plant and equipment hazardous. The extent of regulation will increase in the future only if hospital bills are essentially all paid by third parties. Only the more active and competitive market for hospital care that would result if individuals were financially responsible for more of the cost of their own care is likely to be free enough from detailed government regulation to provide a receptive environment for corporate investment.

NOTES

1. See my proposal in "A New Approach to National Health Insurance," *The Public Interest,* Spring 1971.

Discussion of
Inducements and Impediments for
Private Corporate Investment in the
Delivery of Health Services

Mary A. Wrenn

Mr. Hill's paper reviews the growth in demand for health services, the rising cost of such services and the relevant technological, legislative, and regulatory factors impacting the availability and cost of health care delivery. The author has concentrated on the role that investor-owned entities, especially large investor-owned hospital groups, play in the current health care industry and the intra- and interindustry inequities which impinge on the viability of the investor-owned sector.

In order to assess correctly the desirability of removing impediments to private corporate investment in health care services and the encouragement of the growth of the publicly or investor-owned hospital and other health care delivery agencies, it might be well to:

1. determine the benefits to industry, government and the patients of such public ownership;
2. define objectives of investors; and
3. examine whether and how the health care delivery system appeals to the investor.

The more important reasons for encouraging private corporate investment in the health care delivery system include historical evidence that private enterprise is more efficient in (a) attracting and motivating capable, talented people to operate a business profitably and (b) developing innovative systems to modernize and improve industries.

The increased complexity of business, the costs of conforming to government regulations and the advantages that a company or institution with financial resources and talent has in capitalizing on the advances in communications all favor the large company in almost every industry. This is especially true in a service industry where there is seldom protection of a patented product or proprietary brand name. The challenges facing the health care delivery industry in the United States demand the best talent available to resolve them successfully.

When operated efficiently, the investor-owned company generally establishes standards which can apply to an entire industry. The benefits of such achievements to the public which it serves are illustrated in the records of food retailing with the rise of the supermarket, general merchandising in the development of the discount chain, and the success of the fast food chain in the restaurant industry.

The health care industry is uniquely different from the foregoing examples. However, as the author has noted, the benefits of efficiency of size (bulk purchases, standardization, access to professional personnel) enabled hospital chains to construct hospitals at a cost of approximately $35,000 per bed in 1974 while the average cost per bed for the Hill-Burton financed hospitals was $50,000. Privately owned hospitals are also following the lead of the publicly owned groups in consolidating purchases of supplies and employing professional managers to streamline operations and reduce costs to the benefit of the total health care costs. If these premises are valid, investor-owned health care delivery groups are, and should continue to aid in, containing the cost of health care.

Investor-owned health care delivery groups can also help to meet the escalating capital needs for financing health care in offsetting the declining flow of philanthropic funds for the underwriting of health facilities. Insofar as availability of capital to an investor-owned company is contingent on that company's operating performance, the risk of large capital losses due to internal management errors appears minimized.

The basic objectives of investing, as defined by Graham and Dodd, are the preservation of capital combined with a satisfactory return (i.e., income) or capital appreciation. Capital, in the form of fixed income or debt securities, is made available by the investor to private, government and investor-owned companies. Risk capital in the form of equity financing, however, is available only when the investor expects future rewards to outweigh risks of such investments. Therefore, it is elementary that, to be attractive, common stock investment must be in a company capable of generating profits in order to justify its purchase over other investment alternatives.

The health care delivery industry meets the criteria of an attractive area of common stock investment. The industry's growth, as documented in Mr. Hill's paper, is above that of the economy, increasing at an annual rate that is more than twice that of the Gross National Product. Moreover, the health facilities segment of health care is in a period of transition from a cottage type industry to one which provides opportunities for profit generation through the application of managerial expertise, professional business systems, innovation, and economies of scale to the benefit of both the user (or patient) and the investor. However, unless the regulatory environment is conducive to rewarding the entrepreneur who successfully demonstrates an ability to offer quality health care profitably and at a competitive price, risk capital will not be available to the industry.

The justification for an adequate return on equity in a regulated industry is to attract capital to meet the financial requirements of the industry. If the health facilities industry is not able to accumulate capital and cannot raise it through philanthropy, it must raise it through public borrowing, equity financing or direct government grants. The relevant measure of the security of a debt instrument, absent of a government guaranty, is the prospect for payment of interest and repayment of the principal by the borrower. The proponent of the nonprofit entity in the facilities segment of the health care industry argues that the increased assurance of revenue generation from third party payers, including Medicare, Medicaid, Blue Cross, and private insurers, is sufficient security for the public lender. In providing a base of equity investment for part of its capital needs, however, the publicly owned for-profit hospital improves the security of its debt instruments. Also, because of a more balanced capitalization, it is in a position to obtain credit at a lower interest rate, thus reducing its operating costs and rewarding the purchaser of its stock in the form of earnings and dividends.

Without repeating the detailing of inequities that are outlined in Mr. Hill's paper, I would like to concentrate on the qualitative assessment of the industry under various constraints placed on the for-profit sector of the industry by the changing dynamics of health care technology, by third party reimbursement policies and by government regulation of the type, quality, availability, and cost of health care services.

One of the prime requisites for attracting equity investment in a company is investor confidence in the environment of the industry in which it operates.

The health care industry appears to be on a collision course as government imposes stringent standards for suppliers of health care products and, simultaneously, unrealistic formulas on reimbursement for making such quality products available to the patient. Rapid advances in medical therapy technology, while benefiting the quality of health, are increasing the fixed investment and working capital requirements of the hospital industry and its operating costs. Concurrently, the restructuring of the industry as a result of the National Health Planning and Resource Development Act is disrupting nonprofit hospital operations in areas of overbedding such as New York.

The political appeal to constituents of a broad National Health Insurance program has caused both administrations to advocate its enactment. Such a program will undoubtedly expand the demand for health care and increase the utilization of health facilities. Concern on the part of the investor, as well as of members of the health care community, is that the enactment of such a plan will be based on political rather than economic rationale, thus further jeopardizing the position of the efficient provider of health care, including the investor-owned hospital groups.

The inducements to corporate investment in health services that were mentioned earlier threaten to be nullified by many of the policy areas that are discussed by the author. Certain of these policies appear detrimental to the nonprofit segment of the industry as well. They also tend to discourage efficiency and foster the escalation, rather than the containment, of the nation's total health care bill.

Of these, the most apparent contribution to increased costs to the patient appears to be the costs-plus-a-reasonable-rate-of-return method of reimbursement for services. Such reimbursement provides little encouragement to improve operating efficiency on the part of the administrator of the nonprofit hospital or other health facility.

To the investor-owned company, the interpretation of "reasonable costs" in Medicare reimbursement is particularly burdensome. In all industry, taxes are regarded as a legitimate cost of doing business. The return on equity and on total capital, essential measurements of the soundness of a publicly owned corporation, are determined net of taxes. Failure to consider taxes as a reasonable cost in Medicare reimbursement formulas appears contrary to established guidelines in other regulated industries. If the for-profit hospital is an important contribution to the cost effectiveness of the health care system as it exists today and if, indeed, as the author has noted, the for-profit hospital group is filling a void in the availability of health care by establishing hospitals in localities having no primary care, its existence appears both socially and economically desirable. A change in present reimbursement formulas to include taxes among reasonable costs is necessary for the viability of the investor-owned segment of the industry.

Of equal concern to the observer of the health services industry are arbitrary price controls by national, state, or local governments. Such controls affect the profitability of investor-owned hospitals, resulting in a reduced cash flow, and they discourage new investment in this segment of the industry. Moreover, they reduce the quality of health care that is provided by the entire industry through the inability of hospitals to provide newer, more advanced products and services which improve patient care and, ultimately, reduce total costs by more effective and faster treatment.

Another area mentioned by Mr. Hill where a more progressive posture on the part of government is needed is in the allowable depreciation of equipment. The rapid development of medical technology has tended to obsolete existing equipment, making the present financial life of equipment unrealistic. Not only does this present cash flow and other financing problems for all hospitals, but it also makes the analyst and the sophisticated investor suspicious of the balance sheet of publicly owned companies and acts as a deterrent to investor interest in the industry. Thus, the publicly owned company is in a quandry. To attract patients and avoid threat of malpractice suits it must have the most advanced medical equipment that is demanded by both doctors and patients. If it is not able to recoup the costs of capital equipment, it faces a cash flow problem and weakens its ability to raise funds for growth. An alternative available to the industry, including the for-profit hospital group, is the leasing of equipment with rentals included in operating costs. An added appeal of leasing equipment is that the requirement of a certificate of need for equipment purchases of over $100,000 is avoided. The obsolescence factor in equipment is included in lease rentals, resulting in an addition to reimbursement costs of third party payers. The adoption of realistic depreciation allowances appears more effective in containing the costs of health care and meeting the medical needs of the community, especially with the monitoring under certificate of need and PSRO legislation to prevent proliferation of equipment purchases.

Mr. Hill has also cited other impediments to the profitability of, and resultant deterrents to, corporate investment in the health services area. These include the reporting requirements of regulatory agencies and the growth in the ambulatory care market which is fostered by government support.

Reporting requirements of government agencies and other regulatory authorities are becoming an increasing problem for all industry. Because of the degree of government involvement in health care, resources of health care facilities are particularly burdened by such paperwork. While simplification is certainly desirable, one can also argue that a responsible large corporation is much better equipped to perform such functions at the least cost and, indeed, aid in reducing such costs as are incurred by the nonprofit hospital through providing computer services to the latter for a fee. It thus appears to be a reason for encouraging the trend toward large investor-owned groups.

Outpatient services and ambulatory care appear to be a desirable adjunct to inpatient hospital care, providing that quality of care is maintained. Medical therapy has advanced to where many procedures and patient treatments can be made on an outpatient basis. Such treatment is not only less costly, but, often, less traumatic for the patient than being hospitalized. Large investor-owned hospital companies are excellent vehicles to coordinate outpatient services and ambulatory care clinics with inpatient hospital care and they also lead in the efficient combination of comprehensive care units in the health care complex in localities in which they operate. However, because of their possible adverse impact on the profitability of the total hospital complex, as cited by the author, it may be wiser to have the growth of such centers monitored, to have the conversion evolutionary rather than revolutionary and, possibly, to provide subsidies, where justified, to hospitals which can document that such departments are adversely impacting the profitability of services which it must maintain for the patient who does require hospitalization.

In assessing the attractiveness of the nursing home and home health care market as an area of corporate investment, the greatest impediments today, in the case of nursing homes, are the early abuses, immediately following the enactment of Medicaid, by the publicly owned corporate entity because of unqualified managers and the more recent widespread publicity given to abuses by individual, investor-owned homes. Against this background, it is questionable whether equity investment would be available to the industry even if existing impediments such as inadequate Medicaid reimbursement were removed. If the investor-owned corporate hospital group remains a viable and profitable growth entity in the health service field, ultimate expansion into the nursing home or extended care facility segment of the industry could very well be justified and attractive for both the company and the investor.

While certain health care companies, notably pharmaceutical firms, do operate home health care divisions, it is as yet too early to determine whether the service area of this market is conducive to investor-owned corporate ownerships.

CONCLUSION

The health care industry is dynamic and changing. Producers of health care products, including pharmaceuticals and nondrug items, have a much longer history of corporate ownership and have operated profitably under government health care programs in foreign countries. While the return on investment for such firms has been high and the growth in earnings outstanding, such performance has not been at the expense of the patient, as witnessed by the decline in the prices of drugs that were introduced a decade ago or the average cost increase of all drugs relative to the consumer price index.

Admittedly, the nature of the health services industry differs markedly from that of the pharmaceutical industry in cost composition, capital requirements, community demands, and the limited "market" which each hospital or health facility serves. The health services industry, especially the hospital, has little control over its source of revenues, the patients, who are referred to it by doctors. Moreover, payment for the largest portion of its revenues is by government or other third parties which also regulate such reimbursement.

The escalating cost of health care is primarily due to the demand for, and availability of, more sophisticated quality medical therapy and the rising costs of both professional and other personnel within a hospital. Opportunities do exist, however, to improve the cost structure of the health service industry, particularly within the hospital complex, without impairing the quality of care. Encouragement of the entire medical community to maximize the efficiency of the delivery of health care appears mandatory if the United States is going to provide quality medical care and yet contain the so-called health care cost explosion.

The investor-owned hospital group is supported by private corporate investment in the form of debt and equity. The profit motive has been a strong inducement to advances in other services that are essential to the quality of life. An important role for the corporate form of ownership in the future health services field appears desirable in order to assure benefits to the public from its efficiencies. Proprietary hospitals, following the uneven profit performance of earlier years as an emerging growth industry, are regaining a position as a growth area of equity investment in the stock market with the consolidation among larger, better managed companies. In turn, because of their record, size and proven managerial capabilities, the leading investor-owned hospital groups appear to be the most feasible means of channeling private risk capital in the form of equity investment into the health services field. The removal of impediments to its ability to compete with others for the funds that are available for investment by both institutions and individuals is thus justified, in the writer's opinion, for both social and economic reasons.

Discussion

Dr. Feldstein: We should examine the question of whether for-profit hospitals really are a viable alternative over a period of time in the current environment. Bear in mind that hospital costs rose about 20 percent last year and that this rise has been typical since Medicare and Medicaid. Unless we have a restructuring of financing, the end is going to come in one of two ways. One is going to be direct controls of the sort envisioned by the Talmadge bill, and the other is national health insurance.

We are going to see a change to a system of heavy regulation. Since the vast majority of providers are voluntary, the standards of any new controls will be set to accommodate that segment of the industry, and not the relatively small number of for-profit institutions. I cannot see how, in that context, one can be very optimistic about the rate of return available for for-profit hospitals.

Mr. Lewin: In a recent study that we undertook, we were asked to compare the investor-owned industry with the not-for-profit hospitals. We found that, in general, the cost to patients for comparable service and comparable diagnosis in for-profit hospitals was higher and, even more surprising, that the cost of the unit of care in these hospitals was also higher. These proprietors have chosen to operate in states that have no rate review and, also, in states where Blue Cross is paying charges rather than costs. There is very little incentive for these hospitals to operate differently, so that even though the capacity is there and the managerial skill is there, the fact that charges are not imposed has resulted empirically in less effort to put care on an efficient basis.

Mr. Baker: I have had an opportunity to review that Lewin study that was contracted by the Blue Cross Association. Two outside analysts also reviewed the study and challenged it in terms of sample size and the age of the hospitals.

Mr. Lewin: Even given the analysts' objections, I think that our study still shows that investor-owned hospitals are not efficient. But the real question is not whether they are, but whether they can be, and what incentives are needed. Is a cost-based national insurance system really the only alternative? In fact, we can come up with an areawide pricing system that does provide incentives for efficiency.

Dr. Feldstein: I believe that the social case for for-profit hospitals, as well as the improvement of our hospital care market in general, rests on our ability to change the financing, to restructure insurance and to have more substantial copayment by middle and upper income families.

Right now, the United States government, through the special tax treatment of insurance payments and, in particular, the exclusion of employer payments for health insurance in the calculation of taxable income, provides a subsidy of about $8 billion a year for first-dollar coverage. If we changed our tax laws, wouldn't the unions and the workers want a different kind of insurance? Doesn't the current picture of very comprehensive insurance reflect the fact that, at the margins, employees are choosing between 65¢ after tax in their pocket, or $1.00 spent by their employers on behalf of them in the purchase of health insurance?

Mr. J. Hill: I would agree with much of what Dr. Feldstein says, but we are dealing with the real world and our present hospital system, and I doubt that any new ideology is likely to win out in the near future. Anyone who has had an opportunity to negotiate labor contracts or has had a chance to work with employees knows that coinsurance is a lovely dream. They all want first dollar coverage for everything, from anesthetics to a broken toe, and to try to override that is very difficult, although theoretically, I would love to.

Mr. Lewin: For-profit hospitals tend to be much more luxurious, to offer more amenities, such as offices for physicians on the premises.

Mr. J. Hill: Everybody says that the doctors are omnipotent but we have at least made some progress in this area. In one town where we were building a hospital, the doctors submitted a list of demands. We refused to provide unnecessary services, and most of their demands were turned down. To my mind, that is the name of hospital planning.

Mr. Kelling: Mr. Hill, there was a bill in Congress that would have permitted proprietary hospitals to issue tax-exempt bonds over the $5 million limit to finance new construction, but it did not pass. What effect does that experience have on your future plans for financing construction of new facilities and how do you plan to raise new capital in the debt market for new construction?

Mr. J. Hill: We were terribly disappointed to have that particular provision written out. Where are we going to get the capital? Frankly, we have to pay more money for our long-term debt. Our equity is fairly cheap; we pay only about 9 percent of our earnings in dividends, and the balance of it we use as equities to finance new hospitals. Our debt to equity ratio is 60/40, so as long as we have a real need for hospitals, we can use that remaining equity to finance them. I would have to say that currently there is no real lack of capital for a project that is well conceived, that is needed, that is well planned, and that has reasonable planning approval.

Dr. White: I would hope that the discussion would focus more on the question of how to get capital organized under health care systems that are fully integrated and responsive to the needs of the people. That is where the savings are to be found—in the provision of early treatment, early diagnosis, prevention, the appropriate use of technology and the full spectrum of services. I would argue that there is at least 30 percent fat in the system, and plenty of room to form capital, to reward excellent management, and to get the necessary leverage for change.

Chapter 7

A Survey of the History and Current Outlook of Philanthropy as a Source of Capital for the Needs of the Health Care Field

Joseph V. Terenzio

EARLY HISTORY OF PHILANTHROPY IN HEALTH CARE

Charity, mutual help, and aiding the needy poor are some of the basic principles on which the major world religions were founded. The sick poor were taken care of in fifth century (B.C.) hospitals of Buddhist India, in the temples of Egypt, and in the "sick houses" of Israel. Priests and monks practiced medicine and cared for the sick in early Christian monasteries. These were the beginnings of medical care systems in various parts of the world.

However, this tradition of charity was slow to catch up with the early pioneering spirit of America. Because the early settlers were stubborn individualists and firm believers in hard work, it was not until the development of urban population centers that care of the ailing and the accompanying need to train health professionals led to the birth of voluntary health care facilities as we know them today.

The hospitals founded in America during the eighteenth and early nineteenth century were, by and large, not governmental undertakings.[1] Inspired by the teachings of the noted clergyman, Cotton Mather, Benjamin Franklin, aided by philanthropic support, founded the Pennsylvania Hospital in 1751.[2] The establishment of the New York Hospital in New York City, in 1771, and the Massachusetts General Hospital in Boston, in 1811, followed by the same basic course.[3] Ever since these early beginnings, voluntary hospitals, along with private physicians, formed the basis for the acute-care medical care system of the United States. It should be noted, however, that persons with chronic illnesses were restricted to treatment in the public hospitals of the day. Throughout most of the nineteenth century it was thought that the chronically ill, the "incurable," and the "insane" were not fit for admission into voluntary hospitals. For the chronic patients there was the "workhouse," the "almshouse," or some other publicly funded institution.[4]

As for medical schools, the first three were established at the College of Philadelphia (now the University of Pennsylvania) in 1765, at King's College (now Columbia University) in 1768, and at Harvard College in 1783. However, a proliferation of private "for-profit" schools arose during the nineteenth century. The standard of education in these proprietary institutions was characteristically low, yet their numbers tended to dominate the field throughout the 1800s.

Medical education improved markedly as a result of the Flexner Report of 1910 ("Medical Education in the United States and Canada"), which was commissioned by the Carnegie Foundation for the Advancement of Teaching. In his report, Abraham Flexner condemned the low standards of proprietary schools and criticized the poor quality of education in university-affiliated medical institutions of the day. Due largely to mounting pressure from government, almost all of the proprietary schools closed after the Flexnor Report was made public. Thus, voluntary, university-affiliated, medical teaching institutions of the early twentieth century entered upon an era of preeminence with help from the public sector and philanthropy; we are currently, to a large extent, still witnessing that era of a largely voluntary health care system in America.

SCOPE OF THE PAPER

This paper deals with a survey of the history and current outlook of philanthropy as a source of capital for the needs of the health care field, with due consideration being made for specified changes in federal and state policies. Hospital inpatient care, extended care facilities, physician services, and ambulatory care settings are the main components of the health care system that are considered. Traditionally, philanthropy had a major role in hospitals, medical teaching institutions, and extended care facilities, including nursing homes. These three areas currently constitute more than four-fifths of health care capital investment.

For the purposes of this paper we are dividing the functions of capital formation and usage into three major categories: (1) physical assets, both fixed and movable, (2) working capital, and (3) human resources. Philanthropic giving consists mainly of individual gifts and contributions, endowments and bequests, corporate and foundation grants.

This paper is based on an analysis of data from secondary sources and a nationwide sample survey of health care facilities by questionnaire. The nationwide sample includes twenty hospitals, twelve extended care facilities, and ten medical schools, all voluntary nonprofit organizations (see Appendix 7A).

The conclusion is based, in part, upon discussions with experts in the field of health care financing in the New York City area (see Appendix 7B: List of Discussants).

HISTORICAL PERSPECTIVE

Hospitals, along with physician services, comprised the largest part of our health care system through the early part of this century. As a result of numerous contributions from American industrialists of the late nineteenth and early twentieth century, voluntary hospitals came into existence. There was virtually no significant borrowing or public sector involvement for the general care needs of our nation at that time. In 1929, the last year of the pre-depression boom, philanthropy contributed 50 percent of the capital financing for all medical care facilities, both public and private[5] (see Table 7-1).

Health care capital funding was severely affected by the onset of the depression of the 1930s. In 1935, funding for the construction of medical care facilities dropped to one-fourth, and philanthropic funding to one-tenth of 1929 levels.

The beginning of the Second World War further depressed private and public giving to health care. It took the passage of the Hospital Survey and Construction Act of 1946 (P.L. 79-725) to stimulate the capital funding of health care. The Act, popularly known as the Hill-Burton program, is the most significant event, to date, in the formation of capital for the health care field.

The Hill-Burton program acted as a catalyst in attracting funds from philanthropists. Its requirements of two-thirds financing from nonfederal sources provided an initiative for fund-raisers to seek contributors for capital projects. In just two years, from 1948 to 1950, philanthropic contributions for capital projects increased 277 percent (Table 7-1).

The data (Table 7-2) from the recent United Hospital Fund survey (hereinafter referred to as the UHF survey) also indicate that contributions to private hospitals for capital financing increased from 46 to 53 percent with the passage of the Hill-Burton Program.

The philanthropic share began to decline after the passage of Title XVIII and XIX of the Social Security Act in 1965 (P.L. 89-97). These amendments, popularly known as the Medicare and Medicaid programs, initiated a new era in our nation's health care system. With these programs, the government, for the first time, committed a major portion of its resources to the provision of health care for the aged and the needy poor. The concept, as well as the action, was much needed, but the long-term consequences to the economics of the health care system as a whole proved disastrous. The federal outlay for health care programs increased tenfold in just ten years, from $2.8 billion in fiscal 1965 to $28.5 billion in fiscal 1975. State and local funding also increased threefold during the same ten-year period.[6] Within a short time, Medicare and Medicaid became two of the most controversial publicly funded programs in our brief history of social legislation. One unfortunate consequence of this legislation was a gradual but marked reduction in the granting of Hill-Burton funds, from almost 14 percent of the total in 1967 to 2.5 percent in 1974.[7] Although philanthropic contributions for capital projects increased in dollars from $650 to $775 million between

Table 7-1.   Philanthropic and Federal Contributions to the Construction of Health Care Facilities in Millions of Dollars and by Relative Percentage

Year	Total Cost	Philanthropic Contributions	Percentage Of Total	Federal Contribution (Hill-Burton Grants)	Percentage Of Total
1929	$207	$102	49	–	–
1935	58	10	17	–	–
1940	131	31	24	–	–
1945	139	30	22	–	–
1946	122	*	–	–	–
1947	170	*	–	–	–
1948	349	62	18.1	$74	21.2
1949	679	101	14.9	75	11.1
1950	737	172	23.3	150	20.3
1951	947	209	22.1	85	9.3
1952	867	197	22.7	82	9.5
1953	682	158	23.2	75	11.0
1954	697	168	24.1	65	9.3
1955	673	177	26.3	96	14.2
1956	626	163	26.0	109	17.4
1957	875	202	23.1	123	14.5
1958	990	240	24.2	119	12.0
1959	998	228	22.9	184	18.4
1960	1,102	268	24.3	184	16.7
1961	1,174	328	27.9	184	15.6
1962	1,406	432	30.7	209	14.8
1963	1,546	455	29.4	217	14.0
1964	1,762	599	34.0	216	12.0
1965	1,837	647	34.0	217	11.8
1966	1,903	619	31.0	257	13.5
1967	1,930	650	33.6	267	13.8
1968	2,164	524	24.2	265	12.2
1969	2,500	450	17.9	*	*
1970	3,291	*	*	295	8.9
1971	3,550	*	*	172	4.8
1972	4,081	*	*	*	*
1973	4,145	730	17.6	46	1.1
1974	4,427	775	17.5	110	2.5
1975	4,500	705	15.6		

Sources: Social Security Bulletin, February 1975, Social Security Administration; "Giving U.S.A.," American Association of Fund-Raising Counsel, Inc., New York, N.Y.; Herbert E. Klarman, "Role of Philanthropy in Hospitals," *American Journal of Public Health* 52, 8 (August 1962); and C. Rufus Rorem, "Capital Financing for Hospitals," Health and Hospital Planning Council of Southern New York, Inc., June 1968.

*Note: Blanks in table indicate information not available at time of issuance of report.

Table 7-2. Philanthropy's Contribution to Capital Financing by Percentage 1945–1975: Results of the United Hospital Fund Sample Survey (5/76)

	Before 1945	*1946 to 1965*	*1966 to 1975*
Hospitals	46	53	40
Extended Care Facilities	70	74	53
Medical Schools	50	50	34

those years,[8] their share in total funding dropped from 33.6 percent in 1967 to 17.5 percent in 1974 (Table 7-1).

The recent UHF survey indicates that the share of philanthropic contributions for capital projects in voluntary not-for-profit hospitals decreased from 53 percent in the pre-Medicare period to 40 percent afterwards. Extended care facilities also experienced a drop, from 74 percent to 53 percent during those two periods. Similarly, medical schools witnessed a decrease from 50 to 34 percent (Table 7-2).

PRESENT CONDITIONS AND TRENDS IN THE CAPITAL FINANCING OF HEALTH CARE

The annual budget of the United States has doubled its outlay in the last four years, from around $200 billion in 1972 to $400 billion in fiscal 1976. At this rate of growth, it is expected to reach a trillion dollars in the 1980s. There may be a correlation between skyrocketing health care costs and public sector outlays. Health care expenditures have multiplied from $12 billion in fiscal 1950 to an estimated $130 billion for fiscal 1976.[9] Medical facilities' construction costs have, likewise, escalated from $737 million in fiscal 1950 to an estimated $4.65 billion for fiscal 1976.[10] Surprisingly, philanthropic contributions have kept up with this surge in capital financing costs, increasing from $172 million in fiscal 1950 to an estimated $800 million for fiscal 1976.

For the last four decades, the number of hospitals in the United States has remained fairly constant at around 7,000, but short-term general care beds in community hospitals increased from 470,000 in 1946 to 930,000 beds in 1974.[11] The average community hospital has grown in size and sophistication. Most of these hospitals are voluntary nonprofit organizations. The results of the UHF survey indicate that philanthropy contributed more than 50 percent of capital funds for these voluntary nonprofit organizations, including extended care facilities (Table 7-3).

Most health planning experts feel that the nation has a surplus of hospital beds, though beds are unevenly distributed. As our national attention has shifted toward primary care and local ambulatory care centers, the figures for Hill-Burton funding for fiscal 1974 show that 43 percent of the grants was allocated for out-

Table 7-3. Share of Philanthropic Funds for Capitalization in Institutions According to Responses to the United Hospital Fund Sample Survey

	Percentage of Philanthropy in Capitalization					
	More Than 86%	75-85%	64-74%	50-64%	25-49%	Less Than 24%
Hospitals	7	2	1	2	–	–
Extended Care Facilities	4	1	–	1	–	1
Medical Schools	–	1	1	1	–	3

patient and rehabilitation facilities and public health centers. More than 90 percent of the funds allocated for hospitals was used for modernization rather than for an increase in beds.[12] The results of our survey on capital financing also confirm that hospitals and extended care facilities used a major portion of philanthropic funds to add to, or replace, their plant facilities (Table 7-4). Trends indicate that the modernization of existing facilities and the replacement of old plants will consume a major portion of philanthropic funding in the future. Acquisition of new equipment, research and education will be other areas to be funded.

The UHF survey indicates that there were no significant changes with respect to sources of giving to the health care field as a result of the Tax Reform Act of 1969. Although, of course, the survey is only a modest sampling of the field, the replies tended to be rather uniform from all respondents with respect to this point (Table 7-5).

ALTERNATIVE METHODS OF CAPITAL FINANCING

According to a survey conducted by the American Hospital Association in 1975, 9.8 percent of all of the hospital construction, both public and private, in 1974 was funded by philanthropic contributions.[13] As recently as 1968, 20 percent of all hospital construction was funded by philanthropic giving.[14] At the same time, Hill-Burton grants have tapered off from a high of $295 million in 1970 to $110 million in 1974.

Today, hospitals are increasingly forced to rely on borrowing to finance their capital projects. The share of debt-financing in hospital construction rose from 32 percent in 1969 to 58 percent in 1974.[15] This rapid growth in borrowing is an unfortunate development for the health care field. Table 7-6, showing a capital investment model, illustrates the impact of alternative methods of funding of a project with an outlay of $10 million. The financing alternatives are treated exclusively in order to highlight differences.

It is evident from our comparative capital financing model that the best possible funding sources are, first, philanthropy and then, internal operations. How-

Table 7-4. Outlay of Philanthropic Capital Funds by Percentage, from the United Hospital Fund Sample Survey

	Before 1945	*1946– 1965*	*1966– 1975*	*1976– 2000*
Hospitals				
Construction of New Facilities	48	57	60	49
Modernization of Facilities	27	20	13	24
Purhcase of Equipment	20	17	16	16
Research and Education	5	6	11	8
Other	–	–	–	3
Extended Care Facilities				
Construction of New Facilities	37	50	66	50
Modernization of Facilities	13	14	8	10
Purchase of Equipment	10	8	6	11
Research and Education	2	3	2	3
Other	38	25	18	26
Medical Schools				
Construction of New Facilities	N.A.	28	47	22
Modernization of Facilities	N.A.	13	18	19
Purhcase of Equipment	N.A.	17	18	29
Research and Education	N.A.	40	14	30
Other	N.A.	2	3	–

Table 7-5. Sources of Philanthropic Funds for Capital Financing Projects by Percentage and by Philanthropic Category, from the United Hospital Fund Sample Survey

Type of Institution	*Individual Gifts, En- dowments & Bequests*	*Corporate Giving*	*Founda- tion & Other Giving*
Before the Tax Reform Act of 1969			
Hospitals	83%	12%	5%
Extended Care Facilities	72%	13%	15%
Medical Schools	61%	18%	21%
After Passage of the Tax Reform Act of 1969			
Hospitals	83%	11%	6%
Extended Care Facilities	77%	11%	12%
Medical Schools	53%	28%	19%

Table 7-6. Alternative Methods of Capital Financing: Total Overall Cost to the General Public

Philanthropy	Government Grants	Source of Funding	Debt	Internal Operations
$10 million from donors + approx. $3 million in tax deductions	$10 million in tax dollars	Initial Outlay	$10 million + $0.3 to $0.5 million in debt placing costs	$10 million from internal operations
$1 to $2 million in fund-raising costs	$0.2 to $0.3 million in feasibility and other studies	Additional Costs	$20 million over 25 years at an average interest charge of 8% per year	None
$4 to $5 million (fund-raising costs plus tax deductions)	$10.2 to $10.3 million	Total Overall Cost over 25 Years to the General Public	$30.3 to $30.5 million	$10 million

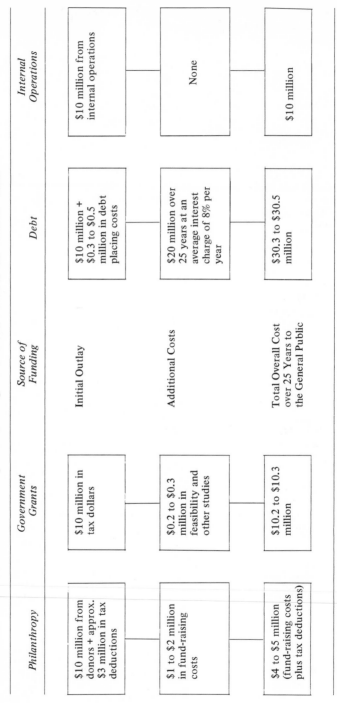

ever, of late, largely inadequate reimbursement rates and inflationary operating costs have made accumulated earnings disappear from the balance sheets of medical care institutions. In 1974, accumulated earnings from internal operations contributed 12.7 percent of total hospital construction costs.[16] More equitable reimbursement rates and controlling the costs of health care are the two items which can have the greatest impact on generating revenues which can be used for financing hospital construction costs. The next best alternative method of financing capital projects appears to be government grants. The Hill-Burton program exemplified the benefits that this method of funding can bestow upon the health care community. It stimulated the philanthropic sector and helped make the United States hospital care system the most extensive one in the world.

Government funding through outright grants has become a part of the history of American health care capital financing. It may yet play a significant role in medical care reorganization under the National Health Planning and Resources Development Act of 1974 (P.L. 93–641). Yet, without the passage of a universal National Health Insurance Act, there is little hope for large-scale contributions by federal and local governmental sources to finance health care construction projects.

The gradual withdrawal of support from government grants and internal operations as sources of funding is leading health care providers to rely on debt-financing to fund capital projects. It is apparent from the UHF study of alternate methods of financing that capital financing by borrowing is the most expensive method of all the alternatives. It is estimated that for every dollar borrowed, the consumer ends up paying three dollars for capital and interest charges over a normal investment life of twenty-five years.

Philanthropy, at the present time in the history of financing of health care projects, appears to be a viable source of capital funding. In the present economic atmosphere, the loss of tax revenue is the only significant cost to government and the consumer. Through philanthropy, capital funds are contributed by donors who can generally afford them. Philanthropic contributions must be considered not only for their monetary nature, but, also for their value in terms of personal commitment to the health care system. Voluntary participation on the part of individuals and communities remains a significant avenue of contribution to the improvement of health care.

CONCLUSION

This section has two basic themes. The first is a series of remarks on the nature of philanthropy as a source of capital funding for the health care field. The second is a policy-oriented look at where we are now in the evolution of philanthropy as a source of health capital and what might be done to improve upon philanthropy's current role.

Much of the following was inspired by discussions with experts on philanthropy and capital financing of health care in the New York City area (see Appendix B: List of Discussants).

Any complete discussion of philanthropy's role in the capital financing of health care should include, at least, a brief discourse of the nature of philanthropic giving. It must be said, first, that philanthropy in the health care industry is not a nationwide phenomenon. There are vast areas of our country in which the role of philanthropy in the formation of health care capital is minor, at best, and often nonexistent. Philanthropic support of health care, which has been most significant in the large cities of the Northeast and the Midwest, is very rare in many regions of the country, notably in the Far West, Northwest, and Rocky Mountain states. In the western-most portions of our nation, health care institutions, since their beginnings, have traditionally received large portions of their support from public sources and, of course, from operating income.

In addition, the nature of philanthropic support varies by location of institution and type of service-area. For example, the suburban community hospital can look with reasonable expectation toward private giving as a source of capital development since suburbanites, who usually possess a high degree of identification with their community health care, feel a commitment to their local institutions and, in turn, give with relative enthusiasm. City-dwellers, on the other hand, have become accustomed to generous government programs and support in the last decade, and tend to feel less of a personal responsibility for financing health care. In addition, there may be several competing health care facilities within walking distance of the city-dweller's home. This situation helps form the illusions of abundance and fiscal self-sufficiency in health care services of our large cities.

It seems that the initiative to give is partially regulated by the degree of necessity that is perceived by the prospective giver. With the increasing role of government in today's cities, it is easy for urbanites to feel that government will take care of the financial needs of health care institutions.

The systematization of giving is another factor which affects the philanthropic public. Over the years, efforts by federated campaigns such as "Community Chests" and "United Funds," have had two basic effects. The first is to increase the volume of philanthropy within the area of operation of the "federation," and to centralize and decrease overall fund-raising cost. This is basically a positive effect. However, the second effect, which is to place the gift in higher abstraction, that is, to remove the giver's feeling of identification with the actual gift, may prove, in the long run, to be detrimental to philanthropy as a source of support.

Again, it is most important that the giver and his family be able to identify with the gift. In this way, the existence of the service or institution which is the recipient of the gift remains a reinforcer of the philanthropic act. This type of reinforcement is likely to encourage more giving from those associated with the original giver. If the object of the gift becomes abstract beyond simple identification, the philanthropic initiative stands to be extinguished.

Another phenomenon which deserves mention is the changing nature of the philanthropic public. Because of changes in the tax laws of our nation, patterns of inheritance, migration of wealth, and the rapid development of federated campaigns, gifts are becoming generally smaller, and from a wider constituency. Legacies of large sums of money from powerful industrialists for use as capital for the health care field are fast becoming a rare phenomenon. As wealth becomes more distributed among the nation's population, so does giving.

Since World War II, the United States has witnessed great change in the financing of its health care. The Hill-Burton program, Medicare and Medicaid, and the growth of the health insurance industry, discussed earlier, were major change agents in the transformation. American philanthropic participation in the health care field, a phenomenon developed well in advance of World War II, has been eclipsed, to a large extent, by the health care reforms of postwar America.

Whether philanthropy in health care is good for the American people is a much debated matter. Those who support the furtherance of philanthropy often present the following arguments:

1. Philanthropy in health care has enabled much research into areas which would have remained untouched if they were left to government financing.
2. Philanthropy brings with it a tradition of moral commitment which transcends the financial aspect.
3. Government officials, especially those in local government, are discovering that the obligation to fund health care through local funds is expensive and is contributing to the fiscal demise of our large cities.
4. Funds obtained through philanthropic sources are, by their nature, least costly to the general public.
5. Philanthropic contribution gives concerned nonhealth professionals an opportunity for input into the health care system.
6. Giving brings with it a feeling of responsibility to those who participate in it. It guards against attitudes of indifference which can be harmful to the quality of life in America.

Those who believe that philanthropy in today's health care environment is not a positive force, offer other arguments:

1. Philanthropy, at least large gift-giving, creates a system of elitism, wherein certain individuals, because of their contributions, stand to receive a better class of health care, than do the "ordinary citizenry."
2. Philanthropists retain a disproportionately large influence over the formation of institutional health care policy, as their gifts are highly sought after.
3. Since most of the funds for the operation of the health care industry are fur-

nished through government and other third party payers, as a result of contributions to general revenues and health insurance, it is inconsistent that the philanthropic interest should be catered to.

4. Reliance upon philanthropic contributions removes the responsibility to provide for the general health of the people from government which, some believe, is the natural repository of that responsibility.

5. Philanthropists often do not contribute to areas of greatest need.

6. Philanthropy is often subject to whim, tax loopholes, stock market prices, deaths in the family, etc. These factors make philanthropy too unstable a resource to use for adequate planning.

It is obvious that there is more than a grain of truth on each side of the issue. Those who take the negative side raise serious points concerning accountability in philanthropic giving. Those who take the positive side properly identify difficulties associated with public funding of health care. Combining these arguments, we can see a question emerging: *Can philanthropy in health care be a viable force in a society of increasing governmental controls and public participation?* If it can, what can be done to improve its quality? The following is a list of possibilities which might be considered toward improving the quality of philanthropy in the health care field in the coming years:

1. Educate the potential philanthropic audience as to the most pressing needs in health care so that its gifts will be best placed.

2. Develop links between health planning and philanthropy so that regional priorities in health care can be best served by philanthropic giving.

3. Develop expertise on the staffs of such federated charities as "United Funds" and "Community Chests," so that distribution of their health care funds serves the best purposes.

4. Develop selective tax incentives so that high-priority items in the health care field receive the greatest share of the philanthropic dollar.

5. Expand the definition of philanthropy to include the donation of valuable time and services by those who have much to offer to the health care system.

6. Explore the creation of regional philanthropic foundations for health care so that the advantages of pooled philanthropic resources in health care can be realized.

7. Develop mechanisms to create public accountability concerning the use of all philanthropic funds for health care, so that the value of the gift is not far exceeded by the costs of upkeep which the public must bear.

8. Create tax incentives for philanthropic participation for those other than the wealthiest among us. If we are to achieve the positive participatory effects of philanthropy to the greatest extent, we must expand the philanthropic audience.

9. Segregate the financing role of government in health care from the role of philanthropic contributors. These two groups should not be in competition for the same territory. Both philanthropy and government have their place in the funding of health care.

10. Design a type of Hill-Burton program to address the health care needs in America today. The maldistribution of health care resources and the sky-rocketing costs of health care can be addressed by programs created through the federal government, furnishing matching-funds or "challenge money" to prospective philanthropic sources. Though the needs of today's health care system are largely "nonstructural," that is, not concerned with the creation of more buildings and beds, there are certainly important national health priorities which need the commitment and funding of private sources. The need for primary care services in our inner cities and rural areas is an example of where philanthropic funds might be channeled.

It is clear that philanthropy remains a valuable source for capital funding of the health care industry. However, if philanthropy is to survive, we must scrap the philanthropic effort as it was known to the "robber barons" of the early American Industrial Revolution. We must work to bring accountability and broad public participation into a field which is often thought of as the province of the rich and powerful.

If something as important as the health care of our nation is to be dependent upon the gifts of a few, philanthropy's future in the health care field is headed for disaster. If, on the other hand, philanthropic giving is incorporated into a system of accountable, rational health planning and resource allocation, the nation stands only to gain from the generous gifts of those who care enough to support all of us.

APPENDIX 7A
UNITED HOSPITAL FUND SURVEY

Methodology in Brief

The nationwide sample to survey the capital financing of health care facilities consisted of twenty hospitals, twelve extended care facilities, and ten medical schools, all voluntary, nonprofit organizations. The survey response was 65 percent (13) for hospitals, 58 percent (7) for extended care facilities, and 70 percent (7) for medical schools. The responses are analyzed into unweighted averages. This method is not meant to yield accurate prediction of national trends. The responses are merely indications and opinions of a sample of concerned professionals.

Survey Sample

Hospitals

Illinois Masonic Medical Center
Chicago, Illinois

Evanston Hospital
Evanston, Illinois

The Presbyterian Hospital in the City
of New York
New York, New York

The Roosevelt Hospital
New York, New York

Sinai Hospital of Baltimore
Baltimore, Maryland

Good Samaritan Hospital
Phoenix, Arizona

California Hospital Medical Center
Los Angeles, California

C.F. Menninger Memorial Hospital
Topeka, Kansas

Methodist Hospital of Indiana
Indianapolis, Indiana

Children's Hospital Medical Center
Boston, Massachusetts

Strong Memorial Hospital of the
University of Rochester
Rochester, New York

St. Joseph's Hospital
St. Paul, Minnesota

Cape Cod Hospital
Hyannis, Massachusetts

Kaiser Foundation Hospital
Los Angeles, California

Providence Medical Center
Portland, Oregon

Swedish Hospital Medical Center
Seattle, Washington

Grady Memorial Hospital
Atlanta, Georgia

St. Paul Hospital
Dallas, Texas

St. Luke's Hospital
Denver, Colorado

Western Pennsylvania Hospital
Pittsburgh, Pennsylvania

Extended Care Facilities

Masonic Home
Wallingford, Connecticut

Scandinavian Home for the Aged
Cranston, Rhode Island

Goodwin House
Alexandria, Virginia

United Church Retirement
Homes, Inc.
Newton, North Carolina

Baptist Towers
Atlanta, Georgia

Tanner Manor and Gardens
Phoenix, Arizona

Home for Jewish Parents
Oakland, California

Lutheran Welfare Service of Illinois
(Region II)
Chicago, Illinois

Villa Clement, Inc.
West Allis, Wisconsin

St. Cloud Hospital
St. Cloud, Minnesota

Riverside Presbyterian House
Jacksonville, Florida

Rocky Mountain Residence
Denver, Colorado

Medical Schools

Stanford University School of
Medicine
Palo Alto, California

Yale University School of Medicine
New Haven, Connecticut

Georgetown University School of
Medicine
Washington, D.C.

Rush-Presbyterian-St. Luke's
Medical Center
Chicago, Illinois

Medical College of Wisconsin
Milwaukee, Wisconsin

Tulane University School of Medicine
New Orleans, Louisiana

Washington University School of
Medicine
St. Louis, Missouri

Albert Einstein College of Medicine
New York, New York

Meharry Medical College School of
Medicine
Nashville, Tennessee

Eastern Virginia Medical School
Norfolk, Virginia

Questionnaire
The Role of Philanthropy in Capital Financing

Volume of Philanthropic Funds

I. What, in your estimation, is and has been the share of philanthropy in your institution's capital financing during the following periods:

A. 1945 and the preceding years (pre-Hill-Burton):
____ (81-100%)   ____ (61-80%)   ____ (41-60%)
____ (21-40%)   ____ (0-20%)

B. 1946-1965 (post-Hill-Burton and pre-Medicare and Medicaid):
____ (81-100%)   ____ (61-80%)   ____ (41-60%)
____ (21-40%)   ____ (0-20%)

C. 1966-1975 (post-Medicare and Medicaid):
____ (81-100%)   ____ (61-80%)   ____ (41-60%)
____ (21-40%)   ____ (0-20%)

II. What would you estimate the philanthropic share of your institution's capital financing to be during the coming 25 years, under the following circumstances:

A. Implementation of the National Health Planning and Resources Development Act of 1974 (P.L. 93-641) and in the event of passage of a Universal National Health Insurance Act:
____ (81-100%)   ____ (61-80%)   ____ (41-60%)
____ (21-40%)   ____ (0-20%)

B. Implementation of the National Health Planning and Resources Development Act of 1974 (P.L. 93-641) but *without* the passage of a Universal National Health Insurance Act:
____ (81-100%)   ____ (61-80%)   ____ (41-60%)
____ (21-40%)   ____ (0-20%)

Uses of Philanthropic Funds

III. What percentage of your institution's capital funds was expended on the following categories:

A. 1945 and earlier years:
____ Construction of new facilities
____ Modernization of existing facilities
____ Purchase of equipment
____ Research and education
____ Other (Please specify) _____
100% TOTAL

B. 1946-1965:
____ Construction of new facilities
____ Modernization of existing facilities
____ Purchase of equipment
____ Research and education

___ Other (Please specify) _____

<u>100</u>% TOTAL

C. 1966-1975:

___ Construction of new facilities

___ Modernization of existing facilities

___ Purchase of equipment

___ Research and education

___ Other (Please specify) _____

<u>100</u>% TOTAL

IV. What would you estimate the percentage of capital funds your institution will be spending on the following categories during the coming 25 years (under the assumption of the implementation of the National Health Planning and Resources Development Act):

___ Construction of new facilities

___ Modernization of existing facilities

___ Purchase of equipment

___ Research and education

___ Other (Please specify) _____

<u>100</u>% TOTAL

Sources of Philanthropic Funds

V. What percentage of philanthropic funds for your institution's capital projects comes from the following sources:

A. Before the passage of the "Tax Reform Act of 1969":

___ Individual gifts

___ Individual endowments and trusts

___ Corporate gifts

___ Corporate trusts and endowments

___ Other (Please specify) _____

<u>100</u>% TOTAL

B. After the passage of the "Tax Reform Act of 1969":

___ Individual gifts

___ Individual endowments and trusts

___ Corporate gifts

___ Corporate trusts and endowments

___ Other (Please specify) _____

<u>100</u>% TOTAL

VI. What is the response rate to the fund raising efforts since the passage of the "Tax Reform Act of 1969":

A. ___ Greater than before the passage

___ About the same

___ Less than before the passage

B. What would you perceive to be the response rate if the "Filer Commission" (Report of the Commission on Private Philanthropy and Pub-

lic Need, "Giving in America: Toward a Stronger Voluntary Sector")
recommendations are enacted into laws:

___ Greater than before the enactment

___ About the same

___ Less than before the enactment

VII. What is the approximate cost of raising funds, expressed as a percentage of total philanthropic contributions to your capital projects:

___ (0-10%)   ___ (11-20%)   ___ (21-30%)

___ (31-40%)   ___ (41-50%)   ___ (51% and above)

VIII. What do you believe is the ratio between government and philanthropic funds for your institution's capital projects:

Govt.		*Phil.*		*Govt.*		*Phil.*
___ 5	to	1	___ 1	to	5
___ 4	to	1	___ 1	to	4
___ 3	to	1	___ 1	to	3
___ 2	to	1	___ 1	to	2
___ 1	to	1			

APPENDIX 7B LIST OF DISCUSSANTS

Mr. Gilbert Bernstein
Director of Development
Church Charity Foundation of
   Long Island

Mr. Donald F. Carrine
Director of Agency Relations
The Greater New York Fund

Mr. Charles M. Forbes
Vice President for Development and
   Public Affairs
Memorial Hospital for Cancer and
   Allied Diseases

Jack C. Haldeman, M.D.
President
Health and Hospital Planning Council
   of Southern New York, Inc.

Hugh Luckey, M.D.
President
The New York Hospital-Cornell
   Medical Center

Mr. Jospeh V. Terenzio
President
United Hospital Fund of New York

Mr. Peter B. Terenzio
Executive Vice President
The Roosevelt Hospital

Frank W. Van Dyke, M.S.
Professor of Administrative Medicine
Columbia University School of
   Public Health

NOTES

1. George Rosen, *From Medical Police to Social Medicine* (New York: Science History Publications, 1974), p.293.

2. Gordon Manser and Rosemary Higgins Cass, "Voluntarism at the Crossroads 1976," Family Service Association of America, New York, N.Y.

3. John H. Knowles, "The Hospital," *Scientific American*, September 1973, pp. 128–137.

4. Rosen, *From Medical Police to Social Medicine*, p. 293.

5. C. Rufus Rorem, "Capital Financing for Hospitals," Health and Hospital Planning Council of Southern New York, Inc., June 1968.

6. Marjorie Smith Mueller and Robert M. Gibson, "National Health Expenditures, Fiscal Year 1975," *Social Security Bulletin*, February 1976, US GPO, Washington, D.C.

7. "Hill-Burton Project Register," Volume II, 1976, U.S. Department of Health, Education and Welfare, Public Health Service.

8. "Giving U.S.A." A compilation of facts and trends on American Philanthropy for the year 1975, 1976 Annual Report. American Association of Fund-Raising Counsel, Inc., New York, N.Y.

9. Mueller and Gibson, "National Health Expenditures (1975)."

10. Ibid.

11. "Hospital Statistics," 1975 Edition, 1974 data from the American Hospital Association Annual Survey.

12. "Hill-Burton Project Register."

13. Sallie Manley, "Sources of Funding for Construction, A.H.A. Research Capsules No. 19," *Hospitals, JAHA* 49 (December 16, 1975).

14. Sallie Manley, "A.H.A. Research Capsules No. 17," *Hospitals, JAHA* 49 (July 1, 1975).

15. Manley, "Sources of Funding for Construction."

16. Ibid.

ADDITIONAL REFERENCES

Andrews, F. Emerson. "Peterson Commission Report." Review. *Foundation News*, November/December 1970, pp. 217–221.

Blendon, Robert J. "NHI: What's to be the Impact on Private Philanthropy?" *Foundation News*, March/April 1975, pp. 15–23.

Calkins, Robert D. "The Role of the Philanthropic Foundation." *Foundation News*, January/February 1970, pp. 1–13.

Fabricant, Solomon. "Philanthropy in the American Economy." *Foundation News*, September/October 1969, pp. 172–186.

Grey, Francis J. "Tax Clinic." *Hospital Financial Management*, February 1973, p. 28.

Heimann, Fritz F. "Developing a Contemporary Rationale for Foundations." *Foundation News*, January/February 1972, pp. 7-13.

Heller, Walter W. "Passing the Buck: Revenue Sharing and Philanthropy." *Fund Raising Management*, September/October 1973, pp. 27–30.

Hobbie, William H. "Nonprofit Hospitals: A Complex Economic Iceberg." *Fund Raising Management*, July/August 1973, pp. 32–33.

Koleda, Michael S., et al. "Federal/Foundation Spending: A Look at Patterns." *Foundation News*, July/August 1975, pp. 28–35.

MacCoun, Malcolm. "Capital Financing in the Health Care Industry." *Fund Raising Management*, January/February 1971, pp. 37–42.

Mahoney, Margaret E. "The American Hospital of the Future: Process of Change." *Fund Raising Management,* July/August 1974, pp. 14–16, 21.

Melnick, Norman. "Health Care of the Future: Where do Foundations Come In?" *Foundation News,* March/April 1974, pp. 10–17.

Morris, Emery W. "Private Philanthropy–Past, Present, and Future." Interview. *Foundation News,* May/June 1971, pp. 110–111.

Mortimer, Charles G. "The Part Philanthropy Can Play in our National Life." *Foundation News,* November/December 1969, pp. 240–242.

Panas, Jerold. "New Tax Law Will Force Foundations to Give More, Maybe to Hospitals." *Modern Hospital,* December 1970, p. 54.

"Perspective, 1970." A selection of articles dealing with the subject of private philanthropy. *Foundation News,* March/April 1970, pp. 45–48.

Peterson, Peter G. "The Role of Private Philanthropy in American Life." *Fund Raising Management,* January/February 1970, pp. 12–17.

Pifer, Alan J. "Revitalizing the Charitable Deduction: An Alternative." *Fund Raising Management,* January/February 1973, pp. 39–43.

Richardson, Elliot L. "Voluntary Ethic: Preserved with Individualistic Vitality." *Fund Raising Management,* May/June 1973, pp. 38–41.

Rimple, H. MacDonald. "Federal Funding Programs for Health Care Systems." *Fund Raising Management,* May/June 1971, pp. 44–46.

Rogers, David. "On Health and Medical Care." *Foundation News,* July/August 1972, pp. 5–13.

Ryan, John T. "Capital Needs of Hospitals: How Will They Be Met in the Next Twenty Years?" *Hospitals,* April 1, 1958.

Sigmond, Robert M. "Hospital Capital Funds: Changing Needs and Sources." *Hospitals,* August 16, 1965.

Smith, J. Kellum. "The Virtues of Diversity in Private vs. Government Funds." *Fund Raising Management,* July/August 1970, pp. 14–16.

"Solicitation of Charitable Funds Act: Model Legislation." *Fund Raising Management,* May/June 1974, pp. 33–37, 53.

Stambaugh, Jeffrey Lynn. "A Study of the Sources of Capital Funds for Hospital Construction in the United States." *Inquiry,* June 1967.

Swartz, William T. "Foundations in the Changing World of Medical Education." *Foundation News,* March/April 1972, pp. 15–23.

Thompson, Kenneth W. "The Future and the Foundations." *Foundation News,* September/October 1970, pp. 183–187.

Towle, William F. "Innovations in Health Care Delivery, Capital Financing." *Fund Raising Management,* July/August 1972, pp. 15–17.

Wardley, Alfred G. "Philanthropic Support for Hospitals: Five Principles." *Fund Raising Management,* July/August 1975, pp. 12–16.

Discussion of
A Survey of the History and Current Outlook of Philanthropy as a Source of Capital for the Needs of the Health Care Field

Michael D. Hernandez

The thrust of Mr. Terenzio's paper is to assess the importance of philanthropic funds as a source of capital financing for the health care industry. He concludes his paper with the question "Can philanthropy in health care remain a viable force in a society of increasing governmental controls and public participation?" To which the answer that is provided is in its essentials—perhaps (but only if giving practices are reformed).

The process of building up to this question and answer includes an analysis of the relative importance of philanthropy in the past as a source of funds for hospital construction. This analysis serves to highlight the difficulty associated with obtaining valid and useful historical data on the capital needs of the health care industry. In the process of analyzing the data, two major points are made with regard to the federal Hill-Burton program which do not seem to be supported by the historical data.

The first point is that "The Act popularly known as the Hill-Burton program, is the most significant event to date in the formation of capital in the health care field." The data on Table 7-1 show that Hill-Burton funds, as a percentage of total health care facilities construction, declined steadily from the program's inception and, importantly, the average percentage for each year for which such funds were recorded was 12.3 percent or about half the same percentage for philanthropic funds over the same period of time. When one considers that these data seem to show only hospital construction and not total capital needs, I must question raising the Hill-Burton program to such a level of importance.

The second major point is that the Hill-Burton program acted as a catalyst in attracting funds from philanthropists. The percentage increases in the volume of philanthropic contributions during the early years of the Hill-Burton program seem, however, more closely related to the statistical phenomenon of a small

259

base number and to the obvious effects that the optimistic postwar economy had on the propensity toward philanthropy rather than to Hill-Burton.

Both of these points, together with other comments in Mr. Terenzio's paper, seem to suggest some causal relationship between government grants and the level of philanthropic contributions. I can see little evidence, in this paper, of such a relationship.

In the next phase of his paper, Mr. Terenzio concludes that philanthropy, internal operations and government grants are far less costly forms of capital than is debt to the community. The comparison does not represent a classical cost of capital analysis and seems to have the following assumptions:

1. There is no opportunity cost over time associated with philanthropic contributions.
2. There is no cost associated with the collection of tax revenues.
3. The effects of taxation and reimbursement are not relevant to the cost of capital provided from debt or internal operations.
4. All sources of capital would be employed in equally efficient health care investments.

I would think that the opportunity exists for further economic evaluation of these alternative sources of capital. Such an analysis should certainly consider the costs to the community, over time, of nonrational capital allocations that are associated with altruistic (principally philanthropic) or political (principally government grants) motives.

A final point made regarding philanthropy seems to me an excellent one. That is that philanthropic funds are not available on a uniform geographic basis. This fact complicates any discussion of philanthropy in relation to the capital needs of the health care industry on a national basis.

In compiling a list of pros and cons regarding the appropriateness of philanthropy, one additional area of discussion would seem to be the indirect impact of philanthropy upon the management of health care institutions. This stems from philanthropic considerations that are associated with the selection of boards of trustees.

I tend to agree with Mr. Terenzio that philanthropic funds represent a form of capital having a low cost to the community as a whole, which makes such capital desirable if it is managed properly. I also agree that such funds are a key point of the voluntary hospital tradition.

I do believe, however, that the much more significant question for this conference is how important philanthropic funds will be as a source of capital for the health care industry in the future and, if such funds are important, how they will affect the health care delivery system. No data are presented which would help to answer this question, but, by doubting the viability of philanthropy as a whole, Mr. Terenzio seems to be suggesting that the importance of philanthropy in relation to capital needs will continue to diminish. Few thoughtful observers of the health care industry would disagree with that suggestion.

A second question that should be pursued is analyzing the nonspecific costs of philanthropy from a human capital perspective. In his introduction, Mr. Terenzio identifies this as a capital requirement. Such an analysis would follow the classical method first suggested by Gary Becker and would attempt to determine the true costs of utilizing philanthropy as a source of capital. It would also attempt to determine, for both the contributors and the hospitals, the costs and rewards of using philanthropy as a source of capital. It must be remembered that there are costs in accepting donations and a rigorous analysis of human capital could show this more clearly than would a simple summing of donations.

Discussion of
A Survey of the History and Current Outlook of Philanthropy as a Source of Capital for the Needs of the Health Care Field

Seymour Martin Lipset

Since I cannot claim any expertise in capital financing and in the operation and funding of hospitals, I will not attempt to comment specifically on the points that Mr. Terenzio makes in his interesting paper. Rather, I would like briefly to place the phenomenon of philanthropy in the health field in America in a wider comparative and historical perspective. It is important to realize, as the article on "Philanthropy" in *The International Encyclopedia of the Social Sciences* points out, that the "expansion of philanthropy . . . has gone further . . . in the United States, than in any other part of the world."[1]

To understand the reasons underlying the greater commitment to philanthropic activities in the United States than elsewhere, it is necessary to recognize that it is linked to the general strength of voluntary associations here. And this strength, in turn has been related historically to the rejection of a powerful, strong central state and of church establishment.

Many communal functions which had been handled in Europe by the state or by state-financed churches were dealt with in nineteenth century America by voluntary associations. The lack of commitment by the state to support communal institutions on the scale fostered by monarchical and aristocratic *noblesse oblige* in Europe has meant that certain institutions have been weaker here. This is most evident in the area of high culture, where opera, symphony, and museums have received much less government backing here, and, as a result, are in worse financial shape. Conversely, however, a variety of other institutions, such as colleges and universities and hospitals, have been widely diffused in this country and are supported by the most extensive pattern of voluntary contributions in the world.[2]

The emphasis on voluntary associations in America which so impressed Alexis de Tocqueville and other foreign travelers as one of the distinctive American traits in linked to the uniquely American system of "voluntary religion." The United States is the first country in which religious groups became voluntary associations. It is the only country the majority of whose inhabitants have adhered to denominations, which never were state churches, particularly the Methodists and Baptists. American ministers and laymen consciously recognized that they had to foster a variety of voluntary associations both to maintain support for the church and to fulfill community needs. As an English visitor to the United States in the 1830s put it: "The separations of Church and State, and other causes, have given rise to a new species of social organization, before unknown in history .. . . Then opened in the American world the new era of the Religious and Benevolent Society system, and summoned into the field an immense body of superior and highly-cultivated talent."[3]

The considerable sums, as well as time, that are contributed to philanthropic works, reaching heights undreamed of elsewhere, are also a consequence of the interrelationship between voluntary religion and secular achievements. Unlike the situation in many European countries, in which economic materialism was viewed by the social and religious establishments—that is, the traditional aristocracy and the church—as conducive to vulgar behavior and immorality, in the United States hard work and economic ambition were perceived as the proper activity of a devout man. Writing in the 1850s, a visiting Swiss theologian, Philip Schaff, commented that the "acquisition of riches is to them [the Americans] only a help toward higher spiritual and moral ends."[4]

The emphasis on voluntarism in both areas, religious and secular, has clearly been mutually reinforcing. Men were expected to be righteous, hard-working, and ambitious. Righteousness was to be rewarded both in the present and the hereafter, and the successful had an obligation to engage in good works and to share the bounty that they had attained. A detailed study by Merle Curti of the history of American giving for overseas purpose stresses the role that "the doctrine of stewardship" played, the belief "that whatever of worldly means one has belongs to God, that the holder is only God's steward and obligated to give to the poor, the distressed, and the needy. From many diaries, letters and other evidence it is clear that this factor was a dominant one in a great deal of giving."[5]

The stress on voluntarism is also related to the dominance of the antistatist, eighteenth century, classical, liberal emphasis in the United States. The American Revolution sharply weakened the *noblesse oblige* collective responsibility values, which had been linked to Tory sentiments, and replaced them with strong individualistic ones. This is evident in the fact that the United States, as H.G. Wells pointed out over seventy years ago, lacks both political parties which favor state responsibility, the Tory and the Socialist. It has been dominated by pure bourgeois, middle class individualistic values. As Wells put it: "Essentially America is a middle-class become a community and so its essential problems are the problems of a modern individualistic society, stark and clear." He enunciated a theory of America as a liberal society, in the classic antistatist meaning of the term, that was to win wide acceptance a half-century later, when enunciated in more detail by Louis Hartz.

> It is not difficult to show for example, that the two great political parties in America represent only one English party, the middle-class Liberal party . . . . There are no Tories to represent the feudal system and no Labor Party . . . .[T] he new world [was left] to the Whigs and Noncon-formists and to those less constructive, less logical, more popular and liber-ating thinkers who became Radicals in England, and Jeffersonians and then Democrats in America. All Americans are, from the English point of view, Liberals of one sort or another. . . .
>
> [My] chief argument . . . is that the Americans started almost clear of the medieval heritage, and developed in the utmost . . . the modern type of social organization. They took the economic conventions that were modern and progressive at the end of the eighteenth century and stamped them there for all time. . . . America is pure eighteenth century. . . .
>
> The liberalism of the eighteenth century was essentially the rebellion of the modern industrial organization against the monarchical and aristocratic state-against hereditary privilege, against restrictions on bargains. Its spirit was essentially anarchistic—the antithesis of Socialism. It was the anti-State.[6]

Scholarly students of the history of philanthropy in the United States empha-size that the underlying support for private philanthropy has been sustained by American "individualistic philosophy and suspicion of government control."[7] Such suspicion not only characterized the sentiments of private entrepreneurs, business men, and farmers, but the American labor movement, both in its mod-erate American Federation of Labor (AFL) and the radical Industrial Workers of the World (IWW) forms, was antistatist, and opposed welfare legislation until the 1930s.

Some indication of the strength of these values may be seen in the rejection by the American Red Cross, in January 1931, of a proposed federal appropria-tion of $25 million for the relief of drought victims. The chairman of the Red Cross central committee told Congress, "All we pray for is that you let us alone and let us do the job."[8] In spite of the growth of the welfare and planning state, since the 1930s, these values are not dead, even on the Left of American life. In 1971, the National Taxpayers Union, a group whose board included three major New Left figures, Noam Chomsky, Marc Raskin, head of the radical think tank the Institute for Policy Studies, and Karl Hess, former editor of *Ramparts,* to-gether with a number of conservative thinkers, advocated sharp cuts in the wel-fare responsibilities of government. To deal with the problem of the "needy recipients such as welfare people," the group advocated "a system of tax credits for any individual or group that provides private support for welfare recipients."

It would allow contributions to be deducted as an outright cut from taxes, rather than, as now, from gross income.[9] The fact that such a proposal could have been made in the 1970s by an organization whose leaders include some of the leading left-wing radicals in America attests to the continued vitality of the American individualist emphasis.

The Protestant ethic and the liberal emphasis on individualism and achievement combined in America, as Max Weber outlined, to provide the values that are most conducive for economic development, and for a democratic polity resting on independent secondary powers separate from the central state, which Tocqueville specified as necessary to avoid authoritarianism. The two sets of factors also helped foster the emergence of an elite which took its communal responsibilities seriously. As early as 1807, members of the Boston elite, in founding the Boston Athenaeum, stated in the founding document that, in their city, "the class of persons enjoying easy circumstances, and possessing surplus wealth, is comparatively numerous. As we are not called upon for large contributions to national purposes, we shall do well to take advantage of the exception, by taxing ourselves for those institutions, which will be attended with lasting and extensive benefit, amidst all changes of our public fortunes and political affairs."[10]

Martin Green, who has called attention to this remarkable statement, notes that "Boston merchants, and to some extent the bankers and industrialists who succeeded them, had the idea that commerce should go hand in hand with philanthropy, and even culture, and should give way to them as soon as the individual had secured himself an adequate sum."[11] In the nineteenth century, they demonstrated the vitality of this sense of responsibility by their support for libraries, the symphony, the Perkins Institute for the Blind, the Lowell Institute, Harvard, and the beginnings of that complex of hospitals which remains at the summit of medical care in America today. The altruistic sentiments voiced by the founders of the Athenaeum were, of course, not the only reasons motivating major contributions by the wealthy. In a fund-raising letter for Harvard in 1886, Henry Lee Higginson, a leading Boston Brahmin, stated, "Educate, and save ourselves and our families and our money from mobs."[12] James Buchanan Duke, the founder of the Duke Endowment, explained his concern for the expansion of health facilities in a newspaper interview in the 1920s saying "People ought to be healthy. If they ain't healthy they can't work, and if they don't work they ain't healthy. And if they can't work there ain't no profit in them."[13]

But though the philanthropy of the American Protestant wealthy had clear elements of self-interest, it is also true that they exhibited levels of generosity that were unmatched by the rich in other nations. John D. Rockefeller, who gave away more in his lifetime than did any other individual, was frequently attacked, and with good reason, for making his contributions for public relations and political purposes, for seeking to clean the image of "tainted money." Yet it must also be noted that, from his days as a teenager on, he would give away a tenth of his earnings to charity. He was a devout Baptist who, in the words of one student of philanthropy, "apparently felt there was some divine cooperation in the construction of Standard Oil Company."

> "God gave me my money," he told an interviewer in 1915. After financing establishment of the University of Chicago, Rockefeller told a campus meeting: "The good Lord gave me the money, and how could I withhold it from Chicago?" In his later years, Rockefeller mused, his wealth was an "accident of history," possible only because of the peculiar circumstances of oil and the nineteenth century, and that he was only its trustee.[14]

The continued linkage of voluntary religion to voluntary giving on a mass level may be seen in the fact that about half of all the monies reported as contributions in tax returns are still given to churches and other religious groups. Education, health, and hospitals are next, but far behind on the list.[15] One study found that "the ratio of gifts to religious organizations to discretionary receipts was remarkably constant over all the income levels covered by this survey."[16]

The Great Depression of the 1930s, of course, brought about a fundamental change in the role of philanthropy. The state increasingly took over responsibility for welfare functions, for hospitals, for higher education, and many other activities. Private contributions have continued to increase in absolute size, particularly since World War II, but they have become a much smaller proportion of the whole, particularly in nonreligious spheres.

The sources of private philanthropy have also changed. Corporations have replaced wealthy individuals as the large contributors. Corporate gifts have come to be recognized as excellent forms of public relations. One student of philanthropy, Aileen Ross, contends that:

> The rise in the contributions of corporations has enabled them to take over the control of raising and alloting money to many philanthropic agencies. Management can determine the amount that will be given, and since the same men are often found on the boards of a number of the larger corporations, they have come to form an "inner circle" which can control both the gifts that are given and the selection of the top executives in the philanthropic agencies and in the more important and prestigious fund-raising campaigns, such as those for hospitals and universities.[17]

It is still true, of course, that a considerable sum continues to come from less affluent contributors. In 1970, it was estimated that seventy million people contributed to charitable causes. Those with incomes under $5,000 gave $800 million, the total for incomes under $10,000 was $1.4 billion, while for people with less than $15,000 the total was $3.14 billion.[18] Still, the overall total collected is seven times the amount given by persons with incomes under $15,000. Most of the contributions of small donors go to religious-related causes.

"Education, mainly colleges and universities, is getting the largest share of corporation giving, followed closely by health and welfare agencies."[19]

In the health and hospital field, which concerns us here, the Great Depression also was a benchmark separating eras. The need for private philanthropic support of major medical costs declined greatly. The Blue Cross and other prepayment insurance schemes took over. By the 1960s, "The numbers enrolled in nonprofit plans, together with those enrolled in related commercial insurance plans, began to approximate the total potential enrollees among the working members of the population and their dependents." The government took over responsibility for the care of the indigent and near-indigent.[20] And after World War II, as Mr. Terenzio emphasizes, the federal government, through the Hill-Burton program, stimulated capital funding. This, of course, did not eliminate private contributions; rather, it resulted in an absolute increase but proportionate decrease. The recent decline in the Hill-Burton program, following on the emergence of the Medicare and Medicaid programs, however, has left a major gap, which philanthropy has not moved to fill.

Hospitals, as Mr. Terenzio notes, no longer are able to satisfy their capital needs from government and philanthropic contributions. They are forced to borrow and, thus, add large interest costs to their increasingly strained operating budgets. Is it possible to increase the role of private giving in an area in which government has become so important? The factors that he cites as necessary to stimulate gifts are valid, but it is doubtful whether the necessary funds can be found. Hospitals can no longer rely on religious motivations to stimulate large and continued giving. Only one road to sharply increased gifts seems open to hospital administrators: to seek to create a greater sense of responsibility in the business community. On the positive side, it may be noted that fund-raisers assume that the public's concern for health is one of the major reasons for donating to United Funds. Although such funds no longer provide important support for the operating budgets of hospitals, they continue to emphasize hospitals in their list of beneficiary agencies. A recent study of giving reports that "failure to list hospitals would hamper fund raising for the other agencies, because donors place the highest priority on giving for health and medical causes . . . . In a full-page advertisement in the New York Times inaugurating a recent campaign of the United Fund of Greater New York, hospitals headed the list of institutions that were to be beneficiaries. . . . In short, the United Funds need the hospitals even if the hospitals don't need the United Funds."[21]

It is doubtful, however, that increased giving will be able to cover the continuing spiral in hospital costs and capital needs. In 1973, the then president of the American Hospital Association concluded that "many large city hospitals are beyond relief by either philanthropy or even greater rate increases. He . . . [added] that nothing short of a complete revision in financing health care with government underwriting will reverse the situation."[22] Mr. Terenzio is pessimistic about the latter alternative for, as he states, "without the passage of a universal National Health Insurance Act, there is little hope for large-scale contributions by federal and local governmental sources to finance health care construction projects." But, since, according to his data, the percentage of the costs of all hospital construction paid for by philanthropy has declined from 34.0 in 1964 to 24.2 in 1968 and 9.8 in 1974, private donations seem an even less hopeful route to go. The realistic alternatives, therefore, appear to be continued debt-financing, with the consequent increase in patient bills, or much greater government aid.

To conclude: the historic, cultural sources of support for philanthropy and voluntary associational activity in America still have vitality for philanthropy generally. Hospitals, however, find religious-linked contributions less important than in earlier eras, as relatively few of them are seen to have effective denominational affiliations or to serve denominational purposes. It is extremely doubtful that hospitals can ever return to the days when they were major beneficiaries of the activities of important voluntary associations. Having become dependent on the state, their future probably lies with state support, with all the problems that such dependence necessarily brings.

Finally, we should not ignore the various critical analyses of hospital costs and financing which point to the ways in which the vast majority of hospitals which are nonprofit and noncompetitive contribute to the profits of others, including those who contribute to them and serve on their boards of directors. It is also argued by many that excess capacity, rather than the need for capital expansion, characterizes the hospital industry. To gain a grip on expanding costs, Victor Fuchs has seriously recommended that "a five-year moratorium should be declared (allowing very few exceptions) on all hospital construction and expansion." He would use this period to "provide incentives to physicians and hospital administrators and trustees to balance costs against potential benefits."[23] The fact that such a serious student of health care and health economics as Fuchs can make this proposal suggests that we may be discussing the wrong issues here. But, as a nonexpert, I will leave that matter to my betters.

NOTES

1. Aileen D. Ross, "Philanthropy," in David L. Sills (ed.), *International Encyclopedia of the Social Sciences,* Vol. 12 (New York: Macmillan Co. and The Free Press, 1968), p. 76.

2. Arnaud C. Marts, *The Generosity of Americans* (Englewood Cliffs, N.J.: Prentice-Hall, 1977), pp. 4–82.

3. An American Gentleman (Calvin Colton), *A Voice from America to England* (London: Henry Colburn, 1839), pp. 87–88.

4. Philip Schaff, *America: A Sketch of the Political, Social, and Religious Character of the United States of North America* (New York: C. Scribner, 1855), p. 259.

5. Merle Curti, *American Philanthropy Abroad: A History* (New Brunswick, N.J.: Rutgers University Press, 1963), p. 625.

6. H.G. Wells, *The Future in America* (New York: Harper and Brothers, 1906), pp. 72–76.

7. Ross, "Philanthropy," p. 76.

8. Robert H. Bremner, *American Philanthropy* (Chicago: University of Chicago Press, 1960), p. 145.

9. David Deitch, "Libertarians Unite in Drive to Reduce Tax Burdens," Boston *Globe,* April 10, 1971, p. 7. See also "What's This?" *Dissent* 18 (August 1971):395.

10. Cited in Martin Green, *The Problem of Boston* (New York: W.W. Norton, 1966), p. 4.

11. Ibid., p. 56.

12. Ben Whitaker, *The Foundations. An Anatomy of Philanthropy and Society* (London: Eyre Methuen, 1974), p. 53.

13. Joseph C. Goulden, *The Money Givers* (New York: Random House, 1971), p. 47.

14. Ibid., p. 28; Whitaker, *The Foundations,* pp. 64–66: Bremner, *American Philanthropy,* pp. 111–113.

15. Edward C. Jenkins, *Philanthropy in America* (New York: Association Press, 1950), p. 91; William S. Vickrey, "One Economist's View of Philanthropy," in Frank G. Dickinson (ed.), *Philanthropy and Public Policy* (New York: National Bureau of Economic Research, 1962), p. 33; George G. Kirstein, *Better Giving* (Boston: Houghton Mifflin, 1975), pp. 59–71.

16. Vickrey, "One Economist's View," p. 45.

17. Ross, "Philanthropy," p. 78.

18. Kirstein, *Better Giving,* p. xiii.

19. Merrimon Cuninggim, *Private Money and Public Service* (New York: McGraw-Hill, 1972), pp. 169–170.

20. Eli Ginzberg, "Hospitals and Philanthropy," in Dickinson (ed.), *Philosophy and Public Policy,* p. 74.

21. Kirstein, *Better Giving,* p. 32.

22. Ibid., p. 88.

23. Victor R. Fuchs, *Who Shall Live?* (New York: Basic Books, 1974), p. 104.

Discussion

Dr. Blendon: In the United States, philanthropy has had an impact on the structure of our institutions. In a number of countries where there has not been a history of philanthropic giving—I am thinking of France in particular—the result is often a series of large public hospitals and very small proprietary ones. By the way, in many of them, the wealthy are cared for in the institutions that have the least technology or specialization.

Dr. Evans: Perhaps you are being overly influenced by France. Canada has not been distinguished by a very high rate of philanthropic giving, but we do not have the kind of situation which you have described. We have some very large public hospitals, but there is certainly not a pattern where the wealthy go to very small private hospitals. As a matter of fact, the very small rural hospital often exists to provide a tax base for the community but the community leaders go to the better hospitals in the central cities for their care. I do not think that your model is fully generalizable.

Dr. Blanpain: I think that the concept of philanthropic giving in this country is being used in a very narrow sense. It is being used in the sense of giving cash, of giving dollars. There are countries around the world where philanthropy as the donation of labor has been extremely important. In the Netherlands, all the hospitals are voluntary hospitals which are based on philanthropy in donated labor, and they are top hospitals, too.

Dr. Evans: In a study on capital sources in the hospital industry, Paul Ginsburg concluded that although philanthropic giving was generally fairly well distributed over the income scale, giving to hospitals was much more highly concentrated among the upper income groups. He went on to argue that the tax deductability that was associated specifically with giving to hospitals was in the neighborhood of 90¢ on the dollar. In other words, most of that philanthropic giving was giving of other people's money, in tax money. If that is the case, then I am doubtful that philanthropy is really another source of funds; it seems to be just a method of enabling people with a lot of wealth to distribute federal government money as they see fit.

Mr. Terenzio: I think that Dr. Evans is referring to Table 7-6 in my paper. We are not talking about one donor giving $10 million; you have to take that into consideration. There aren't very many single donors today giving $10 million to hospitals. That is one of the problems we face.

Mr. Hernandez: Yesterday there was a point made about the problems of poorly administered government-based loan guarantee and other subsidy programs. We in the investment business know that these programs are financing a substantial number of high risk hospitals. How do we know that? Because they are going into default; it is very simple.

Mr. Storrs: I would like to point out the exact default rate in HUD's hospital program which is now eight years old: we insure approximately 120 hospitals and we have defaults on six. That rate is far lower than any of the default rates in any of the housing programs. The mortgagees of five of those six cases have assigned the mortgages to HUD. These five, with the help of HEW, are back in the black and are able to make their payments. The other hospital was in a state where there is no certificate of need, and competition from a private group put us out of business. That we had no control over.

Mr. Hernandez: It would seem that there is an opportunity for philanthropy to be used as a form of venture capital to promote arrangements, organizations and experiments which achieve the goals of thoughtful people in the health care industry. Here is an opportunity for reducing the costs and the uncertainties associated with mergers. A principal reason why hospitals do not merge is that the bigger ones do not want to take the risk. Philanthropy could be a catalytic force in this.

Mr. Ubell: Shouldn't this conference also be talking about capital financing of nonmedical health care facilities? I haven't heard anything about that and perhaps this is the appropriate session, because we are talking about philanthropy which in the past has provided the funds for innovative programs. I am worried that we are ignoring health and, in particular, the nonmedical measures which can be taken to delay or prevent a disease. There is growing up in the private sector a whole series of institutions like Weight Watchers, Smoke Enders, and other health-oriented clubs. If the studies which are being done have any validity, we can expect these activities to increase longevity which will decrease the burden on disease treatment facilities.

Dr. Evans: Some of you may be familiar with my government's white paper on new perspectives on the health of Canadians, published in the spring of '74, speaking to the degree to which the health system as presently constituted has its gun pointed in the wrong direction. That is a very real concern, but I caution against the notion that making people fitter and healthier will really save you any money. I strongly agree with it as a goal, but don't expect it to cap your costs.

✳ *Chapter 8*

A Study of the American Capital Market and Its Relationship to the Capital Needs of the Health Care Field

David C. Clapp
Arthur B. Spector

INTRODUCTION

The growth and the rapidly changing character of the health care industry have been the subject of much discussion and study over the last decade. Nonetheless, there remain a number of areas where the study is incomplete. The purpose of this brief paper is to discuss certain data on capital investment in the health care area, to present certain information about what has transpired, and to provide some interpretation of what has taken place.

Many factors, including shifts in the patterns of utilization of health care facilities, changes in medical technology, the enactment of numerous laws (federal, state, and local) and the establishment of regulations requiring, among others, conformance to certain standards for such facilities, have affected the health care delivery system and have created the necessity for an assessment of the present structure of, and recent trends in, capital investment in the health care industry.

Specifically, we would like to:

1. Provide some perspective by comparing trends in capital expenditures with changes in the Gross National Product;
2. Present a limited data base to show certain statistics and information, mainly about hospital utilization and related trends in construction; and
3. Discuss sources of funds for investment in plant and equipment.

This paper, by its limited nature and scope, is intended to be a basis for further investigation and is intended solely to establish what certain recent trends were and how these trends might be interpreted. It is hoped that this paper will contribute to the important effort to prepare for future changes in, and demands on, the health care delivery system.

CAPITAL AND THE GROSS
NATIONAL PRODUCT

National expenditures for health care construction (bricks, mortar, and equipment only) showed substantial growth from 1965 to 1975. In 1975, approximately $4.5 billion[1] was expended, representing a 145 percent increase over expenditures in 1965. During this same period the Gross National Product increased by 117 percent.

A comparison of the above rates of growth in constant 1972 dollars shows that:

1. From 1965 to a peak level in 1973, the GNP grew 33 percent, but from 1973 to 1975 there was a 9 percent decline—an overall increase of 21 percent from 1965 to 1975; and
2. From 1965 to a peak level in 1972, health care construction expenditures increased by 66 percent, but from 1973 to 1975 declined 17 percent—for an overall increase of 38 percent from 1965 to 1975.

During this period, there were a number of factors influencing health care construction. In 1965, with the advent of Medicare legislation, new impetus was created in the demand for medical services and, consequently, for new facilities. In addition, reimbursement to health care institutions through this program provided a constant and assured source of revenue, which facilitated financing of capital projects. Likewise, the passage of Medicaid legislation injected further revenue and sparked demand for a continuum of health care delivery—from nursing homes to ancillary services. Consequently, health care construction expenditures rose from 0.28 percent of GNP in 1965 to 0.37 percent of GNP in 1972.

At approximately this time, other forces in the economy began to influence trends in the health care industry. Unemployment began to grow and rising prices led to a selective curtailment in consumer expenditures, which included elective health care expenditures.

Although the expansionary influences of Medicare and Medicaid were still exerting upward pressure on the demand for health care facilities in the early 1970s, these forces were affected by the continued constraints upon the industry resulting from the advent of the Economic Stabilization Program (ESP) in 1971. In the latter years of ESP, which finally ended in April 1974, controls were eased or removed in many sectors of the economy. However, controls were imposed upon the health care industry for the full duration of the program. Thus, ever-increasing costs to the industry could not be counterbalanced by increases in charges for services.

In fact, the inability to increase charges created doubt in the minds of lenders and investors about the ability of health care facilities to meet future debt service payments, with the result that many capital projects became either not financeable or perhaps financeable, but only at prohibitive costs. Many projects were postponed and some were entirely abandoned. Relatively few were carried out in accordance with their original construction plans. In any event, the decrease in capital investment in the health care industry in this period was greater than the decline in the Gross National Product during this period. By 1975, health care construction expenditures had been reduced to 0.32 percent of the GNP.

Investment in the health care industry during this period from 1972 to 1975 appears to have been more influenced than was the general economy by increased operating costs and the recession. In addition, technological changes increased the rate of obsolescence of plant and equipment and exerted pressure to spend, modernize, and expand.

Most important, although health care capital investment was affected significantly during the 1972 to 1975 period, the 1965 to 1975 trend, as compared to the GNP, shows that the growth in health care capital expenditure was much greater than the growth in the GNP. This is attributable, at least in part, to the continuing need for the upgrading of facilities, including modernization, replacement, and other construction, to create conformity with federal standards to assure reimbursement to institutions under state and federal regulations.

UNITED STATES HOSPITAL TRENDS

Total United States Hospitals

During the period 1965 to 1974, according to the American Hospital Association, the number of hospitals in the United States declined from a high of 7,172 in 1967 to a low of 7,061 in 1972; thereafter, in 1974, the number returned to the 1967 level of 7,174 (Table 8-1).

Throughout this period from 1965 to 1974, several major categories of utilization declined:

1. The average number of beds per hospital was 239 in 1965 and declined to 211 in 1974—an 11.7 percent decrease;
2. The total number of beds utilized for all hospitals declined from 1,704,000 beds in 1965 to 1,513,000 in 1974—an 11.2 percent decrease; and
3. Occupancy declined from 82.3 percent in 1965 to 77.2 percent. Thus, the average number of beds occupied fell from 196 in 1965 to 163 in 1974—a 17 percent decline.

Table 8-1. Total United States Hospitals

	Number of Hospitals	Number of Beds	Average Beds Per Hospital	Total Beds Utilized	Rate of Occupancy (%)	Admissions	Outpatient Visits
1965	7,123	1,704,000	239	1,403,000	82.3	28,812,000	125,793,000
1966	7,160	1,679,000	234	1,398,000	83.3	29,151,000	142,201,000
1967	7,172	1,671,000	233	1,380,000	82.6	29,361,000	148,229,000
1968	7,137	1,663,000	233	1,378,000	82.9	29,766,000	156,139,000
1969	7,144	1,650,000	231	1,346,000	81.6	30,729,000	163,248,000
1970	7,123	1,616,000	227	1,298,000	80.3	31,759,000	181,370,000
1971	7,097	1,556,000	219	1,237,000	79.5	32,664,000	199,725,000
1972	7,061	1,550,000	220	1,209,000	78.0	33,265,000	219,182,000
1973	7,123	1,535,000	215	1,189,000	77.5	34,352,000	233,555,000
1974	7,174	1,513,000	211	1,167,000	77.2	35,506,000	250,481,000

Source: American Hospital Association.

Nevertheless, two important categories increased from 1965 to 1974:

1. Admissions increased each year from approximately 28.8 million in 1965 to approximately 35.5 million in 1974—a 24 percent increase; and
2. Outpatient visits increased from approximately 126 million in 1965 to almost 251 million in 1974—nearly a 100 percent increase.

In this paper, statistics concerning total United States Hospitals will be classified in the five following categories:

1. Federal hospitals are those institutions directly and solely supported by the federal government, such as those of the Veterans Administration, Department of Defense, and the Indian Health Service;
2. Long-term care hospitals include psychiatric, tuberculosis, long-term general, and other special institutions;
3. Nongovernment, not-for-profit hospitals are community hospitals, both volunteer and religious, short-term general and other special institutions, and hospital units of institutions;
4. Investor-owned hospitals include all proprietaries whether owned by individuals or by a corporation; and
5. State and local hospitals represent all other (nonfederal) governmental hospitals, such as county, city, etc.

In 1974, 42 percent of the 1,362 total hospital construction projects were for modernization projects, 35 percent were for expansion, and the remaining 23 percent for new projects.

From 1965 to 1974, the number of hospitals in the United States remained relatively constant. However, many individual categories did change:

1. Total federal hospitals declined from 443 in 1967 to 387 in 1974—a 12.6 percent decrease;
2. Total long-term care hospitals declined from 944 in 1965 to 810 in 1974—a 14.2 percent decrease;
3. State and local hospitals grew from 1,453 in 1965 to 1,821 in 1974—a 25.3 percent increase;
4. Nongovernment, not-for-profit hospitals declined from 3,426 in 1965 to 3,381 in 1974—only a 1.3 percent decrease; and
5. Investor-owned hospitals totaled 857 in 1965, but declined to 775 in 1974—a 9.6 percent decrease.

Additional information for each category follows.

Federal and Long-Term Hospitals

The average number of beds per hospital for federal and long-term hospitals was greater than for the average hospital in the United States. Specifically, from 1965 to 1974, the typical long-term care hospital was a large institution representing approximately nearly four times as many beds as did the average hospital in the United States. Also, during the period 1969 to 1974, the number of beds for federal hospitals was 1.85 times greater than for the average hospital. (Table 8-2 and Table 8-3).

The average beds per long-term care hospital declined from 835 in 1965 to 549 in 1974 or a 34 percent decline, nearly three times faster than the national average. During the same period, the average number of beds per federal hospital declined from 393 to 351 or a 10.7 percent decrease—slightly less than the average for the typical hospital in the United States.

Possibly of greater interest are the totals for the number of beds utilized for long-term care hospitals and federal hospitals:

1. Long-term care hospitals had 689,000 beds utilized in 1965 versus 357,000 in 1974—a 48 percent decline; and
2. Federal hospitals had 174,000 beds utilized in 1965 versus 136,000 in 1974—a 22 percent decline.

Utilization of federal and long-term care hospitals declined much faster than did the national average.

For these two categories, from 1965 to 1974, occupancy rates were higher than the national average; however, by 1974, they had approached the national average.

Nevertheless, the average number of beds utilized in 1965 for long-term care hospitals was 825 versus 650 beds in 1974—a 21 percent decrease; for federal hospitals, the average number of utilized beds in 1965 was 381 versus 312 in 1974—an 18 percent decrease. In both cases, the decline in average number of beds utilized was much greater than was the national average.

Two major areas increased:

1. Admissions at federal hospitals rose from 1.64 million in 1965 to 1.84 million in 1974 or a 12 percent increase—less than half of the national average; in long-term care hospitals admissions for 1965 to 1974 (723,000) rose only 1.8 percent—significantly below the national trend.
2. Outpatient visits for long-term care hospitals increased from approximately 2.8 million in 1965 to 6.9 million in 1974—a 146 percent increase—much faster than the national average; such visits to federal hospitals grew by only about 60 percent from 30.4 million to 48.7 million—much slower than the national average.

It should be noted that the overall national average was about 35,000 outpa-

Table 8-2. Federal Hospitals

	Number of Hospitals	Number of Beds	Average Beds per Hospital	Total Beds Utilized	Rate of Occupancy (%)	Admissions	Outpatient Visits
1965	443	174,000	393	150,000	86.1	1,640,000	30,393,000
1966	425	173,000	407	151,000	87.2	1,615,000	31,866,000
1967	416	175,000	421	149,000	85.0	1,700,000	34,819,000
1968	416	175,000	421	146,000	83.7	1,766,000	38,426,000
1969	415	170,000	410	140,000	82.7	1,769,000	38,850,000
1970	408	161,000	395	128,000	79.6	1,741,000	42,913,000
1971	407	148,000	364	123,000	83.2	1,788,000	46,504,000
1972	401	143,000	357	114,000	80.0	1,770,000	46,095,000
1973	397	142,000	358	112,000	79.0	1,865,000	47,948,000
1974	387	136,000	351	109,000	80.7	1,841,000	48,682,000

Source: American Hospital Association.

Table 8-3. Long-term Care Hospitals

	Number of Hospitals	Number of Beds	Average Beds Per Hospital	Total Beds Utilized	Rate of Occupancy (%)	Admissions	Outpatient Visits
1965	944	788,000	835	689,000	87.4	709,000	2,769,000
1966	923	737,000	798	660,000	89.6	640,000	3,810,000
1967	906	707,000	780	620,000	87.7	673,000	3,424,000
1968	901	683,000	758	601,000	88.0	723,000	3,616,000
1969	876	653,000	745	555,000	85.0	706,000	3,568,000
1970	856	607,000	709	508,000	83.7	766,000	4,913,000
1971	825	541,000	656	449,000	83.0	733,000	4,798,000
1972	817	524,000	641	431,000	82.3	719,000	6,104,000
1973	835	489,000	586	395,000	80.8	726,000	6,669,000
1974	810	445,000	549	357,000	80.2	722,000	6,961,000

Source: American Hospital Association.

tient visits in 1974 or about 96 a day. For federal hospitals in 1974, it was about 126,000 visits a year or about 395 a day. For long-term hospitals, in 1974, it was 8,000 visits a year or only 24 visits a day.

Nongovernment, Not-for-Profit Hospitals

From 1965 to 1974, there was little change in the total number of nongovernment, not-for-profit hospitals. In 1974, there were 3,381 hospitals of this type. (Table 8-4). However, four major areas differed significantly from the national averages. They were:

1. The average number of beds per hospital was 150 in 1965 and increased to 192 in 1976—a 28 percent increase versus the national average for all hospitals (11.7 percent decrease);
2. Total beds for all such hospitals increased steadily for each year from 515,000 in 1965 to 650,000 in 1974—an approximately 26 percent increase versus the national average (11.2 percent decrease);
3. The rate of occupancy for the period 1965 to 1974 remained at about 77.8 percent, but, because of the increase in the total number of beds per hospital, the average number of beds occupied per hospital increased from 118 in 1965 to 150 in 1974—a 27 percent increase versus the national average (17 percent decline); and
4. Average length of stay remained at about 7.9 days.

Two areas which paralleled the national averages were:

1. Total admissions grew from 19 million in 1965 to approximately 23.4 million in 1974—a 23 percent increase (the national growth was a 24 percent increase); and
2. Total outpatient visits grew dramatically from 59 million to 131.4 million—a 121 percent increase (the national growth was a 100 percent increase).

State and Local Hospitals

Hospitals in this category underwent a constant increase in total numbers from 1965 to 1974, to a total of 1,821 in 1974, representing a 25 percent increase over the 1965 number. (Table 8-5).

Although during this period the total number of beds grew from 179,000 to 211,000 (an 18 percent increase), the actual number of beds utilized increased more slowly—from 131,000 to 148,000 or only a 13 percent increase. The reason for this was that the rate of occupancy actually declined from 1965 to 1974, from 72.8 percent to 70.2 percent. It is worth noting that the average length of stay peaked, in 1967, at nine days and thereafter declined to 7.7 days in 1974.

Two important areas did increase similarly with the national trend. They were:

Table 8-4. Nongovernment, Not-for-Profit Hospitals

	Number of Hospitals	Number of Beds	Average Beds Per Hospital	Total Beds Utilized	Rate of Occupancy (%)	Admissions	Average Length of Stay (days)	Outpatient Visits
1965	3,426	515,000	150	401,000	77.8	19,001,000	7.7	59,233,000
1966	3,440	533,000	155	418,000	78.5	19,263,000	7.9	69,336,000
1967	3,461	550,000	159	439,000	79.7	19,498,000	8.2	73,173,000
1968	3,430	566,000	165	453,000	80.0	19,659,000	8.3	76,428,000
1969	3,428	579,000	169	468,000	80.8	20,338,000	8.2	82,756,000
1970	3,386	592,000	175	474,000	80.1	20,948,000	8.2	90,992,000
1971	3,363	604,000	180	477,000	79.0	21,515,000	8.1	103,016,000
1972	3,326	617,000	186	478,000	77.4	21,875,000	8.0	112,039,000
1973	3,320	629,000	189	489,000	77.8	22,488,000	7.9	120,273,000
1974	3,381	650,000	192	506,000	77.8	23,374,000	7.9	131,394,000

Source: American Hospital Association.

Table 8-5. State and Local Government Hospitals

	Number of Hospitals	Number of Beds	Average Beds Per Hospital	Total Beds Utilized	Rate of Occupancy (%)	Admissions	Average Length of Stay (days)	Outpatient Visits
1965	1,453	179,000	123	131,000	72.8	5,617,000	8.5	29,962,000
1966	1,520	188,000	124	137,000	72.8	5,778,000	8.6	32,850,000
1967	1,568	191,000	122	134,000	72.8	5,646,000	9.0	32,794,000
1968	1,621	192,000	118	142,000	73.9	5,781,000	8.9	33,614,000
1969	1,666	198,000	119	146,000	73.9	6,023,000	8.9	34,216,000
1970	1,704	204,000	120	149,000	73.2	6,273,000	8.7	37,854,000
1971	1,752	209,000	119	150,000	71.6	6,540,000	8.3	40,550,000
1972	1,779	209,000	117	147,000	70.2	6,741,000	8.0	47,103,000
1973	1,814	211,000	116	149,000	70.6	6,939,000	7.8	51,072,000
1974	1,821	211,000	116	148,000	70.2	7,016,000	7.7	54,777,000

Source: American Hospital Association.

1. Total admissions, which rose from 5.6 million in 1965 to 7 million in 1974—a 25 percent increase; and
2. Outpatient visits which grew from approximately 30 million in 1965 to 55 million in 1974—an 80 percent increase.

Finally, the total number of beds did increase from 1965 to 1974, but the average number of beds per hospital declined—from 123 to 116, or about a 6 percent decrease.

Investor-Owned Hospitals

Proprietary hospitals and those facilities which are owned or managed by a hospital corporation accounted for approximately 10 percent of the total number of hospitals in 1974. Although there were fewer investor-owned hospitals in 1974 than in 1965, the total number of beds increased to 70,000 in 1974, representing a nearly 50 percent increase over the 1965 level. Thus, the average number of beds per hospital increased even more rapidly—from 55 in 1965 to 90 in 1974. However, the rate of occupancy was low as compared with the national average or with the average for other categories. The rate of occupancy was 68.6 percent in 1965 and 67.5 percent in 1974. (Table 8-6).

Total admissions grew from approximately 1.8 million in 1965 to 2.5 million—a 39 percent increase. Also, outpatient visits grew from approximately 3.4 million to approximately 8.7 million—a 161 percent increase.

Hospital Trends—Summary

If one analyzes total hospital trends by eliminating the federal and long-term care hospital data from the totals, the results present a very different and important picture of the remaining categories:

1. The total number of hospitals grew from 5,736 in 1965 to 5,977—an approximate 4 percent increase (as compared with the national decline of 11.7 percent); and
2. The total number of beds available increased from 742,000 in 1965 to 932,000 in 1974—a 25 percent increase (as compared with a national decline of 11.2 percent).

As might be expected, long-term care hospitals showed the greatest increase in the number of outpatients served (and total admissions have not grown as fast as the national average). This rise can be explained by the use of ambulatory care facilities, through the use of mental health clinics, and the general acceptance of alternative treatment methods by patients and physicians. Consistent with these new policies and treatment methods, as well as, at least in some cases, the availability of other hospitals, the number of beds for federal and long-term hospitals which were available and utilized has declined, as did the average number of

Table 8-6. Investor-owned Hospitals

	Number of Hospitals	Number of Beds	Average Beds Per Hospital	Total Beds Utilized	Rate of Occupancy (%)	Admissions	Average Length of Stay (days)	Outpatient Visits
1965	857	47,000	55	32,000	68.6	1,844,000	6.3	3,437,000
1966	852	48,000	56	33,000	69.0	1,855,000	6.4	4,339,000
1967	821	47,000	57	35,000	72.7	1,843,000	6.8	4,020,000
1968	769	48,000	62	35,000	73.9	1,837,000	7.0	4,055,000
1969	759	48,000	63	36,000	74.6	1,893,000	6.8	3,859,000
1970	769	53,000	69	38,000	72.2	2,031,000	6.8	4,698,000
1971	750	54,000	72	38,000	71.0	2,088,000	6.6	4,858,000
1972	738	57,000	77	39,000	68.7	2,161,000	6.6	7,842,000
1973	757	63,000	83	43,000	68.3	2,334,000	6.7	7,593,000
1974	775	70,000	90	47,000	67.5	2,553,000	6.7	8,667,000

Source: American Hospital Association.

beds per hospital. It should be again noted that federal and long-term care hospitals, in terms of the number of beds, are much larger institutions than are the national average.

Also, the occupancy rates, which have declined for both federal and long-term hospitals, remain higher than for the national average (although the rates for federal and long-term have declined significantly). Occupancy rates for the other categories have remained relatively stable.

Nationally, the total number of hospitals have been able to handle increasing admissions with fewer beds and slightly lower occupancy by reducing the average length of stay and more effectively utilizing and expanding outpatient facilities.

Other key points about the 1965 to 1974 period are:

1. For nongovernment, not-for-profit hospitals, modernization and expansion of existing facilities had been concerned with the addition of beds as well as ancillary services; also, the average number of beds per hospital utilized basically paralleled the growth in the total number of beds. (These concurrent trends resulted in the occupancy rate remaining basically unchanged.)
2. Nongovernment, not-for-profit, and investor-owned hospitals were the only two categories where average beds per hospital increased.
3. The occupancy rate for the investor-owned hospital was lowest in 1974.
4. The contraction in the total number of beds for federal and long-term hospitals was offset, to a great extent, by the expansion in the three other categories.
5. State and local hospitals are handling many fewer admissions and outpatients per hospital than do the nongovernment, not-for-profit installations.
6. Small, independently owned hospitals have given way to larger corporate institutions. In this category, small hospitals are closing, others are expanding and larger new hospitals are being constructed.

Nursing Home Facilities

Although statistics are more difficult to compile on nursing home facilities, there are trends which can be discerned from 1965 to 1974. In the late 1960s, there was a growing recognition of the need for the construction and modernization of extended care facilities. This recognition was in response to two separate trends in the health care system. The first was the increasing level of demand for specialized nursing home care as an alternative to hospital care, which was partially attributable to the Medicare program support for extended medical care treatment provided in nursing homes. The second significant trend was the movement to develop a continuum of medical care facilities, which included nursing home facilities. Both of these underlying trends are still prevalent today.

From 1965 to 1971, the federal government provided substantial support to the development of these goals, contributing over 10 percent of the medical facilities construction budget to nursing homes and extended care facilities.

However, in the early 1970s, though the government was still persistent in its stated purpose to upgrade nursing homes and extended care facilities, the budget for such activity was almost halved.

Ambulatory Care Facilities

In the early 1970s, the federal government showed a recognition of the need to develop ambulatory care facilities, defined as outpatient departments, clinics, and community centers. The reasons that are cited for this growing need were the increasing cost of health care and the inability of the existing hospital system to deliver services efficiently and economically. The government has maintained a commitment to the development of these facilities through 1975, consistently allocating on the average approximately 13 percent of the total medical facilities construction budget to their development.

SOURCES OF INVESTMENT FUNDS

Throughout this section, we intend to present information on the sources of investment funds for the years 1965 to 1975. Investment sources are to be discussed within the following two major categories:

1. *Private Funds*—including philanthropy, mortgage loans, taxable bond issues, owners' equity, loans from private sources and leases;
2. *Public Funds*—including federal, state, and local sources.

Federal funds include federal appropriations, direct grants, FHA 242 loan assistance, Farmers' Home Administration Loan guarantees, and Hill-Burton loan guarantees and grants. State and local sources include other governmental grants and appropriations, intergovernmental appropriations, tax-exempt bond issues and IRS 63-20 (nonprofit corporation) bond issues.

Private vs. Public Sources

In 1965, private sources provided the health care industry with 64 percent of the total funds for health care capital expenditures. However, by 1975, this proportionate contribution had decreased to 59 percent. Thus, by 1975, there had been a significant increase in the contribution by public funds to 41 percent of the total funds.

1. Private sources contributed approximately $1.2 billion in 1965. This amount grew by 126 percent to $2.65 billion in 1975.
2. Public sources provided $665 million in 1965. This amount grew by 178 percent to approximately $1.8 billion in 1975. (Of the total public sources, state and local sources grew rapidly from $289 million in 1965 to $1.2 billion in 1975.)

Table 8-7. Allocation of Total Sources of Funds, in Percentages**

	Gov't. Grants & Appropriations			Philanthropy			Internal Operations		Debt						
	Fed. Grants	Other Gov't. Grants	Nonre-payable Approp.	Special Fund-Raising	Other Contrib.	Founda-tion Grants	Acc. Earnings	Owners' Equity	Loans	Taxable Bonds	Tax-Exempt	IRS 63–20	HUD 242	H-B[1]	Other*
Total Construction															
Completed 1969	14.7%	17.6%	—	8.8%	5.1%	—	18.4%	—	32.0%	—	—	—	—	—	3.3%
Begun 1973	5.4	1.1	14.3%	6.2	2.9	.8%	14.8	.1%	16.6	4.5%	16.8%	3.1%	4.7%	7.2%	3.3
Begun 1974	2.8	1.1	15.2	4.9	3.1	1.8	12.7	.4	11.5	5.5	28.9	2.1	1.8	8.3	.9
Federal															
Completed 1969	—	100.0	—	—	—	—	—	—	—	—	—	—	—	—	—
Begun 1973	—	—	100.0	—	—	—	—	—	—	—	—	—	—	—	—
Begun 1974	—	—	100.0	—	—	—	—	—	—	—	—	—	—	—	—
Long-Term															
Completed 1969	24.7	61.9	—	1.5	3.3	—	2.4	—	6.2	—	—	—	—	—	19.1
Begun 1973	6.5	.6	41.8	5.9	1.0	1.6	2.1	.1	12.7	—	8.0	—	—	—	—
Begun 1974	2.6	1.1	48.0	1.7	1.0	1.5	2.6	.1	2.9	—	33.7	1.5	—	2.9	—
Nongovernment Not-for-Profit															
Completed 1969	12.4	4.2	—	12.3	5.6	—	21.7	—	39.6	—	—	—	—	—	4.3
Begun 1973	3.8	1.1	2.6	7.1	3.5	.2	17.2	—	21.0	5.7	16.0	2.3	5.3	9.5	2.5
Begun 1974	2.6	1.3	1.0	6.7	4.0	1.9	14.7	—	14.9	7.5	28.4	1.6	2.4	10.6	.8
Proprietary															
Completed 1969	.2	—	—	—	.8	—	30.5	—	62.6	—	—	—	—	—	5.8
Begun 1973	3.7	—	—	—	—	—	4.8	10.3	53.0	17.4	6.4	—	—	—	3.5
Begun 1974	3.4	.9	—	.3	—	—	4.5	24.6	24.6	8.4	27.9	4.2	—	—	.9
State and Local															
Completed 1969	24.0	41.9	—	1.0	5.7	—	12.8	—	13.7	—	—	—	—	—	1.0
Begun 1973	11.4	.1	32.8	2.6	.7	1.7	11.4	—	1.0	.5	25.4	7.2	3.7	.7	—
Begun 1974	3.4	—	38.0	.5	.9	1.1	10.8	—	3.0	.2	34.3	3.1	—	3.3	.8

Source: American Hospital Association.

*Includes Farmers Home Administration, Loans from private sources, and leases.

**All columns add across to 100%.

1. Hill-Burton.

Table 8-8. Allocation of Funds Within Individual Categories in Percentages

	Gov't Grants & Appropriations			Philanthropy			Internal Operations			Debt					
	Fed. Grants	Other Gov't. Grants	Nonre-payable Approp.	Special Fund-Raising	Other Contrib.	Founda-tion Grants	Acc. E.Arnigns	Owners' Equity	Loans	Taxable Bonds	Tax-Exempt	IRS 63-20	HUD 242	H-B[1]	Other*
Federal															
Completed 1969	—	48.1%	—	—	—	—	—	—	—	—	—	—	—	—	—
Begun 1973	—	—	56.4%	—	—	—	—	—	—	—	—	—	—	—	—
Begun 1974	—	—	53.5	—	—	—	—	—	—	—	—	—	—	—	—
Long-Term															
Completed 1969	40.3%	29.8	—	10.1%	21.4%	45.7%	3.6%	—	5.1%	—	14.3%	—	—	—	—
Begun 1973	25.6	33.3	23.6	37.8	19.2	33.3	5.9	1.0%	14.5	—	27.2	14.4%	—	—	76.1%
Begun 1974	21.7	33.3	25.7	18.5	16.9	—	8.0	.4	6.4	—	—	—	—	17.3%	—
Nongovernment Not-for-Profit															
Completed 1969	20.2	2.0	—	83.1	36.4	5.7	32.2	—	32.4	24.2%	28.7	24.2	58.9%	—	38.7
Begun 1973	15.0	61.1	1.5	45.5	67.3	42.3	48.5	—	24.0	46.6	22.8	15.4	100.0	93.1	10.0
Begun 1974	21.7	39.4	.5	72.8	67.8	—	45.1	—	32.8	—	—	—	—	63.1	32.0
Proprietary															
Completed 1969	.3	—	—	—	5.2	—	45.3	—	51.3	73.7	11.5	—	—	—	52.3
Begun 1973	14.6	—	—	—	—	—	13.5	99.0	60.4	52.2	22.4	40.4	—	—	13.9
Begun 1974	28.3	27.3	—	3.3	—	—	13.8	99.6	54.2	—	—	—	—	—	36.0
State and Local															
Completed 1969	39.2	20.1	—	6.8	37.0	48.6	18.9	—	11.2	2.1	45.5	75.8	41.1	—	9.0
Begun 1973	44.8	5.6	18.5	16.7	13.5	24.4	32.1	—	1.1	1.2	27.6	29.8	—	6.9	—
Begun 1974	28.3	—	20.3	5.4	15.3	—	33.1	—	6.6	—	—	—	—	19.6	32.0

Source: American Hospital Association.

*Includes Farmers Home Administration, Loans from private sources, and leases.

**For example, as shown above, of the total funds provided by Federal grants for capital investment in projects completed in 1969, 40.3% went to Long Term Hospitals; 20.2% went to Non-Governmental, Not-for-Profit Hospitals; 39.2% went to State and Local Hospitals and .3% to Proprietary Hospitals.

1. Hill-Burton.

Table 8-9. Expenditures for Health Care Construction by Category[1] (in thousands)

Fiscal Year	Private & Public Total	Private Total	Public Total	Public Federal	Public State & Local
1965	$1,837	$1,172	$ 665	$376	$ 289
1966	1,903	1,162	741	405	336
1967	1,930	1,208	722	344	378
1968	2,164	1,321	843	382	461
1969	2,500	1,557	943	482	461
1970	3,291	2,288	1,003	529	474
1971	3,550	2,227	1,323	541	782
1972	4,081	2,573	1,508	551	957
1973	4,145	2,941	1,204	485	719
1974*	4,427	2,961	1,466	493	973
1975**	4,500	2,652	1,848	634	1,214

Sources: 1. Social Security Administration, Office of Research and Statistics.
2. The Daily Bond Buyer.
*In 1974, $1,292,409 state and municipal Hospital Bonds were sold.[2]
**In 1975, $1,959,019 state and municipal Hospital Bonds were sold.[2]

3. Total funds provided grew from $1.8 billion in 1965 to approximately $4.5 billion in 1975—an increase of 145 percent over the 1965 level.

As indicated earlier, the origin of funds from public sources has undergone important changes during the period of 1965-75. In 1965, the federal government was providing approximately 57 percent of total public funds for health care construction. By 1975, this share had diminished to 34 percent.

In 1975, state and local funding increased to 66 percent of total public funds. In absolute dollars, this was a 320 percent increase as compared to only a 69 percent increase in federal funds over the 1965 funding levels. Clearly, then, the trend toward funds from public sources can be more precisely understood as an increasing dependency upon funds from state and local sources.

The total funds from public and private sources were derived or generated from four areas:

1. philanthropy,
2. internal operations,
3. government grants and appropriations, and
4. debt, private and public.

Philanthropy

Although an institution's level of support from philanthropy is still a very important part of its economic viability, the actual dollar contribution from this source has declined since 1965. In the late 1960s, philanthropy accounted for 13.9 percent of total funding for U.S. hospitals, but only about one-third of the hospitals reporting construction in the early 1970s claimed receipt of any philanthropic funds at all. Nongovernment, not-for-profit hospitals were the major beneficiaries of those funds, claiming some 60 percent of the total. State and local institutions were the only other recipients of any consequence, claiming 22 percent of the remaining funds.

By 1973, the contribution of philanthropy to total capital needs represented only 9.9 percent, a 29 percent decrease from the late 1960s. This level remained relatively consistent through 1974. Nongovernment, not-for-profit hospitals and institutions continued to receive the major proportion of these funds. Throughout the period, special fund-raising (capital fund drives, Community Chest, United Fund, etc.) accounted for the greatest proportion of philanthropic funds.

Internal Operations

During the late 1960s, the decline in philanthropy was partially offset by the increased use of funds from internal operations, mostly depreciation and profit. In 1969, accumulated earnings represented 18.4 percent of total funds expended, a 31 percent increase over 1968. As can be expected, proprietary institutions relied upon this source more than did other categories of facilities. Of the total amount of accumulated earnings used to finance construction in 1969, 45 percent was utilized by investor-owned hospitals; however, nongovernment, not-for-profit institutions also made frequent use of these funds, accounting for 32 percent of the total. It is reasonable to assume that the amount of available internally generated funds was increased as a result of the reimbursement and accounting procedures which evolved in the late 1960s after the passage of Medicare legislation.

However, because of the quantity of capital funds required during the period examined, internal operations were not able even to approach meeting increasing capital demands. In fact, funds from internal operations decreased in their contribution to the total during the period, representing only 14.9 percent by 1973. By 1974, this share had continued to decline to 13.1 percent of the total funds provided.

Government Grants and Appropriations

Government grants and appropriations, federal, state, and local, accounted for approximately 32.3 percent of total funds for construction completed in 1969. By 1973, such participation had decreased to 20.8 percent of the total and by 1974 there was a further decrease to 19.1 percent of the total. Direct federal grants and appropriations represented approximately 46 percent of total governmental funds in 1969. By 1973, grant and appropriation funds had diminished to only 37 percent of the 1969 level and provided only 2.8 percent of the total support for construction that was started in 1974. The institutions most seriously affected by the diminution of federal grants and appropriations were the federal hospitals and those concerned with long-term care. (In 1971, the government had shifted its emphasis in the use of these grants toward the construction of ambulatory care facilities.)

Since 1969, appropriations particularly allocated directly at the federal level, or through state and local authorities, have been a relatively consistent source of funds. Federal hospitals constituted the primary beneficiaries of these appropriations, having received approximately 54 percent of the total for 1973 and 1974. Another 24 percent was allocated to long-term facilities, while state and local institutions received 19 percent.

As indicated, historically, long-term facilities have relied heavily upon governmental monies: in 1969, a full 86.6 percent of construction expenditures were attributable to governmental sources, but by 1974 these funds contributed only 51.7 percent. This same trend was evident for state and local hospitals: in 1969, government sources provided 65.9 percent of construction funds; by 1974, they represented only 41.4 percent. State and local facilities and, to a lesser extent, long-term hospitals have been able to obtain alternative sources for capital, particularly through debt financing.

Private Debt

It is clear that during the period studied, debt—both public and private—has provided an increasingly important proportion of total capital funds to the health care industry and there is every indication that this trend will continue.

In the recent past the most frequently utilized private debt vehicle has been conventional mortgage loans. In 1973, approximately 70 percent of total private debt and some 16.6 percent of total funds were provided from this source. In 1974, mortgage loans decreased to approximately 65 percent of private debt and 11.5 percent of total funds, partially as a consequence of the growth of other sources.

An estimated 57 percent of all mortgage loans issued in the mid-1970s were used to finance construction in investor-owned facilities. Indeed, loans of this type have been the primary source of debt financing for these institutions, providing some 48 percent of their debt structure during the last several years. Nongovernment, not-for-profit hospitals and long-term institutions have been the only other significant employers of this method of debt financing, accounting for approximately 28 percent of mortgage loans issued for health care in 1973 and 10 percent in 1974.

The role of taxable bond issues increased from 1973 to 1974 to 5.5 percent of total funds. Again, investor-owned institutions utilized taxable bond issues to a greater extent than did any other category of facilities. However, in both 1973 and 1974, nongovernment, not-for-profit hospitals financed about 6 percent of their total needs through this source.

Public Debt

For construction completed in 1969, total debt financing, both private and public, represented approximately 35 percent of total construction expenditures. During the late 1960s and early 1970s it appears that most debt financing through public channels was accomplished through Hill-Burton and other governmental loan programs. By 1973, total debt financing represented 56 percent of total sources of funds—a 60 percent increase over 1969. Public debt represented 62 percent of total debt in 1973, the largest portion of which was provided through the tax-exempt bond market.

Tax-exempt bond financing through state and local bond authorities accounted for 48 percent of public debt financing, representing a significant new factor in the market since 1969. State and local hospitals, along with nongovernment, not-for-profit institutions utilized this form of financing most successfully through their respective governmental authorities.

The attraction to debt financing in general continued to increase, representing approximately 59 percent of total funds by 1974. Because of the high cost of borrowing during these years, tax-exempt bond financing and government subsidized loan guarantee programs provided viable and less expensive vehicles to meet capital needs. Coupled with the more widespread availability of state and local bond authorities, the market supported a 72 percent increase in the principal amount of tax-exempt bonds issued during 1973 and 1974. State and local hospitals and nongovernment, not-for-profit institutions continued to be major users of tax-exempts. Unlike in 1973, long-term facilities also took advantage of this form of financing in 1974, deriving 33.7 percent of their total construction expenditures from this source.

The Hill-Burton loan and loan guarantee program was the second most significant public debt vehicle utilized in both 1973 and 1974. These loans became available in 1971 when they were implemented for the purpose of funding construction and modernization at nongovernment, not-for-profit and long term care facilities. In 1973, the Hill-Burton program was responsible for 21 percent of the public debt portion of total capital funds provided; it increased by another 15 percent in 1974. Nongovernment, not-for-profit hospitals were the most prominent utilizers of these loans and loan guarantees (93.1 percent of available funds in 1973 and 63.1 percent in 1974). (Long-term institutions did not benefit noticeably from this source until 1974.) Finally, state and local facilities were more frequent utilizers of these loans in 1974, using almost 20 percent of all available monies (up from 7 percent in 1973).

Mortgage Loan Insurance through the Department of Housing and Urban Development (the FHA Section 242 program) accounted for 13 percent of all public debt in 1973, being utilized most frequently by nongovernment, not-for-profit and state and local institutions. The role of this financing vehicle declined in 1974 to 31 percent of its 1973 magnitude.

Tax-exempt financing through state and local issuers authorized under IRS Ruling 63-20 (nonprofit corporation bonds) and other debt instruments, both public and private (such as loan guarantees through the Farmers Home Administration, loans from private groups, and leases), did not contribute more than 5 percent of total debt during the 1965-1974 period.

PURCHASERS OF DEBT

Insurance companies, through both their mortgage departments and their investment departments, have been among the most active investors in the health care industry. An analysis of the portfolios of the insurance companies surveyed reveals that these institutions have approximately 1.8 percent (on the average) of their mortgage portfolios and approximately 1.4 percent (on the average) of their investment portfolios invested in health care. Their loans to the industry include conventional mortgages as well as a variety of government guaranteed mortgages. A recent analysis showed that the portion of their portfolios that was invested in health care was approximately 28 percent in tax-exempts, with the remainder being held in taxable bonds. Most of the tax-exempt instruments are held in the portfolios of casualty companies, although many mutual companies benefit from tax-exempts and are holders. A survey of insurance companies shows that they have invested in hospitals, both not-for-profit and proprietaries, nursing homes, group practice facilities, extended care facilities and HMOs.

Commercial banks are also major investors providing for health care capital needs. These institutions are primarily interested in shorter term loans and participate most prominently in construction financing and equipment financing. Tax-exempt bonds are held in banks' bond portfolios because of their attractively high yields. However, health care bond issues represent a small portion relative to their total tax-exempt holdings, due to their limited liquidity and marketability and due to the fact that banks may not, as a matter of law, underwrite most hospital bonds. There was an estimated $150 million in hospital bonds held by commercial banks in 1975.

Bond mutual funds account for a large proportion of the tax-exempt investments in health care. A recent portfolio analysis of the two major bond mutual funds revealed that they held approximately 20 percent of all tax-exempt hospital bonds. It is believed that another 10 percent can be attributed to remaining mutual funds active in the bond market. These funds are sold to individual investors, so that, in reality, this represents an extension of the individual investor contribution to health care capital financing. The proportion of health care debt held by individuals can, at best, be only estimated. A sampling of investment bankers who were surveyed believed that the major portion of taxable bonds are purchased by individuals. In addition, a large percentage of tax-exempt bond issues are purchased directly by individuals (rather than through the mutual fund device).

Debt Vehicles Preferred by Investors

In the late 1960s and early 1970s mortgage loans were the most popular debt instruments for investors in the health care industry. It is not surprising, in the light of investors' apprehension toward assessing health institutions as real estate, that most of these loans were made to investor-owned facilities which could demonstrate the profitability of a going concern. In addition, investors felt that they could lend on the credit and performance of the owner.

For similar reasons, taxable bond issues have provided a steady source of capital to the industry. In order for an institution to market these issues successfully, it must be capable of exhibiting sufficient economic viability to warrant a competitive credit status.

With the various problems caused by the economic turmoil of the early 1970s, the cost of borrowing became prohibitive for many institutions and, thus, severely limited the number of institutions able to enter the market for their financing needs. The viability of health institutions was affected, not only by high interest rates, but also by tightened regulations under ESP as mentioned earlier.

It was within this framework that the tax-exempt market began to grow. Tax-exempt bonds provided the institutions with an affordable method of borrowing. In addition, these instruments found a willing and expectant market in those lenders who were willing to forego taxable yield for tax-exempt interest. Casualty companies, bond funds, and individuals became the most significant investors.

Rising interest rates in the early 1970s affected not only the not-for-profit institutions, but also impacted upon the borrowing capacity of the proprietaries. It was during these years that the hospital corporations began to move into the area of contract management. Significant benefit was realized by the corporations, since not-for-profit institutions also had access to financing through IRS Ruling 63-20.

Industrial Revenue Bond financing has been frequently used as a conduit by the hospital chains and it is not surprising that many are anxious to see this vehicle more fully developed. Many investors who are in the tax-exempt market find IRBs as safe as, or safer than, the bond issues of not-for-profits.

Despite the national market which tax-exempt financing provides for the health institutions, investors have found the secondary market for these vehicles to be limited, although there are a number of major investment banking firms who offer a market in these securities. The most active investors, therefore, are those who are purchasing bonds to hold for a long period.

The factors which continue to prohibit the flow of investment from the private market are related to the concern of many investors about the industry, rather than about tax-exempt financing itself. The tax-equivalent yields that are offered and required by many investors to mitigate the perceived risk of hospital bonds are often not competitive in the current market. However, the level of risk that is perceived by investors could, itself, be reduced through a greater understanding of the credit involved.

There are some investors, most notably those whose assets are sufficiently large to allow significant portfolio diversification, who strongly believe that government guarantees would adversely affect investment. For these investors, the credit of health institutions would, in effect, become too safe, and these investors would lose interest in the lowered yields.

Although proposed revenue changes to FHA Section 242, which would compel institutions to meet their 10 percent financing requirement with cash rather than with the traditional letter of credit, and would impact adversely upon the issuing facility, investors would not be affected. Likewise, although the pending replacement of IRS Ruling 63–20, taking the issuing authority away from hospitals, would be of no consequence to investors, such action would most likely effectively terminate any further use of this financing vehicle by the health institutions.

Attitudes Towards Investment in Hospitals

With the growing trend toward debt financing and, most particularly, tax-exempt financing, the health care industry has experienced an increased dependency upon the capital markets.

The dilemma for some investors in supplying health care capital lies in their inability to assess the investment comfortably. Although there is a growing recognition that hospitals, nursing homes, and other health facilities can, and should, be viewed on a full credit basis, a significant number of investment decisions are still being made solely in the mortgage departments of prominent lending institutions.

The difficulty with designating health facilities as real estate is, of course, that they are single-purpose buildings and, as such, they offer little to mitigate the investors' fear of adequate remedy in foreclosure. In most cases, a sound credit analysis reduces the investors' overdependency upon the real estate value of the facility. Since the passage of Medicare, health institutions and, most particularly, hospitals, are perceived increasingly as more reliable sources of revenue. Perhaps just as important, reimbursement programs also impacted upon health institutions by encouraging them to initiate a more precise system of cost accounting. This system forced hospital managers to exercise greater control over their operations and was instrumental in the elimination of many inefficiencies. Also, the quality of management is viewed by many to have improved possibly even faster than in other institutions across the country.

It is, therefore, far more feasible today for an investor to determine the economic viability of a health care facility than it was ten years ago. Today, investors require, and look for, a sound financial history, current stability and a bright future. Feasibility studies which attempt to ascertain the future solvency of an institution are being utilized by investors and are almost universally required in any credit determination. Many feel that the quality of these studies has improved and that they are extremely useful. In addition, many investors will generate their own projections to supplement the formal studies. The projection of a given level of debt coverage is a primary concern.

An appraisal of the economic value of a health institution must include an examination of factors other than the financial feasibility. Many investors carefully evaluate the geography and demography of the region where the facility is located. Geographical preferences can be predicted based upon several factors. A regionally diverse portfolio is fundamental to many investors. Medical complexes in our society are evaluated on the basis of their growth potential. States which do not have reliable state agencies to certify need may increase the doubt of some investors. Demographic information is essential in reviewing the utilization patterns and projected patterns for a facility, as well as in projecting sources of revenue and reimbursements. Estimation of the competition which a facility confronts, or will confront, is a consideration. In many cases, the level of community support for the facility is thought to be a strong indication of the probability of its success. Such support is generally reflected in its board of directors. Many investors believe that the prestige of the institution and of the members of its board will ensure financial viability in difficult times. The quality of the medical staff is, of course, very important.

The mix of services which the institution does, or will, provide is an influential criterion in the investment decision. In some cases, the performance of profit centers is measured and compared. The more active investors in health care facilities prefer a diverse combination of specialty units, including provision for ambulatory care. They are also concerned with the implementation of increased efficiencies, such as the sharing of services and high technology equipment. There is also a significant interest in teaching and research facilities, since many investors feel that the existence of high quality services will assure a more reliable and larger source of users.

Investor Concerns

Some investors are wary of investing in the health care industry. They have a number of concerns, including, but not limited to:

1. Can Medicare and Medicaid payments be assured as a reliable source for hospitals or will there be restrictions and delays?
2. Will the certificate of need programs be effective and prevent proliferation?
3. Might increased regulation of rate structures be myopic and not provide adequately for future capital needs?
4. May technological change make institutions and equipment obsolete in such a way as to affect the financial viability of the institution?

Nevertheless, despite all of these concerns, investments in hospital financing have grown dramatically and continue to grow.

National health insurance is a significant unknown. There is no consensus as to when, or even if, such legislation will be enacted, or what form it will assume. Few will dispute that a national insurance plan will ensure a source of revenue to health institutions and resolve the differences now existing among the states' reimbursement plans. Many also believe that the possibility of lower net revenue per patient would be compensated by the increased utilization that such a plan would effect.

However, a common reaction expressed by some investors is that the government will not recognize debt service as a reasonable cost and that sources of income such as philanthropy will not be perceived as separate from operating income.

Many investors believe that national health insurance is unnecessary. They point to the fact that only 15 percent of the population is not already covered by some form of health insurance and recommend that only these individuals be considered for a new plan. These investors suspect that national health insurance will become an inefficient and inflationary alternative as well as a costly program.

The Future of the Proprietaries

The role and future of proprietary hospitals and other profit-oriented facilities has become an area of growing interest. When many investors discuss the potential of proprietaries, they are referring to the future of hospital management corporations. The history of these chains has been one of response to market developments and to changes in the industry.

When the availability of third party revenues fashioned an industry in which hospital ownership could be profitable, the corporations entered the business—basically within the last ten years. At a time when not-for-profit institutions were experiencing difficulty in establishing credit and in locating viable financing vehicles, the corporations were able to flourish through the issuance of common stock and debt. In the early 1970s, however, the chains were also adversely affected by certain factors in the economy. The rising cost of borrowing led many chains to consider seriously the contract management business as an alternative to ownership. In that way initial capital outlays could be avoided. At the same time, tax-exempt financing became available through Industrial Revenue Bonds, IRS 63-20 and state authorities.

As mentioned earlier, there are fewer individual investor-owned facilities today than there were in 1965. Corporate ownership has increased, as has the number of corporately-managed facilities. The chains are also contemplating the extension of their market beyond hospitals into the management of outpatient facilities and HMOs.

The reaction of investors to the growing strength of proprietaries in the industry has been mixed. However, a growing number of investors have been impressed by the ability of the chains to deliver comparable quality services at competitive prices and to maintain a strong profit line.

Hospital corporations are addressing many of the current problems in the industry. The chains can diversify their risk geographically and be equally effective in those rural regions where the raising of capital may be more difficult. They have also been successful in some cases in utilizing resources more efficiently by, for example, the sharing of services.

There are two avenues of thought which place the future of the proprietaries in question. Some investors fear that the climate of increasing regulation will limit their profitability through the imposition of price controls. Others believe that costs in proprietaries and not-for profits and the quality of many services are converging, so that the narrowing of differences may reduce the attractiveness of the corporations as investments.

CONCLUSION

In preparing this paper we were most concerned by the lack of relevant and reliable data. In almost all cases some information is available, but there is no one place where reliable data have been gathered, evaluated, and kept up to date. A strong recommendation would be to commission a truly exhaustive study into the subject of how much money has been spent on health care, where and how it has been spent, and what were the sources of that money.

For our purposes here, that much detail has not been necessary for us to draw certain conclusions. It seems clear that capital funds can be provided to meet the growing capital needs of the health care industry. In fact, whether in an expanding economy or during recession, there is no evidence that there has been any significant gap between the capital needed and the capital provided. The sources of funds have shifted and are continuing to shift: philanthropy and traditional internal sources have given way, first to mortgages and grants and similar sources, and then to bond issues with mortgages and leases.

Economic factors, not really measured or studied here, and a variety of other factors which apply to the nation as a whole, have contributed to the shift from one source of funds to another. For instance, the health care industry is not alone in experiencing a decline in the percentage of assistance being provided by philanthropy.

Of striking note to us in the course of our research was the fact that, despite the Economic Stabilization Program, the recession, and the fact that the ten-year period just concluded saw constant regulatory bickering and change (beginning with Medicare-Medicaid debates and ending with P.L. 93-641), nevertheless, inflation in health care capital costs and the ability to expand capital were similar to the rest of the national economic experience. It is true that inflation was greater for health care during the earlier part of our study period, but we believe that a new push behind hospital construction was caused at that time by the need to construct and to modernize in order to meet the regulatory and other demands of Medicare and Medicaid. It is also true that construction slowed and inflationary pressure lessened in the latter part of the study period, but this was the ESP period and was consistent with national policy and goals.

It appears that this nation, at least for the time being, is willing to countenance a situation where health care construction and related costs occupy a greater portion of the GNP than was historically the case. Social legislation (more accurately, politics), beginning in about 1960, no doubt contributed to this fact. But it seems to us that increased dollars available for capital from investment institutions, advancing technology which produces hardware and systems that need to be sold, and increased expertise and communications which constantly seek to improve and alter health care delivery (and which, on balance, exert additional growth pressures) have been of greater significance to the relative position of health care expenditures for construction and the size of the GNP.

The number of hospitals in the country has remained relatively static. The need for services and refinements in thinking relative to the type of services needed have produced shifts away from large federal hospitals and very small country hospitals to facilities with greater ambulatory care capability and to institutions owned, or owned and operated, by private, nonprofit organizations and for-profit investor-owned corporations. In sum, there is an increasing participation by the private sector, whether at the nonprofit or for-profit level. This may seem ironic in an age of increasing governmental regulation. But we believe that the responsibilities and fiduciary duties carried out by nonprofit hospital boards of trustees, and the efficiency needed to produce profits in the case of proprietary institutions, are elements which produce, or will produce, the best atmosphere and the most hope for the health care consumer. The patient, after all, is positioned between management and regulator, and he is dependent upon them to create a system where he can be cared for at a reasonable cost.

The patient, however, has had small direct influence on capital expenditures during our study period. Rather, market considerations appear to be way out in front as the single most influential factor relative to the amount of money spent on health care since 1965. Changes in regulation, ESP considerations and all other similar factors seem to be elements which have been discounted by the market place rather than serious hindrances to the ability to finance health care construction. The market requires a rate of interest as compensation, and if that rate is available, or if a rate in excess of acceptable levels may be obtained, then the financial institutions of this nation will provide capital.

This is not to say that, in all events, any capital project may be financed. Proper security, in the form of pledges of real property and revenues and additional security to be derived through subordinations and covenants against future dilution, are required, in some form, in order to accomplish financings. In addition, projections of revenues, including studies of demand and the analysis of competing facilities, are now used to increase the lender's understanding of the projects and to enhance the contention that the hospital borrower is creditworthy.

Yet, in the final analysis, all but the most risky hospital credits are able to borrow for capital needs. This borrowing may involve either governmental or private sources. Well-known default situations which have occurred in various parts of the country have not appreciably slowed the ability of institutions to borrow. When there are investment funds available, they must be invested, and quickly. That is how the market works. The main question then becomes the cost of borrowing. Here, again, overall trends in the money market are the key, and not various new health care regulations or the relative merits of health care institutional credit.

However, it is true that hospitals and related facilities remain among the most costly to finance, primarily because many institutional purchasers of debt simply do not fully understand the business of hospitals, so that the risks inherent to them require that they be compensated with higher rates of interest.

For this reason, and because costs of borrowing contribute significantly to health care costs, and because the market appears to be there for such borrowing at such high costs, it would seem that regulation should concentrate not only on defining which construction should take place, but also on creating an atmosphere where the creditworthiness of hospitals can be better assured. More assured systems of reimbursement, through national health insurance or otherwise, based on approved projects and with specific reference to costs of financing, would reduce interest and other costs of financing health care. In addition, all methods of financing, including tax-exempt, should be made available to approved hospital and related projects, whether such projects are for charitable or for profit institutions.

In circumstances where regulation appropriately recognizes and gives better assurance of the repayment of debt for health care projects, it seems that the long range prognosis for controlling health care costs will be optimistic. In a generally expanding economy (and it would appear that the United States meets this description), regulation should be carefully geared, not only to restrict and guide the construction of certain facilities, but also as a means whereby available funds for investment might be prevented from being directed, in ever increasing amounts, into the health care field. If this goal is not accomplished, then, in most cases, the money will be invested to assist in the proliferation of unwanted facilities.

With an appropriate amount of brick and mortar in place or in progress, the day may come when available funds could be used to improve certain personnel compensation related to health delivery, to find better solutions to the problems of inequitable distribution of available facilities and for the growing capital needs which will be associated with the creation of facilities for health maintenance.

NOTE

1. Social Security Administration, Office of Research and Statistics.

Discussion of
A Study of the American Capital Market
and Its Relationship to the Capital Needs
of the Health Care Field

Karl D. Bays
(Presented by
Richard Williams)

INTRODUCTION

The study on "Capital Investment in the Health Care Industry" which is being presented at this conference, highlights several important trends in generating and financing capital projects.

Before I begin my analysis of the present capital market, let me summarize the major trends covered in the conference paper.

1. In both real and nominal terms, total capital expenditures in the health care industry are rising at least as fast, and probably faster, than either the Gross National Product or total business capital spending.
2. The total number of hospital facilities has remained relatively constant over the last ten years although there has been some shift in the composition of the total.
3. Both the total number of beds and occupancy rates have decreased over the last ten years.
4. Regular admissions are up slightly, and outpatient admissions have almost doubled in the last ten years.
5. Philanthropy and retained earnings (equity funds) have both decreased their relative positions as a source of funds for financing capital expenditures.
6. Borrowed capital has risen from just under 40 percent to 65 percent of all sources of capital financing in the last seven years. On a current basis, this means that almost $4 billion is needed in debt financing this year.

Several implications may be drawn from these facts. I will discuss them in two categories: first, implications for the demand for capital expenditures, and second, implications for raising funds. Afterwards, I will offer some recommendations for specific actions.

CURRENT DEMAND FOR
CAPITAL EXPENDITURES

The trends which I have just outlined clearly point to a change in the nature of capital spending over the last few years. The relative constancy in total facilities, the decrease in occupancy and the decrease in average stay in the hospital, along with the overall increase in expenditures, imply that more money is being spent per patient. Some of this rise is due to inflation; however, it also is due to shifts in technology and in the nature of health care delivery. There is every reason to believe that these trends will continue and, consequently, we should observe a continuing pressure for new capital.

Further, there is what might be called an unrealized demand for capital expenditures due to the current payment mechanisms used in the delivery of health care. Many knowledgeable people have argued that the public utility sector overspends on capital goods because the ultimate rate of return depends on the assets employed in the utility industry. Similarly, it might be argued that the health care industry is undercapitalized because many reimbursement schemes allow a larger percentage of direct costs to be passed through than they allow capital costs to be recovered.

This undercapitalization due to cost reimbursement has several consequences. One is that the reimbursement schemes may discourage the use of the most cost-effective method of delivering a particular patient service. This can happen when the more capital intensive costs would be lower but not recoverable in full. Thus, there is a direct increase in the total health care costs to society due to this built-in inefficiency.

Any change in reimbursement schemes which are designed to remedy this problem will stimulate the demand for cost-effective systems and place an additional pressure on the health care industry to finance new capital expenditures.

CURRENT FINANCING OF HEALTH CARE
CAPITAL EXPENDITURES

The continued growth in the need which we foresee for capital expenditures implies a continued need for raising new capital in the health care industry. The current situation shows a clear trend toward more debt financing and less equity financing.

If the financial health of the industry is to be maintained, the trend toward ever more debt financing must be reversed at some point. The temptation is strong to continue outside borrowing because it quite often provides the most expedient method of raising funds. However, as debt levels increase, the convenience will disappear, making future borrowing increasingly difficult.

For every borrower, there must be a lender. The main concern of every lender is the ability of the borrower to repay interest and principal in a timely fashion. Health care institutions compete with the federal government, state and municipal governments, and private businesses for funds in the capital markets. If other classes of borrowers are offering a more secure promise to repay, they will have first access to funds generated in the capital markets.

Lenders to the health care industry will scrutinize the financial and operating records of the health care facility in the same manner that they analyze other borrowers in making their investment decisions. The criteria that they will use include historical coverage of past debt servicing, capital structure, and current management practices.

In addition to analyzing the current and historical record, investors may ask for additional security in the form of collateral. If the financial prospects and/or the collateral are deficient relative to other classes of borrowers, capital will simply not be made available to the health care institution. Further, that capital which is forthcoming will demand a large price or high interest rate to compensate for the larger perceived risk incurred in making the loan.

However, several health care trends that I have mentioned are at odds with a picture of increased reliance on debt financing. The shift from "bricks and mortar" expenditures works against the most traditional type of hospital debt, that of mortgage loans. Mortgages, or collateralized loans, become much less viable as the capital expenditures shift from general site construction to more specialized buildings and more specialized equipment expenditures.

Thus, the traditional investor reliance on collateral to augment the safety of principal and interest will have to be replaced by an increased reliance on current operations to provide a sound basis for generating funds. From the investors' point of view, this increased reliance on current operations means cash flow projections to provide coverage of debt service as well as debt to equity ratios which are in line with those of other classes of borrowers.

The only alternative to this increased financial soundness of the borrower is a reliance on government, preferably the federal government, for a guarantee. If debt were backed by the government's promise to pay, it would have the same degree of risk in the minds of the lenders as that of the government guarantor. In the current capital market, many state and municipal governments are not viewed with great favor by the lending institutions. This leaves the federal government as the guarantor of choice.

We will not dwell on the implications of federal government guarantees for private health care debt financing. Suffice it to say that increased financial soundness of the health care industry is the only alternative.

While I believe that a trend toward ever more debt financing is not a viable future for health care institutions, some reliance on debt financing must remain. In that case, increased financial soundness, represented by respectable coverage ratios and leverage ratios, will not only provide access to the capital markets but also access at reasonable prices.

One measure of the market's view of the ability to pay interest and principal in a timely fashion is represented by the ratings that are given to various health care borrowers by the two most widely used rating agencies, Moody's Investors Service and Standard & Poor's. It is widely recognized that the combination of coverage ratios, leverage ratios, and a general assessment of management are the main components of the ratings assigned by these agencies. The higher the historical debt service coverage, the lower the debt-equity ratio and the stronger the management is perceived, the higher the rating.

To see what difference the rating can have in borrowing costs, a recent analysis of seventy-two hospital tax-exempt bond issues showed a spread of 338 basis points (3.38 percentage points in interest paid) between the highest rated borrower (Aaa) and the lowest rated borrowers (BBB-Baa).

For example, a $10 million bond issue placed at the highest rating will save $6.76 million in interest over a twenty-year period, as compared with the same $10 million bond issued at the lowest rating, assuming the 338 basis point spread. Thus, substantial savings may be realized by achieving financial soundness, at least according to the criteria employed by the rating agencies.

GENERAL SUGGESTIONS FOR INCREASING FINANCIAL SOUNDNESS

There are many areas which might be examined for improving the overall economic condition of a hospital. The four prime areas that I would like to discuss are pricing and dealing with diverse reimbursement policies, operating efficiencies, structuring debt issues, and alternate financing methods.

In the area of pricing and dealing with reimbursement schemes, hospitals are not always free to collect a fee for services based on the market price of the services. Reimbursement, especially by government or quasi-government agencies such as Medicare and Medicaid, often follows formulas which do not allow full recovery of costs for all services.

In many respects, the problem of pricing and reimbursement lies at the heart of any discussion of raising capital funds. As I have pointed out, the two most important elements in the investor's assessment of the borrower's ability to repay interest and principal are the debt service coverage and the capital structure of the borrower.

This means that the hospital must show sufficient cash flow to cover debt service by a multiple of three to five times, and it must show a substantial portion of its assets backed by equity. In each case, revenue generation is the key to providing the necessary financial picture for competing favorably in the capital markets.

Pricing must be such that there is some profit in the system to provide funds to support a substantial portion of new capital expenditures. This equity base may be viewed as supporting the debt financed portion of new capital raised.

Again let me point out that a sound financial picture of the hospital allows not only entry to capital markets, but, also, entry at reasonable prices.

The profit in the system may be viewed in another way. It can be regarded as the return or repayment of the capital that is invested by the hospital, and, as such, it is just as necessary as payment of the wage bill. In other words, sufficient funds must be generated to repay existing debt in order that new debt be fundable.

The current system of medical reimbursement is a hindrance to the generation of retained earnings and the return on capital that is necessary to promote a competitive position in the financial markets. In fact, to the extent that less than full reimbursement is made by government agencies, a tax is placed on the hospital. This tax could easily be larger than the corporate income tax on private firms. In addition, it is quite arbitrary, since it depends on the percentage of patients covered by Medicare and Medicaid.

Current reimbursement methods have the effect of minimizing the direct charges to the insurer. However, this method of holding down costs is illusory. It promotes less than the most efficient combination of capital and labor for accomplishing many tasks and raises an ever increasing barrier to raising additional capital.

Also, current methods of reimbursement shift onto the uninsured patient the burden of inflated costs which will ultimately either drive that patient out of the health care delivery system and into the uncollected statistics or force him into an ever widening government-backed insurance system. In either of these events, the uninsured patient will not remain a viable source of recovering costs.

What is needed is reimbursement of full economic costs as opposed to reimbursement of only certain accounting costs. Included in full cost reimbursement would be an implicit return on capital at least as large as the inflation rate, depreciation charges based on replacement cost, and an allowance for uncollectable charges or charity cases.

A hospital is a complex organism providing a multiplicity of economic and social services. Its main business is to provide health services. In providing these services, it performs several auxiliary economic functions.

The hospital is a hotel, a dining facility, a warehouse, a parking lot, a billing and record-keeping service, and so forth. All of these separate economic functions must be so managed as to be cost-competitive with similar private single-purpose business entities. If they are not, the overall cost-revenue generation will not provide the basic financial position to make the hospital competitive in the capital markets.

From Adam Smith onward, specialization has been the basic tenet in our economic system. Thus, taking advantage of specialized services can increase the hospital's operating efficiency.

The use of contractual services to provide many of the nonmedical functions of the hospital is one such use of specialization. Contracting outside housekeeping, plant engineering, and dietary services not only may provide increased economic efficiency, but, also, has the extra benefit of freeing funds for medical-related projects, because capital which had been tied up in nonmedical facilities will be provided by the private suppliers of the services.

Along with specialization, the concept of economies of scale plays an important role in providing increased efficiency. Many facilities have scale economies which may be realized only at a scale of operation larger than could be provided by one hospital. Thus, to realize the economies of scale several hospitals might need to share facilities.

For example, a central computer facility for billing and record keeping might serve many hospitals. In this way, the duplication of both hardware and software could be avoided. Similarly, centralized clinical laboratories might eliminate duplication of the purchase of expensive batch processing equipment and the employment of specialized technicians.

If outside support for laundry and dietary services is not contracted, these facilities could be shared by several hospitals. Warehousing and inventory control systems might also be shared by several hospitals.

While the idea is simple in concept, implementation of shared facilities requires a good deal of managerial skill. Cooperation and problem-solving, especially among competing institutions, does not arise unless thoughtful planning and careful negotiating take place. Here, then, is an area in which direct management talent can increase the financial soundness of the hospital.

Concerning the structuring of debt issues, there are several types of debt instruments which may be issued by hospitals. Debt may be publicly issued or privately placed. It may be taxable or, in certain cases, it may be tax-exempt.

Within these categories, the debt may be purchased by several different classes of lenders. Both institutional investors and private investors may purchase the various hospital debt offerings.

To a large extent, the hospital chooses its lenders by its financial structure. In other words, the choice of loan terms, covenants, and conditions determines the choice of investor. In structuring the financing, the health care institution should try to retain maximum flexibility for future offerings.

Besides future flexibility, costs differ among various types of debt. Taxable publicly issued bonds will usually have a higher issuance cost than will privately sold bonds due to costs associated with underwriting risks, sales commissions, legal and printing costs, and the like. Further, due to the small relative size of the typical issue and the fragmentation of the hospital debt market, underwriting costs may be higher than for comparable industrial bonds. All but the largest issues will not have the size to provide liquidity for a secondary market, and this typically raises the risk to the underwriter, who will then need additional compensation.

A 1 percent front end underwriting charge on a 9 percent taxable bond maturing in twenty years raises the effective rate to 9.15 percent. A private placement of the same issue might have avoided this front end charge.

Tax-exempt bonds have the obvious advantage of paying a smaller coupon rate. There also is a relatively strong and well-developed market for tax-exempt securities. Typically, tax-exempt issues are sold as the debt of some public authority which acts solely as a conduit, provides the tax-exempt status and usually imposes conditions on the bond covenants to protect the bond holders.

Some restrictions and impositions of public agencies provide interesting management challenges. For example, debt service reserve funds which are sometimes required by bonding authorities offer the possibility of interest arbitrage in favor of the hospital. In certain cases, advance refunding also offers opportunities for the hospital manager actually to increase revenues from financially related transactions in the tax-exempt area.

The use of FHA Section 242 loans, or loans insured by the Government National Mortgage Association, also provides possibilities for lower interest terms through the credit standing of these agencies. The costs are typically severe restrictions placed in the covenants of the loans and the time involved in securing necessary permissions and approvals. Again, interesting possibilities arise from solid management reviews of these instruments, especially with the advent of the Chicago Board of Trade market for the Government National Mortgage Association securities.

Thus, good management practices and solid review and discussion of the various possibilities for structuring a debt issue may substantially decrease or offset the costs that are involved in borrowing funds.

Leasing productive capital may also be a viable alternative to competing for funds in the capital markets. This is espeically relevant in the current environment that is constrained by cost-based reimbursement and federal and state regulatory laws.

However, to employ leasing as a rational alternative, the hospital administrator must understand the types of leasing arrangements available and, especially, the effects of leasing within a system of cost reimbursement.

If a lease arrangement is deemed to be a rental and not a purchase of equipment, the lease payments are considered a current expense and are reimbursed under cost reimbursement formulas. Under many such formulas, costs that are associated with equipment which is debt financed are limited to operating costs, depreciation expense, and interest expense. Whenever the loan repayment period is shorter than the depreciable life of the asset, the cash flow that is generated by the cost reimbursement will not be sufficient to cover repayment of interest and principal.

Leasing also relieves the hospital of the risk of technological obsolescence of equipment. Any equipment which needs to be replaced prior to its full depreciable life will lose its revenue generating power under cost reimbursement formulas. With leasing, the risk of obsolescence is borne by the lessor. Of course, a charge sufficient to compensate for this risk may be included in the lease payment schedule. This charge is then included as part of the reimbursable costs and is passed on to the insurer, rather than being absorbed by the hospital.

Leases may also allow hospitals to avoid certain direct regulation, such as federal (P.L. 93-641) and state certificate of need laws which require that all purchases over $100,000 be subject to the approval of regional planning agencies.

The hospital administrator must exercise care and good management judgment in entering a leasing arrangement. Some leases require a prepayment of the last several periods of the lease contract. Third parties will reimburse the hospital for these lease payments only during those periods for which they actually apply. Thus, working capital is encumbered for the duration of the lease. Substantial use of such leases would generate severe working capital problems for the hospital.

In addition, the lease arrangement has a substantial bearing on the degree to which lease payments may be reimbursed. A financial lease is typically characterized by full recovery of the purchase price of the asset by the lessor over the life of the asset and the transfer of ownership to the hospital at the end of the lease period. A rental lease usually does not imply ownership rights to the hospital and quite often does provide full cost recovery by the lessor.

If the asset does not retain any future service potential at the end of the lease period, the hospital may be considered to have owned the asset in substance. Under a financial lease, the equipment will be carried as an asset on the hospital's balance sheet, together with an explicit recognition of the lease as a liability. In this case, cost reimbursement may be treated like a debt financed project. I should also point out that with a financial lease it is imperative that the lease contract explicitly state the interest charge so that it may be eligible for reimbursement.

Leasing, its implications for cost reimbursement and its effect on the financial condition of the hospital is a complicated subject. However, good management can utilize leasing to increase the total financing potential of the hospital and to increase revenues and decrease costs.

To summarize, a hospital is a purposive economic unit which must compete with private business and with the government for scarce resources, such as capital, technical personnel, and managerial talent. To compete effectively, hospitals must take advantage of the same managerial skills as those employed in private business and structure their financial positions to attract investors.

Hospitals must take advantage of specialization, the economy of scale and outside expertise when necessary skills are not available internally. Also, they must not be hampered by government regulations which have the effect of promoting inefficient operations.

Only under these circumstances will the cost of medical care administered by hospitals move with the general level of economic activity.

Discussion of
A Study of the American Capital Market
and Its Relationship to the Capital Needs
of the Health Care Field

Barry Bosworth

Mr. Clapp and Mr. Spector have compiled a useful set of data concerning the pattern of capital spending and financing within the health care field. I believe that I would also agree with their conclusion that there is not a capital market problem which is specific to the health care industry; private markets should be adequate to serve the future needs of the industry.

In their examination of past trends, they emphasize the role of the price controls program in accounting for the decline in construction activity after 1972. Given the perspective of their own data, I am surprised that they do not place a greater emphasis upon the evidence of excess capacity as a result of previous overbuilding. I also do not share their concern about the growth of debt financing. Since these facilities last for a long period and serve a local population which changes over time, I think that future users should be required to finance a portion of the cost through amortization.

The interest cost of capital financing has increased substantially, but this is a reflection of a general rise in interest rates and is not specific to the health industry. These rates, in turn, reflect the acceleration of inflation to which medical care has been a major contributor. I think that it is unfortunate that these higher interest costs should be used as a justification for greater reliance upon loan guarantees and tax-exempt bond issues.

Except in those situations where they are aimed at correcting specific capital market imperfections, loan guarantees are highly undesirable. The sorting out of good and bad investment projects is one of the most valuable functions that the capital markets perform, but the existence of a guarantee leads a lender to be indifferent about the quality of investment projects and the result can be an enormous waste of resources and defaults which must be paid for by the taxpayer. In this case, there is no reason to believe that the capital markets cannot correctly evaluate the relative merits of investment in the health care area.

The increased reliance upon tax-exempts is equally undesirable, from a general, public policy point of view. It is a very inefficient form of subsidy, since nearly half of the tax loss accrues to high income individuals rather than to the subsidized sector. The proliferation of these forms of subsidies is one of the major barriers to the effective use of capital markets to allocate a limited amount of savings.

The evidence of the Clapp-Spector paper implies an industry with excess capacity where future investment should decline. I see little reason to try to prevent this trend through credit subsidies.

The investment problems of the health-care industry result from rapid increases in capital goods prices and from high interest rates. These problems are general to the whole economy and result from inflation rather than from specific capital market difficulties. As a major contributor to the inflation, the health care industry would be best served by addressing the inflation problem directly rather than by trying to avoid its costs through new capital market subsidies or the expansion of old ones.

The primary future concern for capital formation in the health care industry would seem to revolve around the probability of a national health insurance program and its impact upon the growth in demand for health care facilities. This issue is not addressed directly in the paper, but the data, indicating substantial underutilization of facilities, would seem to imply that a considerable surge in demand could be met without a shortage of facilities. However, the type of program that is enacted may sharply affect the composition of demand and, thus, strain physical facilities in some areas.

There has been some concern about a general "crisis" of capital formation in the United States which could impinge upon the health care industry, but recent developments and studies have tended to reduce it. Studies of capital "needs" indicate that future increased requirements for energy investment and pollution abatement are not of sufficient magnitude for a sharp increase of the economy—wide ratio of investment to GNP. Private savings have been very stable as a share of GNP, with substantial increases over time in household saving rates. Recently, the downward trend in business savings has also reversed, with the implication that business financing in the capital markets will be moderate in future years.

Instead, the "capital crisis," I believe, should be seen more properly as simply a reflection of the more basic problems of inflation and recession. The shortage of capital is one of composition rather than overall magnitudes, as industries have been led to make serious capacity planning errors because of the cyclical instability of demand in the last decade.

In addition, the structure of our capital markets, with intense emphasis upon fixed interest debt instruments and highly liquid deposit accounts for savers, is poorly suited to a world of inflation. However, evolutionary changes are taking place to moderate these problems.

The equity market is becoming an important source of new investment funds and financial institutions are broadening the structure of both their assets and their liabilities. Most of these changes can be accomplished without the need for significant government actions. Thus, I would conclude that a "capital crisis" is not a significant problem for the health care field.

Discussion

Mr. Ziegler: Depreciation is designed for debt service and, as investment bankers, I think that we should tell the borrower that he is wrong if he wants to use it for some other reason. Depreciation should be used for what it is designed for and it is our responsibility to make sure that it is.

Dr. Bosworth: I see nothing wrong, in principle, with the notion of subsidies. If the federal government wants to subsidize, it should go through state, local, or federal budgets or through taxation. I think it inappropriate to shift resources for such social projects through the capital market where the burden falls on other capital market projects. We have to recognize that every time that we finance a hospital through the financial market, instead of saying that all Americans in general should bear some reduction in their current level of consumption and make those resources available for hospital care, we shift the burden to the housing industry and to small business.

Mr. Van Nostrand: Since HRA is currently reviewing the future of the loan guarantee programs of Title XVI of the PHS Act, as well as the FHA loan guarantees, I think that credit subsidies should be carefully reviewed to determine if they are useful or are, in fact, a detriment to proper capital formation. If there truly is excess capital in the health care industry, there needs to be further consideration as to when credit subsidies should exist and how they can be targeted to areas where the capital markets are imperfect.

Dr. Bosworth: Loan guarantees lead to an excessive focus of capital intensity in the choice of the particular type of inputs that hospitals, or any other type of industry, should choose to put into the production process. One may argue that there are regulatory measures and other features that lead to distortions in the opposite direction, but the answer is to try to correct those distortions and not to pile one set of distortions atop another.

Dr. Evans: I think that Dr. Bosworth's comment is one of the clearer statements that we have had so far and I very much agree with him. But one thing that does worry me a bit is his objection to loan guarantees on the grounds that one of the primary objectives of the capital market is to try to allocate funds in response to some kind of underlying economic structure. It seems to me that one of the key problems in the health care sector is that funds are allocated in the expectation of generation of cash flow, and that this has little to do with health care needs.

Mr. Spector: I certainly do not find any evidence to indicate that the capital market as we know it is responsive to changed priorities or the problems of the inner city. Even so, they are subject, in some degree, to local public policy. The community identifies the need for capital in an area and expresses public policy. I think that it is important to link planning and public policy objectives with the question of capital formation.

Mr. Schwab: Whether a particular capital project is appropriate or desirable from a health policy perspective is a question having little impact or role in "external" investment decisions. The policy issues, consequently, would seem to be: who determines the appropriateness of such capital projects; how is this determination most effectively undertaken in the context of a participatory planning process; what analytic basis should underlie such a determination, given the current "state of the art"; and, once such determinations have been obtained, what alternative forms of financing, including those offered by the capital market, are themselves appropriate for respective capital projects.

Dr. Cain: When the Health Planning Act was going through the Congress, there was one provision that was discussed that would have required the Health Planning Agency to review all existing institutional services for their "appropriateness." I understand that the private capital financing community became very concerned over that kind of provision. From what I understand, the result of such a provision would be a rise in interest rates because of the increased risk.

Dr. Ginzberg: Do investment bankers get requests for relatively small amounts of money which are aimed at changing the ratio of capital to human resources? In many industries, part of the labor is replaced with new capital equipment, with the intent of lowering costs. Do present reimbursement systems discourage people who would want to open up ambulatory facilities from coming into the capital markets? This is again a question of appropriateness. The capital market in this area seems to operate in terms of cash flow or salability as distinct from serviceability.

Mr. Clapp: We do get requests for systems relative to equipment and other items which, in our business, we call small leases. But, in the hospital industry new equipment tends to create more jobs, even though the equipment is more efficient.

If you are making the point that the vast majority of capital providers have not yet tackled the question of appropriateness, that is so, and I don't think that they will until such time as the communication between groups such as this convinces them of the importance of this issue, and that there is the kind of regulation that prevents them from investing in inappropriate facilities.

✳ *Chapter 9*

The Projected Response of the Capital Markets to Health Facilities Expenditures

Robert S. Kelling, Jr.
Paul C. Williams

INTRODUCTION AND SUMMARY

The purpose of this paper is to project and evaluate the response of
the capital markets to future demands for debt and equity financing
for health care facilities over the next five-year period. We shall examine the
ability of the diverse funding sources to meet the anticipated increases in financing requirements. Special attention will be given to the market for tax-exempt
hospital revenue bonds. Further, we shall take into consideration recent changes
in federal and state legislation and policy as they will affect the supply and
demands for funds. Finally, we shall conclude with commentary on proposed
legislation as it may effect the capital funding process.

The private debt market has emerged as the leading and most rapidly growing
source of funds over the past fifteen years. This development may be associated
with the advent of Medicare and Medicaid and the broadening enrollment of
private health insurance plan coverage. Third party reimbursement plans have
laid the foundation for securing debt financing, thus shifting the burden from
philanthropy, government grants, and internal sources. Within the past five years,
there has been a dramatic change in the composition of debt financing, with the
result that tax-exempt debt financing is now providing more than half of the
new funds raised to finance community hospital construction, replacement and
remodeling. In a period of mounting inflation, there is an expectation that capital

The authors wish to acknowledge the contribution of Elizabeth Berman, research assistant, who gathered and evaluated much of the background and supportive data for this
paper.

319

needs could far surpass funding sources, which is heightened by the fact that the health care sector now places a critical dependence upon tax-exempt financing.

Will there be a "capital gap"? What will be the impact of national health insurance on hospital utilization and the demand for funds? Our research addressed these questions, among others, and we have derived the following conclusions.

We do not foresee a "capital gap" for bricks and mortar construction. While it is true that the visions of hospital administrators and trustees will always surpass, in the aggregate, their ability to finance projects, we believe, for a variety of reasons, that implemented construction programs will not place an inordinate strain on the capital market . . .

Most of the recent increase in expenditures is explained by inflation. In terms of constant 1967 dollars, there has been no increase in real spending since 1970. According to Department of Commerce construction data, real spending has actually declined slightly since 1972. The intent of recent legislation (most notably the Social Security Amendments of 1972 and the National Health Planning and Resources Development Act of 1974) is to rationalize the hospital facilities planning process. The result has been to slow down or to queue the implementation of hospital capital construction and to improve utilization. While national health insurance, if enacted, may result in a new surge in hospital care expenditures, comparable to the Medicare/Medicaid surge of the late 1960s, we do not believe that it will induce a concomitant surge in capital expenditures. Unlike in the late 1960s, the health care community is now moving away from the idea that "more is better," and the emphasis is clearly being placed on improved utilization, the merger of institutions, renovation, replacement, and outpatient care.

There appears to be a flurry of financing and construction activity prompted by the desire of hospitals to beat inflation and to build before more stringent regulations are effected, but this anticipatory construction will soon expire.

While we believe that there will be no "capital gap," in projecting over the next five years we see a number of potential developments which could seriously inhibit the ability of many health care institutions to raise funds in the capital market. We are frankly concerned that certain features of potential laws and regulations, which are intended to contain health care costs, will inadvertently impair debt security, in both a real sense and in the perception of the investment community which will be expected to accept future hospital loans.

DEFINITIONS

In developing our projections, we have defined health care facilities and capital funding in terms of physical assets and dollars. Our discussion is limited to those investments made by health care institutions to construct, expand, renovate, and equip the physical plant of the nation's health care delivery system. Given the data that were available and could be assembled for this paper, we have divided our definition of health care facilities into the following categories:

1. Community hospitals: nonfederal, short-term acute care hospitals
   a. nonprofit
   b. local government-owned
   c. proprietary or investor-owned
2. Extended care and nursing home facilities
3. Major equipment.

Throughout this paper, references to hospitals will mean community hospitals which serve most of the acute care needs of the nation. According to the American Hospital Association, the breakdown is as shown in Table 9-1. Federally-owned and-operated hospitals and state mental health facilities are not included in the scope of our analysis.

Due the paucity of data, we could not provide further breakdowns for ambulatory outpatient clinics or health maintenance organizations. As of this writing, the data obtainable for nursing homes and equipment expenditures is quite general and approximate.

Health care facilities are financed, as a general rule, from permanent funding sources, including philanthropy, governmental grants, debt, leases, and internally generated surplus cash flow. The discussion of financing requirements and funding sources is limited to permanent funding; thus, for example, interim or construction financing which ultimately will be refinanced with a mortgage loan or a bond issue is not included in our computations.

Table 9-2 delineates the funding sources and methods; it outlines the market structure and institutional relationships through which health care institutions obtain capital funds. Using an index rating of 1-5, we have assigned values to identify the relative importance of a particular financing vehicle within the total institutional framework. The left side of the chart shows the relative importance of a particular financing vehicle to a particular use or purpose. The right side of the chart depicts the relative importance of each source of funding.

For example, lease financing is used virtually exclusively for major equipment and it is placed almost exclusively with banks. Other market channels have not been substantially developed. On the other hand, tax-exempt revenue bonds are a very important source of financing for nonprofit community hospitals and these bonds are placed with five categories of investors—banks, trusts, insurance companies, individuals, and bond funds. The bond funds are the most important

Table 9-1

Community Hospitals—1974	*Hospitals*	*Beds (000)*	*Average Beds*
Nonprofit	3,381	650	192
State and Local Government	1,821	211	116
Investor-Owned	775	70	90
Totals	5,977	931	

Table 9-2.   Health Care Facilities Financing Institutional Structure

| | Uses | | | | | | | | Sources | | | | | | |
| | Community Hospitals | | | Extended Care & Nursing Home | Major Equipment | Internal | | | External–Market Channels | | | | | | |
Financing Vehicle	Non-Profit	State & Local	Propri-etary			Cash Flow	Endow-ments	Corpora-tions & Founda-tions	Govern-ment	Banks	Trusts	Insur-ance Co.'s	Pension Funds	Indi-viduals	Bond Funds
Depreciation	2	2	2	2	4	5									
Net Income	2	2	2	2	4	5									
Philanthropy	1			3	1		2	5						4	
Taxable Bonds	3			2	3					2	2	3	3	5	1
Mortgage Loans															
a) Conventional	3			4	3					5	1	5	1		
b) FHA Insured	1			2	1					5	1	5	5		
c) HEW Guaranteed & Subsidized	1				1				2	5	1	5	5		
Tax-Exempt Bonds															
a) Revenue Bonds	5	1	2	5	5					3	2	3		3	5
b) Tax-supported		5		1	1					5	3			4	1
c) HEW Direct Loan	1			1	1				5						
Common Stock			1									5	2	5	
Bonds & Debentures			5									5	2	5	
Lease				5	5					5					

Scale of Relative Importance
1—Very Minor
2—Minor
3—Moderate
4—Important
5—Major Factor

market sector. Trust purchases are very minor, since trust accounts tend to buy tax supported bonds. Pension funds, though they represent enormous accumulations of capital, do not need tax-exempt income and, with few exceptions, do not purchase tax-exempt bonds.

While it was not possible to quantify the flow of funds for each financing vehicle and source, we were able to establish estimates of aggregate money flows for certain market channels.

CAPITAL EXPENDITURES AND HEALTH CARE FACILITIES

The time horizon for our quantitative projections is five years, to 1981. We anticipate that developments over the next five years will largely reflect the momentum of current trends as they may be modified by recent legislation and policy actions. To identify those trends, it is useful to recapitulate the historical pattern of the past ten years. This backward glance reveals how supply and demand relationships have changed, how quickly they have changed, and what factors should be considered in looking to the future.

HISTORICAL PERSPECTIVE

Between 1966 and 1975, total health care expenditures increased from $44.9 billion to $122.3 billion, nearly threefold, at a compound rate of 10.5 percent. Statistics compiled by the American Hospital Association show that hospital care expenditures also increased slightly more than threefold, from $14.2 billion to $46.6 billion during the same interval. Construction expenditures (the demand for construction funds) kept pace with total spending increases. Construction reports prepared by the Department of Commerce indicate that private hospital construction (value put in place) increased from $1.2 billion to $3.4 billion between 1966 and 1975. Most of the increase over the past decade is explained by inflation. In terms of constant dollars, however, based upon a construction index in which 1967 is the base year, real aggregate expenditures have increased from $1.54 billion to $1.83 billion, by approximately 18.8 percent. Over the past four years, real expenditures have declined slightly.

Table 9-3 shows the distribution of construction expenditures by the five basic categories.

Factors Behind the Trends

The average annual rate of growth in hospital care expenditures between 1965 and 1970 was 14.5 percent and between 1970 and 1974, 12.5 percent. Most of the increase in spending resulted from the introduction of Medicare and Medicaid between 1965 and 1970. Federal and state contributions to health care expenditures increased 24 percent a year during that period. Hospital utilization expanded commensurately.

Table 9-3.   Distribution of Capital Expenditures (000,000s)

	1976 (est)	*1974*	*1968*
Community Hospitals			
Nonprofit	$2,500	$2,400	$ 850
State and Local	700	680	175
Proprietary	180	170	75
Nursing Homes	800	750	275
Major Equipment	900	700	300
	$5,080	$4,700	$1,675

Source: American Hospital Association.
Data adjusted by John Nuveen & Co., Incorporated.

During this period, expenditures under the old Hill-Burton program reached a peak and then quickly declined. In 1968 and 1969, general hospitals built over 20,000 beds with the aid of Hill-Burton grants and locally generated sources. By 1971, this activity had dropped to 6,600 beds and has declined steadily since then.

Over the past ten years, the average bed complement for all community hospitals has increased by 20 percent from 129 to 156. Admissions increased from 26.4 to 32.9 million, and inpatient days from 205 to 225 million. Utilization rates and average length of stay (ALOS) in the aggregate remained virtually constant. The nationwide average length of stay reached a peak of 8.4 days in 1968 and then dropped steadily back to 7.7 in 1974 as Medicare/Medicaid reimbursement changed and as utilization and review had begun to take effect. Of all categories of service, outpatient visits underwent a remarkable increase, from 106 million to 194 million between 1965 and 1974, reflecting the extension of reimbursement to include outpatient services, the general decline of family practitioners and the substitution of outpatient for inpatient procedures.

Several observations are pertinent: First, combining inpatient and outpatient services, total utilization has increased considerably, while the composition of services has changed. This may be observed not only in admissions but in statistics on surgical and laboratorical procedures. Second, there has been a dramatic change in medical equipment technology. Third, the average age of the nation's hospital plant system has probably remained constant, while design and operations standards have escalated substantially. A major portion of the system has been rendered obsolete or nonconforming.

These trends, along with shifts in the geographic distribution of population, have changed the pattern of demand for capital. We reviewed the official statements for twenty-five hospital financings involving $475 million in construction and $545 million in tax-exempt bond financing over the past two years. In the aggregate these hospitals expanded the total bed complement by 4.35 percent, from 8,545 to 8,917 beds. Approximately $70 to $75 million, or slightly more than 15 percent of project costs were devoted to new beds or completely new facilities; the balance provided for replacement beds, renovation and remodeling, and expansion of outpatient, surgical, and ancillary facilities. Hospital expansion projects were largely confined to suburban areas of large metropolitan areas or to rapidly growing communities. The pattern of capital spending appears to relate to changing demands and practices.

Table 9-4 shows how the distribution of funding sources for hospital construction has evolved between 1968 and 1974.

The emphasis of hospital capital programs has changed substantially over the past ten years, reflecting changes in utilization patterns, the obsolescence of physical plant, advances in medical technology and service standards. It further reflects an important shift in federal policy away from new bed construction. Nineteen seventy-one marked the first year in which replacement and remodeling surpassed new bed construction. Since 1971, replacement and remodeling—updating the physical plant—have become the primary determinants of the demand for capital funds. This change may be directly related to the sudden drop in Hill-Burton sponsored projects, but it also reflects recognition in the health care industry of the serious potential economic consequences of overbedding. Further, the dramatic increase in outpatient activity has necessitated rapid expansion of emergency facilities, clinical labs, and other ancillary services.

During this period, according to the AHA survey, aggregate expenditures increased 193 percent, from $1.1 billion to $3.2 billion. During the same period, government grants and guaranteed loans increased 76 percent and philanthropy only 44 percent. Most of the difference was provided through debt financing, which increased 305 percent.

Between 1968 and 1974, expenditures for nursing home construction were estimated to grow from $275 million to $750 million. It was not possible to quantify the diverse sources of financing for these facilities, although we can report that a small portion, between $25 and $40 million, has been provided through tax-exempt general obligation (tax-supported) and revenue bond financing each year, except for New York which, through the Housing Finance Agency, raised over $100 million between 1970 and 1975 for nursing home construction. Elsewhere in the country, tax-exempt financing for nursing homes

Table 9-4. Distribution of Funding Sources Community Hospitals (000,000s)

	1974		1968	
	$	%	$	%
Internal Operations	423	13.1	160	14.5
Debt	1,874	58.0	371	33.7
Government Grants	617	19.1	350	31.7
Philanthropy	317	9.8	220	19.9
	3,231	100.0	1,101	100.0

Source: American Hospital Association.

is done under local auspices. For example, communities in Minnesota have made extensive use of tax-supported bond financing, while small communities in Wisconsin have used both tax-supported and revenue bond debt. Most of the nursing home construction (80 percent), we believe, is financed through mortgage loans that are provided by banks, with substantial equity contributed by owner-operators, developers, and limited partnership arrangements.

Major equipment was estimated to increase from $300 million to $700 million between 1968 and 1974. Historically, the funds for equipment expenditures have been provided from internal operations—operating margins and depreciation recapture. Over the past five years, the use of lease financing for hospital equipment has expanded rapidly as the cost and sophistication of this equipment has increased and hospital administrators have become more conscious of conserving their cash flow for other projects and have become aware of the advantages of "true leases" from the point of view of cost based third party reimbursement. Leasing also permits hospitals to reduce the risk of technical obsolescence. As of this writing, we do not have a reasonable basis for estimating the volume of lease transactions for equipment.

One of the most significant changes in capital financing has been the emergence and growing use of tax-exempt revenue bonds to provide funds for facilities construction. Table 9-5 traces the rapid growth of tax-exempt financing which has occurred over the past five years.

Demand for Funds

We have prepared a baseline projection of future expenditures for health care facilities—short-term, acute care hospitals, nursing homes, and major movable equipment. These projections are presented, not with the purpose of estimating to the last dollar what we believe future expenditure will be, but, rather, to show the relative magnitude of the expenditures.

The assumptions and premises for our projections have both a quantitative and impressionistic basis. Recent trends in health care facilities expenditure were analyzed and extrapolated, taking into consideration the most current changes in

Table 9-5. Tax-Exempt Bond Financing for Hospitals 1971-1976 (000,000s)

	Revenue	Tax Supported	Total
1971	189	73	262
1972	435	90	525
1973	415	194	650
1974	1,057	235	1,292
1975	1,700	276	1,976
1976*	905	185	1,090

*First six months.
1975-1976 *The Bond Buyer.*

rates of growth. In extending the growth curves, we modified rates of growth, where appropriate, to accommodate certain developments which we think will affect health care spending within the next five years. Thus, for example, implicit in our baseline projection is the belief that the HSAs authorized under the National Health Planning and Resources Development Act (P.L. 93-641), once they become operational, will slow the rate of capital formation. This impact is defined as the impact of legislation in place but not yet fully manifest.

Several other assumptions and considerations warrent attention. First, the emphasis of hospital facilities development will continue to be on renovation, replacement, ancillary, and outpatient facilities. It is anticipated that the total number of community hospital beds may even decline over the next five years by as much as 5 percent to 10 percent. This will be the logical outgrowth of the process of consolidation and merger already underway as well as of shifts in population. Utilization and review practices will result in reducing the average length of stay perhaps by as much as one day, from 7.7 to 6.7 days. This drop will be reinforced by the trend for certain medical procedures to be shifted from inpatient to outpatient basis. Further, the demand for nursing home and extended care facilities will be buoyed as economic pressures mount to relocate semi-acute patients from high cost acute care facilities. Finally, we assumed that construction costs would increase at a rate of 5-6 percent per year.

The baseline forecast does not assume the implementation of a specific national health insurance program. In addition, we have not explicitly attempted to incorporate the potential impact of prospective rate setting upon the utilization of the health care facility system. The importance of these developments requires separate treatment. Finally, we have assumed that there will not be a dramatic change in the mix of sources of revenue, i.e., there will be no significant shift toward cost base reimbursement which will result in a dramatic decline in aggregate operating margins (net operating income after depreciation and fixed charges). It is anticipated, however, that the gradual decline in operating margins which has been experienced over the past decade (from 4.4 percent to 3.3 percent between 1968 and 1974) will continue.

Table 9-6 summarizes our total projections in terms of expenditures incurred in the year in which permanent financing is arranged. To derive this table, we assumed a one-year lag between financing, takedown, and construction in place. The data for project initiation exceed Value-Put-in-Place. We converted the data to coincide more closely with our projection for the demand for funds in the capital markets.

Supply of Funds

The overall rate of growth in expenditures projected for the next five years averages about 6.6 percent per year. This is a conservative estimate which assumes an average rate of inflation of approximately 5 percent. The tabulation in Table 9-7 shows projections of supply of funds (see also Figure 9-1).

Table 9-6. Projected Capital Outlays 1976 to 1981 (000,000s)

	1976	1977	1978	1979	1980	1981	Compound Rate of Growth %
Community Hospitals							
Nonprofit	$2,625	$2,809	$3,005	$3,216	$3,441	$3,680	7.0
State and Local	740	787	836	889	945	1,000	6.3
Proprietary	190	203	217	231	247	265	6.8
Nursing Homes	815	853	892	933	976	1,020	4.6
Major Equipment	1,000	1,076	1,158	1,246	1,340	1,440	7.6
	$5,370	$5,728	$6,108	$6,515	$6,949	$7,405	6.6

Demand for Tax-Exempt Revenue Bonds

Based upon the projection of funding sources for construction, we have derived a projection for the demand for tax-exempt revenue bonds.

Year	Par Value (000s)
1976	$1,875,000
1977	2,090,000
1978	2,335,000
1979	2,605,000
1980	2,910,000
1981	3,250,000

From surveys of numerous hospital financings, it may be observed that a hospital sells $1.17 in par value of tax-exempt bonds for every $1.00 of construction outlay. (This relationship is explained more fully in the next section.) We used this ratio to calibrate our projection of the demand for financing on the basis of estimates of future construction.

THE TAX-EXEMPT BOND MARKET AND HEALTH CARE FACILITIES FINANCING

Until the 1960s, debt financing for private, nonprofit hospitals consisted primarily of taxable bonds and mortgage loans. Publicly-owned county and municipal hospitals and nursing homes were largely financed through the issuance of tax supported general obligation bonds, sale and lease-back financing where the lease was secured from tax monies and, finally, limited tax special fund obligations. Prior to 1963, with few exceptions, private nonprofit hospitals had virtually no access to the tax-exempt market.

Table 9-7. Community Hospitals* Construction Outlays Actual and Projected Funding Sources 1974 to 1981 (000,000s)

	Actual 1974	Projected 1976	Projected 1977	Projected 1978	Projected 1979	Projected 1980	Projected 1981	1976-1981 Compound Rate of Growth %
Internal Operations	$ 425	$ 300	$ 295	$ 290	$ 285	$ 280	$ 275	(-1.8)
Government Grants	200	100	100	100	100	100	100	0
Philanthropy	325	350	364	378	393	409	425	4.0
Debt								
Taxable Bonds	250	250	259	269	279	289	300	3.7
Mortgage Loans	350	300	318	337	356	378	400	5.9
Tax-Exempt Bonds	200	300	318	337	356	378	400	5.9
Tax-Supported Revenue	1,100	1,600	1,786	1,994	2,226	2,485	2,775	11.6
Insured and Guaranteed	300	300	277	255	235	217	200	(-8.5)
Equity Financing	50	50	54	59	64	69	75	8.4
Total	$3,200	$3,550	$3,771	$4,019	$4,294	$4,605	$4,950	6.87

*Insufficient date for allocating funding sources for Nursing Homes and Major Equipment.

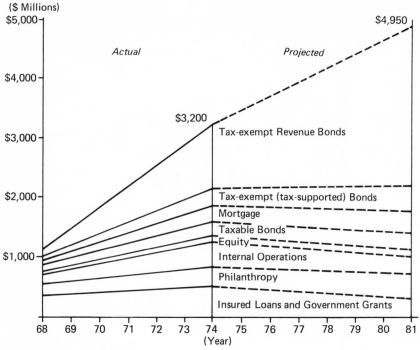

($ Millions)

Figure 9-1. Community Hospitals Capital Funding Actual and Projected Funding Sources 1968 to 1981

Source: John Nuveen & Co. Incorporated

In 1963, the Internal Revenue Service promulgated Ruling 63-20, which was used as the basis for private hospitals to issue tax-exempt bonds, with the proviso that title in the financed project would ultimately revert to a municipality (or other public entity) upon final repayment of the debt.

In 1966, the state of Connecticut established the Health and Education Facilities Authority to act as a financing vehicle for private not-for-profit educational and health institutions. In February 1968, the Connecticut Authority issued its first hospital revenue bonds in the amount of $9,300,000 on behalf of Middlesex Memorial Hospital. Over the past ten years, many states (Arizona, Idaho, Illinois, Maine, Maryland, Massachusetts, Michigan, Missouri, New Hampshire, New Jersey, New York, Rhode Island, South Dakota, Vermont, and Washington) have followed suite by creating special authorities to make tax-exempt financing available, bypassing certain features which were considered cumbersome in "63-20" financing and, more importantly, permitting title to the hospital facility to remain with, or revert to, the hospital corporation. Other mechanisms are available. In some states, statutes have been enacted to permit the creation of local hospital financing authorities (for example, Alabama, Michigan, and Indiana). In other states, previously enacted industrial revenue bond statutes have been broadened to provide tax-exempt financing for private hospitals (for example, Iowa, Minnesota, and Wisconsin). In the case of not-for-profit institutions, these financings have been exempt from the $5 million limit on industrial aid financing.

What has prompted the shift to tax-exempt financing? Essentially, four reasons may be offered. First, lower rates. Because the interest is exempt from federal income taxes, tax-exempt bonds typically sell at 1 1/2 percent to 2 percent lower interest rates than do comparable taxable bonds. Second, longer term to maturity. Mortgage and taxable bond financing is typically restricted to a fifteen- to twenty-year term to maturity, whereas tax-exempt financing may be structured to mature over twenty-five to thirty years. The combination of the longer maturity schedule (which more closely coincides with the expected useful life of the project), coupled with lower interest rates, results in substantial reductions in annual debt service requirements with tax-exempt financing. Third, no equity is required. While all categories of fixed income investors consider equity as a positive factor, the tax-exempt market does not impose a standard equity requirement as typically found in the taxable mortgage and bond market. It is not uncommon for the par value of a bond issue to supply virtually 100 percent of the project costs. Fourth, there is income orientation. Tax-exempt bond investors look primarily to the income generating capability of a health care institution. They place great importance upon the feasibility study prepared by an independent accounting or consulting firm and the analysis of patient demand, competitive position of the hospital, the composition of third party reimbursement, and the medical staff and management of the hospital. This approach to security analysis is based on the tradition of municipal analysis of public revenue-supported enterprises or public utilities in which the quality of the income stream is preeminent, since the mortgages provided by public enterprises have nonforeclosable provisions.

Several principles of municipal utility financing have carried over into hospital revenue bond financing. Included among these are the ability to set rates freely in order to secure sufficient revenues to pay the principal and interest on the bonds. Equally important, if not more so, is the notion of providing a monopoly of service or maintaining a franchise. While most hospitals exist in a competitive environment, investors have shown a preference for "sole provider" facilities. Further, many investors felt that the certificate of need requirement under the Social Security Amendments of 1972 reinforced the franchise concept.

Over the past ten years, the advantages of tax-exempt financing have become more widely appreciated. Other sources of funding have either declined or have not grown at a rate nearly comparable with the increasing costs of projects. The legal mechanisms available for financing have proliferated and the expertise to assemble a financing, while still quite concentrated, has become more widespread. Further, while the tax-exempt market has been extremely volatile, it has nevertheless, grown substantially over the past decade and has, thus far, demonstrated the ability to absorb largely the dramatic increase in the volume of financing.

Some Facts About the Municipal Market

First, we conducted a survey of twenty-five recent tax-exempt financings for hospitals, aggregating $545 million. Table 9–8 shows the percentage allocation of the sources and uses of funds in the aggregate for these twenty-five financings. We believe that this breakdown is representative of those hospitals that use tax-exempt financing.

On average, total requirements were $1.40 for every $1.00 of construction outlays. This includes professional fees, funded interest during construction, and a reserve fund. Bond proceeds, among the projects surveyed, provided $1.17 out of the $1.40 of total requirements. The balance required, approximately 15 percent of the total, was derived from internal operations, philanthropic contributions and government grants. Other forms of debt financing generally require much greater equity contribution. Further, this use of tax-exempt financing has enabled hospital administrators to channel cash from internal sources to equipment purchases and small incidental replacement and remodeling.

Second, the debt service requirement generally averages between 10 percent and 20 percent of the last year's operating and maintenance expenses prior to the financing. From the feasibility studies, we find that debt service requirements, as a percentage of operating expenses, is projected to range between 5

Table 9–8. Aggregate Sources and Uses of Funds 25 Hospital Projects 1975 and 1976

Uses	% Total Project Cost	% Par Value of Bonds
Project Costs	73.1	87.2
Refinancing Debt	7.7	
Net Interest During Construction	6.9	
Debt Service Reserve	7.7	
Fees and Expenses	4.6	
Total Project Costs Financed:	100.0	
Sources		
Cash Flow	10.0	
Philanthropy	2.4	
Government Grants	3.8	
Revenue Bonds	83.8	
Total Sources:	100.0	

percent and 15 percent of projected operating and maintenance expenses during the first full year of operation after the completion of the projects. These projected ratios typically assume a 7 percent to 8 percent inflation rate in hospital expenses generally. If a lower rate were realized, the ratio of debt service requirements to total expenses would be somewhat greater. At the extreme, in the case of a new facility construction project, debt service was projected to be slightly over 15 percent of total expenses.

By comparison with other municipal utilities, the ratio of debt service to operating expenses in community hospitals is low. That of a power plant is 35 percent to 40 percent, a water utility 45 percent to 50 percent and, at the extreme, a hydroelectric dam is 75 percent to 80 percent. Thus, while the dollar amount of health care facility financing appears enormous, it is still quite clear that hospital care remains, at this time, a "labor intensive" activity.

The Market

Over the past five years, tax-exempt revenue bond financing for hospitals has grown rapidly. Between 1972 and 1975 it grew by 376 percent. The results for the first half of 1976 show an increase of approximately 10 percent over last year, not including refinancings of outstanding tax-exempt debt.

In 1975, according to statistics prepared by the *Daily Bond Buyer,* there were 146 financings totaling $1.96 billion. They consisted of 46 tax-supported issues of $276 million and 110 revenue bond issues (almost exclusively for private nonprofit facilities) totaling $1.7 billion. The results of the first half of 1976 are shown in Table 9-9.

We estimate that, at current levels of activity, approximately 3 percent to 3.2 percent of the private nonprofit hospitals in the nation will enter the tax-exempt market in 1976 to furnish their principal sources of financing. If we assume that the hospital plant in place in the nation's health care system has an average useful life of twenty to twenty-five years and, therefore, an annual replacement rate of about 4 percent to 4 1/2 percent, then we can see that tax-exempt financing has already become the predominant source of funds for nonprofit facilities. The exceptionally rapid changeover to such financing appears already to have taken place. The increase of it will not be as dramatic over the next five years as it was between 1972 and 1976.

Table 9-9. Tax-Exempt Hospital Financings First Half—1976 (000,000s)

	Par Value	# Issues	Average Size
Revenue Bonds	$ 905	68	$13.3
Tax-Supported Bonds	185	50	3.7
	$1,090	118	

The Distribution of Tax-Exempt Hospital
Revenue Bonds

While there is no "typical" tax-exempt bond issue, for purposes of generalization we shall try momentarily to live with such a fiction. So far, in 1976, a typical revenue bond issue has a par value of $13.3 million and a term to maturity of about twenty-five years. For purposes of marketing, the maturity schedule is typically divided into two parts with 40 percent of the bonds maturing serially, commencing after the completion of the project and through about fifteen years, and the balance of the bond issue, or about 60 percent, bearing a term maturity of twenty-five years, which it is anticipated will be amortized annually from a special sinking fund. The majority of financings are patterned after mortgage financing since debt service payments are level each year. Based on our tabulations of sales data for over $100 million of revenue bond financings placed in 1976, we estimate the distribution of hospital bonds to be as shown in Table 9-10.

Since bond funds are ultimately distributed to individuals, we see that over 60 percent of the hospital revenue bonds are ultimately purchased by individuals. At this time, this is consistent with data compiled by the Treasury Department and the Federal Reserve Bank which shows that households (or individuals) are the fastest growing sector of municipal bond buyers. Over the past three years, households have purchased an average of nearly 60 percent of the net increase in long-term municipal debt.

We draw a distinction between bond fund purchasers and individual purchasers because bond funds function like investment institutions. The investment decisions are heavily concentrated, and the blocks of bond purchases range from $500 to $5 million and even $10 million. Bond funds have aided the efficiency of distributing hospital bonds. More important, the growth of hospital financing has correlated very closely to the growth of tax-exempt bond funds.

Insurance companies (primarily casualty companies), according to our esti-

Table 9-10.   Estimated Distribution of Tax-Exempt Hospital Revenue Bonds*
January through June 1976

	Esti- mated *% Share*	*Estimated Par Value ($ million)*
Bond Funds	40	365
Individuals	22 ½	205
Insurance Companies	12 ½	110
Banks	25	225
	100	905

*Estimated by John Nuveen & Co., Incorporated.

mates, purchase about 12 1/2 percent of the new hospital revenue bond issues. This is about equal to the ratio of their purchases of new municipal issues; however, it is below the ratio of their investments in long-term revenue bonds. (During 1974 and 1975, casualty insurers, traditional buyers of long-term municipals, reduced their purchases due to insurance underwriting losses and poor profitability.) It has been our experience that the acceptance of tax-exempt hospital bonds by insurance companies has been restrained at best, though it may increase as their spending for tax-exempt bonds increases this year.

Bank investment in hospital bonds is typically restricted to the shorter maturities—the serial bonds. By and large, banks limit their purchases of hospital bonds to facilities constructed in their locale because they are more familiar with the credit and they are willing to support local institutions. There is only a select group of preeminent institutions, such as Massachusetts General Hospital, the University of Pennsylvania, Rush-Presbyterian, St. Luke's, or Northwestern University, whose obligations have been accepted by banks nationwide.

Because of the restrained acceptance of hospital revenue bonds by insurance companies, the dependence upon individual purchasers and bond funds and, also, the entrenched belief that, somehow, hospital bonds entail more risk than, for example, the electric utility revenue bonds, the interest rates assigned to hospital bond financing have typically been substantially higher than for other forms of revenue bond financing. The spread between coupons and yields on hospital bonds and electric utility bonds, of a comparable investment grade rating, ranges between 1 percent and 1 1/2 percent. Further, since interest rates are very much dependent upon supply and demand relationships in a more narrow marketplace, we have witnessed considerable volatility in prices.

The pricing of hospital bonds at this time depends, primarily, on the demand expressed by tax-exempt bond funds. We estimate, on the basis of our knowledge of bond fund buying behavior, that the current stable capacity for hospital revenue bonds is on the order of $150-175 million per month. When the volume of financing substantially surpasses that level, adjustments are required in interest rates to provide additional yield and encourage increase in demand for bonds.

It appears that market conditions have changed over the past six months and the capacity of the market to absorb hospital revenue bonds has improved. The total volume of financing has increased. The onset of the managed bond funds, in addition to the unit investment trust bond funds, has tapped a new supply of money. Also, casualty insurers appear to have increased their purchases.

In 1975, total bond fund volume was $2.17 billion. During the first half of 1976, it was $1.38 billion and approximately 20 percent of its aggregate volume consisted of hospital bonds. We anticipate that, in 1980, aggregate bond fund volume will be on the order to $4 to $4 1/2 billion. The capacity of bond funds to absorb hospital financing will increase commensurately, assuming that nothing substantial happens to impair the confidence of the investment community for this type of investment.

IMPACT OF FEDERAL POLICY UPON DEMAND
FOR CAPITAL INVESTMENT

A multitude of articles and reports have been written in recent months addressing themselves to the influence of federal health care policy upon the demand for capital investment. We shall examine some of the more important of those policies and their impact.

1. *Certificate of Need.* Section 1122 of the Social Security Act provides that reimbursement for depreciation, interest, and other costs that are associated with a project costing in excess of $100,000 may be denied if the project is not approved by the designated planning agency. Thirty-seven states have contracted with the U.S. Department of HEW to conduct Section 1122 reviews. In nineteen states, similar types of provisions connect Blue Cross reimbursement to project review by planning agencies or the Blue Cross plans. In all states, eligibility for capital investment subsidies through the Hill-Burton program requires planning agency approval, and participation in construction financing programs requires such approval in forty-two states.[1] The two major federal programs, Section 1122 and P.L. 93-641, were promulgated within the past four years and all but five of the existing certificate of need laws were enacted after 1970. It is felt that the certificate of need approach will soon emerge as the predominant form of investment control. Of the fourteen states which did not participate in the Section 1122 program, nine already had certificate of need laws, and their lack of interest in the program was based on a belief that 1122 review would not add to their existing authority or would conflict with state administrative practices.[2] The National Health Planning and Resources Development Act of 1974 (P.L. 93-641) added to the public health service act a new Title XV, "National Health Planning and Development" and a new Title XVI, "Health Resources Development." Among other things, the new Title XV authorizes HEW to enter into agreements with eligible entities for the designation of health system agencies (HSAs). Among the specific duties required of HSAs by Title XV is that they perform reviews of proposed new institutional health services to be offered or developed in their respective areas and that they make recommendations to the appropriate state health planning and development agencies respecting the need for such services. The proposed rules promulgated on March 19, 1976, and which are out for comment, list as those "new institutional health services subject to review" by the HSAs the following: (a) the construction, development or establishment of a new health care facility or HMO, (b) any expenditure by, or on behalf of, a health care facility or HMO in excess of $150,000 (or lesser amount as the state may specify), (c) a change in the existing bed complement of a health care facility of HMO.

There is not a clear consensus among the researchers as to the effect of a certificate of need program upon demand for capital investment. Salkever & Bice present the conflicting arguments. Some have argued that a certificate of need program, merely by its existence, may discourage construction and capital expenditures by causing an anticipatory reaction on the part of providers. Others believe that the certificate of need process actually stimulates hospital construction by causing applicants to accelerate their plans in order to preempt others. Following a regression analysis, Salkever & Bice conclude that, while certificate of need seems to have controlled expansion and bed supply, it has stimulated other types of investment, such as ancillary services and equipment and, therefore, has had little effect on total investment expenditures. However, the new federal regulations propose a review for *any* capital expenditures in excess of $150,000 and are designed to prevent this displacement from continuing into the future. Assuming the adoption of regulations which provide substantially the same as the proposed regulations, it is reasonable to assume that certificate of need and its related programs will have a definite negative impact upon future demand.

2. *Professional Standards Review Organizations (PSROs).* Public Law 92-603 creates a nationwide network of locally-based physician groups to review the necessity, quality and appropriateness of institutional care that is made available under requirements of the Social Security Act. These physician groups are designated as PSROs. The original legislation enacts two provisions of major importance: (a) preadmission screening and (b) length of stay review.

The researchers of this topic seem to be in total agreement that the PSROs will have a dramatic operational and financial impact on hospitals. The most important, from our standpoint, is an expected decrease in inpatient utilization (by as much as 10 percent) because of change in length of stay.[3] This decrease should result in a drop in the demand for bed construction which should, in turn, result in less pressure for new capital investment in that sector. There is not enough evidence at this time to attempt to quantify this impact of PSRO on new and replacement bed construction other than to say that the impact is decidedly negative.

3. *Health Maintenance Organizations (HMOs).* The HMO Assistance Act of 1973 (Public Law 93-222) has given encouragement to the growth of comprehensive prepaid health plans. The objective is to convert the delivering of many aspects of care from an inpatient to an outpatient basis.

The extent of the effect upon the demand for capital investment would depend primarily upon the type of prepaid health plan that would be in effect in a given hospital service area, i.e., whether or not such plan contracts for both ambulatory and inpatient services. In the case where the plan would not contract for inpatient services, there should be a decidedly negative effect upon utilization in the hospital's service area. If such a plan does contract for inpatient services, then the evidence still points to a negative impact on utilization, but to a lesser degree. For example, during the years 1968 through 1970, Blue Cross subscribers were averaging 896 hospital days per 1,000 persons while subscribers to the Kaiser plan were averaging 490 days.[4] Nevertheless, HMOs, whether contracting for inpatient services or not, should have a negative impact on new or replacement bed construction and the demand in the service area for that particular component of capital investment.

4. *National Health Insurance.* There has been no clear-cut indication from Congress as to which type of national health insurance plan is supportable. There are many issues to be resolved, including the type and extent of benefits, the method and place of administration of the plan, and the method of financing. A number of national health insurance plans have been proposed over the past few years. A proposal backed by the AMA uses tax credits to encourage greater coverage under private health insurance plans. The Long-Ribicoff proposal would replace Medicaid with a federal plan for the poor but would cover catastrophic expenses for everyone. Plans sponsored by the current administration, the American Hospital Administration (the Ullman proposal) and the Health Insurance Association of America all rely heavily on the purchase of private health insurance through employer groups. A compromise plan (Kennedy-Mills) relies primarily on public insurance financed by payroll taxes and federal and state general revenues. The Health Security Act (backed by the AFL-CIO) replaces private insurance with a federal program covering virtually all medical bills.[5]

The topic of national health insurance is very complex, especially if one is attempting to examine the net effect of the "cost" of a particular program. The component of any such plan that is of most interest to us is the extent of benefits that it affords. All of the proposals would cover both inpatient and ambulatory services. All would cover skilled nursing-home care. All, except the AMA and Long-Ribicoff plans, would cover prescription drugs. The Health Security Act would provide for free care for virtually all medical services. At the other end of the spectrum, the Long-Ribicoff plan would require those meeting an income test to pay for the first sixty days of hospital care and to contribute towards coinsurance. The other plans all provide for moderate direct patient contributions, except by low-income families.

A Rand Corporation Report (1974) analyzed the impact of national health insurance on demand for hospital services, utilizing two protocol plans: one that provided for full coverage (without coinsurance) and one that provided for a maximum of 25 percent coinsurance. The conclusion of the report was that there would be only a small increase in demand for hospital services (as contrasted to ambulatory services) primarily because approximately 90 percent of total hospital costs currently are covered by some type of insurance. The report also estimated an increase in demand of 5 to 15 percent with a full coverage plan and 5 percent with the 25 percent coinsurance plan.

IMPACT OF FEDERAL POLICY UPON SUPPLY
OF FUNDS FOR CAPITAL INVESTMENT

The supply of investment capital (more fully discussed earlier in this paper) is divided into four major sources—government grants and appropriations, philanthropy, internal operations, and debt financing. Debt financing, in turn, is subdivided into four categories—taxable mortgage loans, taxable bonds, government loans and guarantees, and tax-exempt bonds. In 1975, of the $3.3 billion total capital investment, debt financing provided approximately 65 percent. If we look at the projected year 1981, debt financing is expected to provide 82 percent of the total. It becomes obvious that, for purposes of this paper's inquiry into the impact of future federal policy upon supply of investment capital, the focus should be upon those policies which impact debt financing.

We will first examine those considerations which were also encompassed by the demand side of the equation, namely, certificate of need, PSROs, health maintenance organizations, and National Health Insurance. In addition to these considerations, we will examine others which, we have discovered, will also impact the supply of investment capital.

Certificate of Need. While certificate of need has had a negative effect upon the demand side of the capital investment equation, it becomes a positive factor upon the supply side. From the investor's standpoint, the competitive climate in which the hospital operates is of utmost importance. Investors tend to favor hospitals which are "sole providers" in their service areas and, in their absence, prefer hospitals which are not subject to intense competition from others nearby. With the advent of certificate of need, the investor was given the additional comfort of an independent third party conducting a determination of the need for the project, particularly where it concerned the addition of new beds. The investor looks at certificate of need as a form of franchise or license to operate within the service area and places reliance upon the fact that (a) there is a current demonstrated need for the project and (b) that another hospital will not be allowed to construct a similar project at some future time solely or primarily for the purpose of competing within the existing hospital's service area. It is our opinion, based upon discussions with investors, that certificate of need was one of the primary factors that induced many of them to begin purchasing hospital debt obligations. To the extent that certificate of need is finally implemented in all fifty states, we can expect that investor acceptance of hospital obligations will be furthered.

Professional Standards Review Organizations (PSROs). As already discussed, the establishment of the PSROs is expected to have an impact on inpatient utilization. With a drop in utilization, we should expect the net review also to decrease, causing potential investors to attribute more risk to the investment and, therefore, to expect a higher interest rate. If the net revenue of the hospital decreases to the point where coverage of debt service cannot be attained, then the hospital will not have access to the market. "Coverage" is an investment term that indicates the margin of safety for payment of debt service on the hospital's debt, reflecting the number of times or the percentage by which net revenue (before depreciation and fixed charges) exceeds debt service payable for such period. A decline in utilization which causes a decline in coverage also signifies that internally generated funds, one of the components of the supply of investment capital, will also be decreased. A hospital will then have to rely more on debt financing than on this traditional form of "equity" financing for its source of capital.

National Health Insurance. As already discussed, it is expected that National Health Insurance will have the effect of slightly increasing (between 5 and 15 percent, depending upon the type of benefit) the demand for inpatient hospital services. This increase in demand would presumably be translated into increased utilization and, potentially, an increase in the revenue of the hospital. On the other hand, the proposed plans provide for a variety of methods and levels of reimbursing providers of medical services, ranging from the liberal features contained in the AMA bill to the fairly restrictive provisions of the Health Security Act (AFL-CIO bill). The remainder of the bills provide for more moderate forms of reimbursement which attempt to allow hospitals about the same level of reimbursement as they currently earn.[6]

The source of investment capital most directly affected by National Health is internally generated funds, and it appears logical that the level of reimbursement, rather than the benefits provided, will have the larger impact.

Health Maintenance Organizations (HMOs). As discussed earlier, the establishment of HMOs is expected to have a negative impact upon the utilization of a hospital's inpatient services and, consequently, on its occupancy. This, in turn, would reduce internally generated funds available for capital investment and require the hospital to debt-finance a larger portion of the project. Because of increased reliance on debt financing, accompanied by decreased coverage, investors will tend to place it in a higher risk category and will demand a higher interest rate for the hospital's obligations.

Prospective Reimbursement. Studies by the Department of Health, Education and Welfare indicate that in varying degrees, 25 percent of the nation's 7,200 hospitals are involved with varying types of prospective reimbursement. Involvement at the state level has been through special legislation, Blue Cross plans and certain voluntary programs offered by Blue Cross, state hospital associations, and a nonprofit corporation. Under a prospective system, the rate to be paid to a particular hospital is established prior to the period for which the rate is to be applied. Rates can be established in a number of ways, such as by negotiation, by formula or by review of a proposed budget. Payments are then made according to the established rate, independently of what actual cost the hospital incurs. The theory of the prospective system is that, because the hospital is put at financial risk, it will be prompted to operate in a more efficient manner.

From an investor's viewpoint, one must try to anticipate what prospective reimbursement will do to the hospital's ability to generate adequate coverage. If efficient hospitals are lumped together with inefficient ones, then we can assume that, at least over the short term, the efficient hospital will benefit financially. Over the longer term, however, if inefficient hospitals are induced to become more efficient through prospective reimbursement, then we can expect that any benefits to efficient institutions would slowly diminish to the point where, finally, no hospital would benefit at the expense of another. It also seems reasonable to assume that, under any prospective reimbursement system, efficient hospitals would not be allowed to reap "windfall" profits and, on the other hand, an inefficient hospital would not be forced out of business while in the process of attempting to become more efficient. The net effect, then, should be that prospective reimbursement will eventually have a negative impact upon a hospital's internally generated funds. This will place a heavier reliance upon debt financing and, in doing so, upward pressure upon interest rates on hospital debt obligations will be exerted because: (a) the total supply of hospital debt obligations has been increased and (b) the security for hospital obligations has been diminished by reason of decreased coverage.

Prospective Review. From an investment standpoint, one of the more controversial elements in health planning is the requirement of P.L. 93-641 for reviews of the appropriateness of institutional health services. Section 1513 of the Act provides that each health systems agency (HSA) shall, on a periodic basis (but at least every five years), review all institutional health services offered in the health service area of the agency and make recommendations to the State Health Planning and Development Agency as designated under Section 1521. Section 1523 provides that the state agency shall complete its findings with respect to the appropriateness of any existing institutional health service within one year after the date that a health systems agency has made its recommendation under Section 1513.

During the development of the National Health Planning and Resources Development Act of 1974 (P.L. 93-641), the Senate version was S. 2994 and the House version was H.R. 16204. The report of the House Committee provided for periodic HSA reviews of all institutional health services and recommendation of a continuing need for reviewing such services. In the House floor debate on H.R. 16204, an amendment was passed which removed periodic review of institutional health services for *need* and substituted the language now in the law. The objection was that to permit a review for need constituted recertification where a certificate of need had already been granted. The House representative who proposed the amendment stated, with respect to initial certification, that "once a facility is approved, there should be no further doubt as to continued governmental approval in terms of anticipated longevity. The possibility that a service of that a whole institution might be eliminated will make long term financing of that service or institution much more expensive if not altogether impossible." In the Senate, the discussions of S. 2994 emphasized that the ability of a reviewed institution to incur debt must be taken into consideration when findings are made on the need for services. In the Senate, an amendment was offered and passed exempting from periodic reviews for need those facilities and services subject to review for Section 1122 and certificate of need purposes. In the conference committee, when representatives met to resolve the differences between H.R. 16204 and S. 2994, the Senate amendment which would have exempted from periodic review the facilities subject to Section 1122 and certificate of need reviews was dropped. The House amendment for reviews for appropriateness was adopted.

Much is still left unsaid about review for appropriateness, such as the meaning of the word "appropriateness," how the review should be initiated and conducted, and what, if any, actions and sanctions would result from such reviews.

From the standpoint of an investor, one is concerned with reviews for appropriateness to the extent that the initial investment decision is based upon the hospital's having obtained the necessary certificate of need for the project. If the hospital (or certain services provided by the hospital) can be curtailed or shut down by prospective review, then an investor must initially assign a higher degree of risk to the investment and expect a higher rate of return, or perhaps even avoid making the investment. If review for appropriateness, then, is ultimately cast as a regulatory function, rather than as a planning function, a solution to this problem might be that where a hospital is shut down or curtailed by prospective review, provision would be made for the retirement of any affected debt obligations.

Federal Grants, Guarantees, and Subsidies. During the 1960s, the Hill-Burton grant program, which provided for outright grants to hospitals for new construction, was the only major financial assistance program sponsored by the federal government for short-term hospitals. In June 1970, the Hill-Burton Loan Guarantee with Interest Subsidy program was enacted as part of P.L. 91–296, which program became operational with the publication of regulations on January 6, 1972. The program is divided into two categories, the "Loan Guarantee Program" and the "Direct Loan Program." The former provides for a guarantee by the Department of Health, Education and Welfare (HEW) of mortgage loans which loans would then be placed with private lenders. In addition, the interest rate is subsidized by 3 percent. The Direct Loan Program was enacted so that hospitals using tax-exempt financing could also take advantage of the subsidy. Under the Direct Loan Program, HEW purchases from the issuer a par amount of bonds equal to the allocation that the hospital has received. The coupon rate is equal to the FNMA four-month auction rate adjusted by the 3 percent subsidy. The bonds purchased by HEW are then either sold to FNMA or packaged and sold on the open market as taxable securities. Congress authorized $1.5 billion of such loans for the period 1971–1973 and the allocations were made to Hill-Burton state agencies on a formula basis. Although the net effect upon the supply of funds for capital investment by these programs has been minimal, hospitals taking advantage of the Loan Guarantee Program have benefitted from a lower interest rate. Furthermore, allocations made under the Direct Loan Program have had the effect of taking off the market an equivalent amount of tax-exempt bonds. Assuming a meaningful volume of this type of financing, the effect would be to decrease the supply of tax-exempt bonds and, to reduce upward pressure upon interest rates. In addition, since the interest rate is subsidized, the internally generated funds of the hospital would increase. It has been our experience that hospitals which have elected to utilize tax-exempt bond financing will use the Direct Loan Program only when the FNMA rate (less the 3 percent subsidy) is below the rate obtainable in the tax-exempt market. Otherwise, there is no benefit. As far as the Loan Guarantee and Subsidy Program is concerned, the problem has been that a hospital will receive an allocation which is less than the borrowed amount. Unlike the Direct Loan, the Guaranteed Loan cannot easily be separated and becomes somewhat of a hybrid, i.e., a loan that is only partially guaranteed and subsidized. The borrowers who fared the best in the market were those who received an allocation to cover the entire borrowed amount which enabled them to place a *fully* guaranteed and subsidized mortgage loan. Currently, because of the lack of significant appropriations, there is very little activity in either of these programs.

Another problem of federal assistance is mortgage insurance for nonprofit hospitals. The Housing and Urban Development Act of 1968 added a new Section 242 to Title II of the National Housing Act which authorized the Department of Housing and Urban Development to insure mortgage loans to finance the construction and rehabilitation of nonprofit hospital facilities, and the purchase of equipment for them. These loans are commonly referred to as FHA insured loans. More recently, these loans have been accompanied by a guarantee by GNMA which places them in the category of a full faith and credit obligation of the United States. There is no subsidy involved. Because a hospital can generally sell obligations in the tax-exempt bond market at a lower interest rate than the rate on insured (and even GNMA guaranteed) obligations, the activity in this program has been primarily limited to two instances: (a) when, because of its credit rating, the hospital could not otherwise obtain financing at reasonable rates in the tax-exempt bond market or (b) when interest rates on tax-exempt bonds occasionally have risen above FHA rates.

Another program which is currently under much discussion in Congress is the "taxable bond option" which would give prospective issuers of tax-exempt bonds the option of issuing taxable securities coupled with an interest subsidy by the federal government. The amount of subsidy under discussion is in the 30 to 35 percent range. It is difficult to predict what effect, if any, this program, if enacted, would have upon the supply of funds for hospitals. It would most likely impact supply much in the same way as the HEW Direct Loan Program does, and, in situations where the interest rate attainable in the tax-exempt market would be lower than the taxable subsidized rate, the hospital would opt for tax-exempt financing. There is still a question as to whether taxable hospital bonds beyond the traditional fifteen- to twenty-year maturity range are readily marketable. If a market can be established for these securities, then the result would be to decrease the supply of tax-exempt bonds which should reduce upward pressure upon interest rates in that sector of the market. Since the subsidy is merely making up the difference between the tax-exempt and taxable rates, there should be no appreciable effect upon internally generated funds.

CONCLUSIONS

In this paper we have not sought to forecast precisely the aggregate demand for capital for health care facilities or to predict exactly the relative mix of funding sources. Rather, our intention has been to extend current trends in the supply and demand for capital financing, to identify the principal sources of funding and to discuss those policy issues that are likely to have an impact on future developments. Our conclusions are briefly summarized below:

1. Between 1966 and 1975, hospital construction expenditures (value put in place) increased by 283 percent from $1.2 billion to $3.4 billion. This rapid growth for the first five years reflected the surge in spending resulting from Medicare and Medicaid and strengthened by the Hill-Burton Grant Program. Since 1971, however, all of the increases in expenditures are explained by inflation. In terms of constant dollars, real expenditures over the past four years appear to have declined slightly.

2. During the next five years, from 1976 to 1981, we anticipate that projected capital outlays for health care facilities will increase at an average annual rate of 6.6 percent. This assumes an inflation factor of 5 percent. Total capital expenditures will increase from $3.5 billion to $5 billion for community hospitals, aggregating $25 billion over the period.

3. There has been a dramatic shift to debt financing over the past ten years. Between 1968 and 1974, debt financing increased from 33.7 percent to 58 percent of the total supply of funds, as reported by the American Hospital Association. By 1981, debt financing from all sources is expected to provide over 80 percent of total community hospital capital outlays. For the years 1976-1981, the aggregate amount (par value) of tax-exempt hospital bond financing will exceed $15 billion and by 1981 will account for more than two-thirds of total debt financing.

4. We believe that the private capital market has the capacity to expand to accommodate future financing requirements. Based on our analysis of the patterns of distribution of hospital revenue bonds, we believe that the tax-exempt market, in particular, will have the greatest capacity to expand. Approximately 40 percent of the par value of tax-exempt hospital revenue bonds is currently purchased by bond funds. The bond fund market appears to have the potential for growing between 40 percent to 50 percent over the next five years, at a rate which should be sufficient to absorb future demands.

5. As the standards under certificate of need become more stringent, this

trend will further restrain the demand for capital funds. We believe that this will encourage capital investment (supply) because certificate of need enhances the fundamental security for debt financing by strengthening the franchise and public utility concept in hospital financing.

6. Professional Standards Review Organizations (PSROs) will tend to depress inpatient utilization. This will encourage mergers and discourage bed-for-bed replacement financing. The overall impact on the demand for funds will be negative. To the extent that actions of PSROs depress hospital earnings and cash flow, the supply of investment funds could be negatively affected.

7. National Health Insurance will increase facility utilization and should increase the demand for capital. The magnitude of such changes will depend upon the array of benefits afforded by the plan that is finally adopted. The impact of NHI upon the supply of funds will depend principally upon the method and level of reimbursement that is contained in the plan that is adopted.

8. Health Maintenance Organizations (HMOs) are expected to reduce inpatient utilization, thus discouraging both demand and supply for capital.

9. Prospective Reimbursement could have a serious impact on the supply of private capital, because it creates uncertainty as to the adequacy of future cash flow for coverage of debt service requirements.

10. Prospective Review of services could also discourage the supply of funds by creating uncertainty with investors as to the future need for facilities and services that are currently being financed.

Cost containment is a preeminent objective which must be achieved, but, in reaching that objective, careful consideration must be given to those policies which simultaneously discourage private capital investment in health care facilities. Over the next five years, we will be in a period in which health care financing will rely more than ever before upon the private market.

NOTES

1. David Salkever and Thomas Bice, "The Impact of Certificate of Need Controls on Hospital Investment," *Health and Society*, Spring 1976, pp. 185–214. The statistics are as of April 1, 1974.

2. Ibid.

3. C. Havighurst and J. Blumstein, "Coping with Quality Cost Tradeoffs in Medical Care: The Role of PSROs," *Northwestern University Law Review* 6 (1975):1970.

4. First Report of the Special Senate Committee to Make an Investigation and Study Relative to the Establishment of a System of Community Medical Centers (established by Massachusetts Senate Order No. 1484, 1971).

5. For a comprehensive analysis of these plans, see Karen Davis, "National

Health Insurance: Benefits, Costs and Consequences," The Brookings Institution, 1976.

6. Ibid.

ADDITIONAL REFERENCES

American Hospital Association. *Guide to the Health Care Field,* 1975.

American Hospital Association. *Hospital Statistics,* 1975.

American Hospital Association. *Marketing Profile of U.S. Hospitals.* Chart No. 2M-11/75-4628, 1975.

Bicknell, William and Diana Walsh. "Critical Experiences in Organizing and Administering a State Certification of Need Program." *Public Health Reports,* 91, 1 (1976).

Cooper, B. and N. Worthington. "National Health Expenditures, 1929-1972." *Social Security Bulletin,* 36 (GPO, 1973).

Ellis, C. "Prospective Reimbursement: Pain or Panacea?" *Modern Health Care,* May 1976, p. 31.

Federation of American Hospitals. "Statistical Summary." *Review,* June 1976.

Foster, Richard and Dorothy McNeil. "How Hospitals Finance Construction." *Hospitals,* July 1, 1971, p. 47.

Hanft, R.S. "National Health Expenditures, 1950-1965." *Social Security Bulletin,* 30, 2 (GPO, 1967).

Harmer, Harold H. *The Hospital Industry.* Chicago: Becker Securities Corporation, Investment Research Department, January 19, 1976.

Internal Revenue Code of 1954. Proposed amendment to the income tax regulations (26CFR Part 1) to revise the regulations under Section 103 (a). 41FR 4829.

Lewin & Associates, Inc. *Evaluation of the Efficiency and Effectiveness of the Section 1122 Review Process.* Washington, D.C., September 1975.

Manley, Sallie. "Sources of Funding for Construction: A.H.A. Research Capsule No. 19." *Hospitals,* December 16, 1975, pp. 104-109.

Manley, Sallie. "A.H.A. Research Capsule No. 17." *Hospitals,* July 1, 1975, pp. 82-84.

Medical Electronics Industry Report. San Jose: Creative Strategies, January 1976.

Talmadge, Herman E. Opening statements of hearing on S.3205, legislation for Medicare/Medicaid reform, July 26, 1976.

U.S. Bureau of the Census. *Statistical Abstract of the United States, 1975.* 96th Edition, Washington, D.C., 1975.

U.S. Bureau of the Census. *Construction Reports, Value of New Construction Put in Place, February 1976.* Series C30, April 1976.

U.S. Department of Commerce. *U.S. Industrial Outlook 1976.* Ch. 38: Medical and Dental Instruments and Supplies; Ch. 42: Health and Medical Services.

U.S. Department of Health, Education and Welfare, Facilities Engineering and Construction Agency. *Representative Construction Costs of Hospitals and Related Health Facilities January to October 1970.*

U.S. National Center for Health Statistics. *Health Resources Statistics,* 1974.

U.S. National Center for Health Statistics. "Current Estimates, 1971." *Vital and Health Statistics,* Series 10, No. 79, 1971.

U.S. National Center for Health Statistics. "Health Facilities as Reported from the 1971 MFI Survey." *Vital and Health Statistics,* Series 14, No. 12, p. 7.

U.S. Social Security Administration, Office of Research and Statistics. *Medical Care Expenditures, Prices and Costs,* September 1975.

U.S. Social Security Administration, Office of Research and Statistics. *Research in Health Care Financing,* Publication No. 76–11912.

U.S. Social Security Administration, Office of Research and Statistics. *Research and Statistics Notes,* Number 1, SSA Publication 75–1101, February 19, 1975.

U.S. Social Security Administration. *Social Security Bulletin,* January 1975.

Winders, John J. "Hospitals' Use of Tax Exempts Tops $1.9 Billion." *The Daily Bond Buyer,* January 12, 1976.

Discussion of
The Projected Response of the Capital
Markets to Health Facilities Expenditures

H. Robert Cathcart

In the very helpful introduction and summary the authors indicate that they do not anticipate a "capital gap" for the construction of hospitals. They then go on to add, "While it is true that the visions of hospital administrators and trustees will always surpass, in the aggregate, their ability to finance projects, we believe, for a variety of reasons, that implemented construction programs will not place an inordinate strain on the capital market." The fact of the matter is that hospital administrators, trustees, and medical staffs are really reacting to the demands of society to provide the best possible current medical services that are available. They are not creating the demand, they are reacting to it. Failure to respond would have created a crisis causing many other problems that could have resulted in a change of the system to some other kind of ownership.

Understanding and agreeing that the providers of the services are not creating demand, but reacting to it, is of fundamental importance. A substantial majority of the population in the United States now has some type of hospital insurance. The data indicates that between 77 and 83 percent of the population is currently covered for hospital expenses. Also, 149 million Americans (approximately 70 percent) have some form of catastrophic benefits.[1] Whether they have paid for this insurance personally, or have had a governmental or employer source pay, they have a strong vested interest in obtaining full value from this "earned investment." Obtaining this full value and receiving what has been promised, by either the employer, the union, or the government official, has become a challenge that is placing record-breaking demand on the system. How this over-promised demand works and how to control it is not fully understood. The authors have properly considered what might happen to this demand as controls known as certificate of need, professional standards review organizations, health maintenance organizations, prospective payments, health planning legislation (P.L. 93-641), and a variety of other controls are introduced into the system. But, these controls are so new and untested that it is dangerous to assume that they will cause the system to react exactly as forecast. We know that the system is not well balanced and controlled and, thus, it is impossible to predict precisely how it will react to these controls.

Perhaps a safe way to approach this consideration is to recognize that there is a great demand for health services, a demand that comes from society, and that there are various new controls that should function in a certain manner. To some unknown degree they will function as expected, but, in doing so, a variety of unexpected new influences will be released. The impact of these new influences is difficult to anticipate and measure. The only certain factor is that the consumer has been promised health services by his employers, his union, or his government. He will want to collect on these promises and in this way will continue to stimulate demand which the defined controls may or may not manage. If the health providers are able to cope adequately with this demand, and one part of this coping will be the capital financing of health care facilities, the organizational pattern of the present health care system will survive. If not, there will be a major reorganization, which might be most traumatic to the system and to those who have supplied capital for the facilities in the system.

It will be important for public policymakers to recognize that health care facilities are now incurring substantial, new fixed costs. Kelling and Williams point out that between 1968 and 1974, the aggregate capital expenditures for community hospitals increased 193 percent, from $1.1 billion to $3.2 billion. "During the same period government grants and guarantee loans increased 76% and philanthropy only 44%." The difference was provided through debt financing, which increased 305 percent. As these new fixed costs were accepted, so were new management rigidities. Most health care facilities will accept a responsibility for servicing this debt as one of their highest priorities. Thus, when, and if, arbitrary limits on payments are imposed, as they have already been tried in New York State, and as they have been suggested by the president of the nation and by several leading lawmakers, there may well be profound changes in the quality and, perhaps, the quantity of service that is available to the consumer, since it is assumed that fixed charges will probably be financed before the introduction of new or innovative patient services will be. As part of his budget proposal for 1977, President Ford had legislation introduced that would place a 7 percent ceiling on the increase in federal payments for hospital services. The bill was not enacted. Representative Rostenkowski, in an effort to assemble his committee's form of Medicare Reform Amendments, asked committee members to consider a number of issues, including the imposition of a 9.5 or 10 percent ceiling. As of September 25, 1976, specific legislation has not yet been drafted. The only way of providing for these innovative and high cost limited demand services will be to create a loophole type of policy permitting a total pass-through of approved debt service cost. Without this loophole those institutions with considerable debt cost will be placed at serious competitive disadvantage with those institutions that have avoided these fixed costs, assuming, of course, that it is possible to find any debt-free institutions.

Some health care economists and national policymakers will advise, and strongly work, against the acceptance of any cost pass-through mechanism for debt service, while institutional health providers will advocate it. How this issue will be resolved is difficult to predict. This give-and-take does merit careful monitoring as well as active participation on the part of those who feel identified with either of the positions.

During the past ten years, the increased complexity of financing the daily operations of health care facilities, dealing with the variety of third party payers, understanding complex reimbursement regulations, and having to maximize revenues has made it essential that these institutions have competent financial executives to deal with the challenges. The current swing toward debt financing of capital projects, as documented by Kelling and Williams, reinforces this need and makes it apparent that such expertise is essential. Without it, the ability of health care facilities to provide cost effective and currently accepted health services will be compromised. The industry, then, will have to attract an ever increasing number of individuals with excellent financial management talent. As this type of informed manpower is assembled within the health care facilities, it will have increased influence and will slowly give the institutions an orientation where prudent financial input is more welcome and of great influence in overall policy. As this shift takes place, hospitals will become more attractive to those who wish to make capital investments.

When defining the market for capital investment the paper has excluded consideration of health care facilities serving patients with mental health problems. This had made the management of the subject easier and is supported for this reason. However, such exclusion does tend to mask a large capital market of psychiatric health care facilities which have a great potential. The figures in Table 9D-1 confirm the market size.

It is true that a significant part of the psychiatric health service market is now controlled by state and local governments. Ninety-five percent of the beds, 76 percent of the admissions and 95 percent of the inpatient days are controlled by the local and state governments. However, there is also a slowly accelerating trend away from the use of governmental facilities. With the growth of greater prepaid insurance coverage for psychiatric services there might well be a significant swing of patients from state and local governmental units to local public hospitals, nonprofit institutions and investor-owned units. For example, short-term inpatient treatment services are increasingly covered by voluntary health insurance. Astrachan et al.[2] report that some "states insist on such coverage in new policies. Currently, three quarters of the population has some coverage for the general hospital and 63% has some inpatient coverage for psychiatric illness." This trend

Table 9D-1

	Hospitals	Beds	Average Daily Census
Short-Term General Hospital Beds	6,186	1,025,246	769,794
Short-Term Psychiatric Hospital Beds	151	13,103	9,061
Long-Term Psychiatric Hospital Beds	419	344,257	280,041
Total Psychiatric Beds	570	357,360	289,102

could also be fostered because of the impersonal and obsolete facilities of many governmental psychiatric facilities. Since the local and state government psychiatric facilities serve such large numbers of patients, movements of patients in 5 or 10 percent increments could establish staggering new demands for development capital, upsetting all previous estimates of demand, including those in the Kelling paper. It would not be advisable to hold your breath while waiting for this trend to materialize. On the other hand, there are important factors that could cause a sharp movement of psychiatric patients into local units. These facilities would be forced to depend upon debt financing to meet such a demand. Large demands could seriously influence the availability and the cost of funding of other non-psychiatric units. These are possibilities that should be carefully followed.

Robert S. Kelling, Jr. and Paul C. Williams have provided a stimulating and useful paper. As noted earlier, it will be useful for all policymakers. It deserves wide distribution and discussion. It will provide answers to many questions, cause other questions to be asked and prompt more research and thinking about this important subject.

NOTES

1. *Health.* United States, 1975, Department of Health, Education and Welfare, Public Health Service, Human Resources Administration.

2. Boris M. Astrachan, Daniel J. Levinson, and David A. Adler, "The Impact of National Health Insurance on the Tasks and Practice of Psychiatry," *Archives of General Psychiatry* 33, (1976):785–793.

Discussion of
The Projected Response of the Capital
Markets to Health Facilities Expenditures

Lawrence A. Hill

When one is asked to deliver a commentary on, or discussion of, a paper, it is usually fortunate for the discussant if the paper is a bad one. Then the discussant can ape the literary or drama critics and produce a blistering, perhaps colorful, and even humorous piece which leaves the reader or listener in no doubt concerning the identity of the true expert.

In this case, however, no such circumstances prevail. The paper by Kelling and Williams is thoughtfully done, draws reasonable and, in my view, correct conclusions and, furthermore, is comprehensive in scope, omitting no major pertinent considerations. Having said that, what does one do by way of a commentary? The only obvious answer is amplification of some issues within the paper. I have, therefore, chosen as my text the final sentence in the "Introduction and Summary." "We are frankly concerned that certain features of potential laws and regulations, which are intended to contain health care costs, will inadvertently impair debt security, in both a real sense and in the perception of the investment community which will be expected to accept future hospital loans."

It is my belief that this concern is eminently valid and perhaps understated in the paper. It is a concern which has received some national attention, but which is not yet truly a national problem. As a problem it shows up most clearly in the northeastern part of the country where hospitals are subject to the most severe scrutiny and regulation, especially by state government.

By and large, the existence of the threat to capital acquisitions that is posed by regulation is not recognized at the state level, but it is recognized, to some degree at least, in the United States Congress as evidenced by the debate leading to the passage of P.L. 93-641, the so-called Planning Bill. A key provision in the drafts of the bill was recertification of facilities on a periodic—say, three-year— basis. Under this provision, a hospital could have been granted permission, by the appropriate planning authority, to build a facility or to add a service. It might finance this construction with debt capital and then, three years later, that same planning agency could come back and declare the facility or service no longer necessary and order it closed. How, then, is the hospital to repay its debt? During the congressional debate, testimony by the financial community convinced the committee that recertification could kill the supply of capital for hospitals. Thus, the provision was deleted from P.L. 93-641, but the idea is not dead. It may appear in modified form in the amendments which, undoubtedly, will be attached to the law when it comes up for renewal in 1978. Further evidence of federal awareness of this issue is apparent in the exclusion of capital costs in the ceiling calculations that are embodied in section 223 of P.L. 92-603 and, also, their exclusion from ceiling calculations in the proposed Talmadge bill.

Such awareness, however, does not appear to be present within certain state regulatory authorities. By and large, state efforts are aimed at control over hospital expenditures without much regard for the capital structure of the hospital, of its working capital needs or its ability to secure debt financing. Again, however, it should be stressed that this phenomenon is found largely in the northeastern states and, therefore, is, as yet, a localized issue. Localized or not, however, the threat posed by legislation and regulation to the ability of hospitals to attract capital is real. And if hospitals are unable to attract capital within the private sector, there can be only one outcome. Because the nation must have hospitals, they will not be allowed to dry up and blow away; they will be "saved" by the government and, eventually, will become governmental enterprises.

Having commented in general terms, I will now be more specific. As a practicing hospital administrator who, in a highly regulated setting, is faced with needs for physical plant improvements, perhaps my contribution to this conference can be best made in the form of a case study. At this point it is possible to relate only part of the case, because the story is only in the early stages.

My hospital has filed with the state an application for a certificate of need to replace a pediatric inpatient facility, to replace obsolete operating rooms and laboratories and, also, for ambulatory care space to be used by the full-time medical staff and faculty. The price tag attached to this proposal is $51 million. The planning of this project was carefully done and step-by-step consultation with the state's A & B agencies was a major factor in producing the final product. Nevertheless, at the last step, the state certificate of need agency voted 3-2 to deny the certificate. The hospital appealed the decision. The appeal was upheld by an appeals board which ordered that the case be reconsidered. As of this writing, a request for a rehearing has been filed by the hospital and we are awaiting a response.

In the meantime, however, the state has written a batch of new administrative regulations governing the administration of the certificate of need program. These were issued on September 29, 1976, retroactive to September 1. Further, paragraph 40 of the regulations states that any applications filed but awaiting action will have to conform to the new regulations. Because these demand new and different kinds of data to support any application, no application that was written to conform to the old regulations can meet the new ones. Therefore, in essence, the deck has been swept clean. The state hospital association is going to court to enjoin the new regulations, so that, at this time, the issue is in doubt. This chapter of our case is cited simply to make the point that a CON program, operated under ever-changing regulations that are promulgated with little notice and with retroactive force, and whose decisions have been called capricious by an appeals board is probably not a program which would inspire much confidence from financing agencies.

While it is true, as Kelling and Williams state, that a certificate should imply a public charter and, thus, encourage capital, that is true only if the certificate of need program is credible and if other state agencies recognize its decisions and are willing to live with them.

Judging from indications in our own case, it is not at all clear that achieving a certificate would be a positive influence on the ability to acquire capital financing. Under existing regulations, the certificate of need agency can place certain conditions on the certificate granted. These, in turn, can, in my judgment, inhibit the ability of an institution to finance a project for two reasons. The first is that the agencies could issue a certificate allowing only a part of a given project to be built. It is entirely possible, therefore, that a certificate could be so worded that the economic viability of the entire institution could be placed in jeopardy, given the limitations of the certificate itself. For example, at the first hearing in which my hospital was denied a certificate the agency demanded that we draw up a schedule of priorities among these facilities, the clear implications being that the council might grant a certificate for a portion. The operating facts of life are such that, if the hospital were granted a certificate to build, say, just pediatric beds without any of the other services, the operating costs involved in a fragmented project with inevitable built-in inefficiencies would probably destroy the financial viability of the institution and make the project impossible. If debt financing were required, the ability to pay that indebtedness would be in question. Such a fact would not be lost on those asked to lend the money and, therefore, it is doubtful that financing would be available.

The second reason for concern in our case is that the certificate of need agency has given evidence to show that, in granting a certificate, it also wishes to impose conditions describing the operating costs and "bottom line" outcome of any new facility. Given the fact that, from the date of granting the certificate until substantial new construction is up and operating, several years elapse, guarantees concerning operating results are risky, at best, probably foolhardy, and certainly not designed to inspire confidence in any lending agencies. Therefore, while I would agree, in general, with Kelling and Williams, that a certificate does imply public approval and support for capital expenditures, the behavior of the agency itself and the conditions which it attaches to a certificate can encumber a certificate to a point where, rather than being a potential factor in achieving financing, it could be negative and even destructive.

The second element of control that appears at the state level, again primarily in the northeastern states, is so-called cost control legislation. While the details of such legislation vary among the several states, they clearly have one objective, which is to slow down the rate of increase in reimbursement to hospitals. Clearly, constraints on the amount that hospitals can charge for their services and the amounts which they can collect for services rendered have a direct effect on their profit and loss statement. It is ridiculously obvious that a poor P&L statement discourages prospective lenders.

Beyond the aggregate effect of controls on charges and collections, state rate-setting legislation and regulation have shown a distressing tendency to intrude into internal management questions within the institution. It seems that state regulators are not content to deal with aggregates or with broad parameters but wish to exercise controls on the detailed analysis of operating departments within the hospital. In so doing, the usual method is to compare the operation of a given department in one hospital with that of a whole group of hospitals, to strike an average and rule that the average is all that the state will pay for that particular service. This process usually becomes bogged down in a meaningless mass of statistical data that cause confusion for the controllers as well as for the controlled. The outcome is almost certainly financial uncertainty. Again, the process tends to discourage lenders because the hospital cannot, with any certainty, state its financial condition or its prospects for the future.

To return to our own situation. Two controls are being proposed by the state which could prove disastrous to any hospital seeking funds in the money market. The first of these relates to certificate of need. Here the state is proposing that a hospital that wishes to take any beds out of service for thirty days would have to apply in advance, in writing, to the state or it could not reactivate those beds without permission from the state. This would mean, for example, that a hospital hoping to renovate a nursing unit might lose the ability to use that unit, once renovated, with obvious effects on hospital revenues. It would also mean that a hospital which (because of location in a resort area) might incur substantial seasonal census variations and which economized by closing units during the off season, could no longer do so without the risk of being refused permission to reopen the units. Again, the financial consequences are not insignificant and are certainly not designed to inspire confidence among those with money to lend.

A second proposal states that all depreciation funds that are collected by the hospital should be put in a statewide pool to be doled out by the state agency when certificates of need are granted. Clearly, again, the institution which has to give up control over this segment of its operating costs and revenues would be financially weakened and a much poorer credit risk than one which was its own financial master.

These examples, some real and some proposed, some stated generally and some stated in a more specific way, are intended to reinforce the fact that governmental regulations, primarily at the state level, and regulations that are aimed at operating finances could have the effect of rendering hospitals so financially risky that lenders in the market would not want to touch them, or that hospitals would be such a high risk venture that loans would carry a very high rate of interest so that the hospital would be unable to carry the financing costs and still live within rates set by state agencies.

It is my hope that state governments will follow the federal example and recognize that to stop capital sources for hospitals is not in the public interest. Perhaps they will, and perhaps my own views at this time could be considered alarmist. Nevertheless, while Kelling and Williams do allude to these dangers in their paper, it is my judgment that they are more real, closer and more important than the treatment given to them in their paper.

Philanthropy

Perhaps a word about philanthropy could also be added to the Kelling and Williams considerations. They point to the fact that third party payment does provide for securing debt financing, thus lifting a burden from philanthropy. This statement is undoubtedly true, but once again it is not the whole story. Third party reimbursement, as found in much of the country, is cost-related, which means that the institution which, through operating efficiencies—or some type of magic—decreases costs is rewarded by an equal decrease in reimbursement. Therefore, there is really no way, in a cost-related system, to achieve surplus funds through operations. Philanthropy, then, is about the hospital's only source of acquiring money which can be used in a discretionary fashion. When faced, therefore, with a major capital expenditure, the hospital may well select debt financing, assuming that the costs that are involved can be recovered through the normal reimbursement channels without using philanthropic funds. If they are used, philanthropic funds only decrease the cost of financing the project, decrease allowable hospital costs and, therefore, decrease reimbursement. Philanthropy, therefore, is not an economically sound way for a cost-reimbursed hospital to finance major capital projects.

In summary, the conclusions made by Kelling and Williams are substantially correct, but they understate, in my belief, the clear and present dangers that governmental controls represent to the financial viability of the hospitals and, therefore, their ability to tap a capital market which indeed does, at this time, contain ample supply for the future.

Discussion

Mr. P. Williams: Investor-owned hospital securities are becoming more and more sophisticated in terms of the ultimate source of payment and in the way that the hospital derives its revenues. In fact, the hospital is becoming more and more like a public utility. Since the investor does not feel that the mortgage or equity has any practical value, he cannot see himself foreclosing a hospital. It is becoming more common, therefore, for hospitals to finance facilities with debt in excess of 60 or even 70 percent of its total capitalization.

Mr. Needleman: The ability to obtain capital may be affected by some kind of rate review, prospective reimbursement, or negotiated rate structure. Still, there seems to be a growing sense that reimbursement systems are going to have to be changed. What safeguards ought to be built into the system to help overcome the potential hazards of prospective reimbursement?

Mr. L. Hill: I am an advocate of prospective reimbursement. What I would advocate, however, is that when my budget is negotiated with appropriate groups, that it then be reimbursed. Medicare does not reimburse full cost. I have no argument with prospectivity; I feel that it is a matter of risk taking. But if I, in behalf of an institution, am willing to take that risk, then the state also should be willing to take a risk, and reward me if I beat the system.

Mr. Cathcart: I want to stress the need for a realistic appeal process. Most providers of services would feel comfortable if the appeal process were not in the hands of the same agency of government that is paying the bills. There should be some insulation between the payer and the regulator.

Mr. Kelling: We have not had very much experience yet with prospective reimbursement, and it is going to take a while for us to determine its impact. At this point we are dealing with layer upon layer of uncertainties, and prospective reimbursement is only one of them. We are all in favor of cost containment, but many of the solutions have built-in problems that must be carefully weighed against the benefits.

Dr. Evans: I am concerned by the implication that we are all in favor of cost containment. We are not; most of us have a direct stake in keeping those costs moving up. There is a line in Mr. Cathcart's discussion paper in which he claims that the demand on this industry is exogenous and that he is simply responding to that demand. As long as we take that linear view of the industry, we are implying that the industry and all of the people in it have a direct economic stake in its expansion. I would say, however, that the trend is growing towards a more sophisticated interpretation of the evidence; we are realizing that this is a very complex interdependent industry in which patterns of utilization do not reflect demand in the normal economic sense.

Dr. Ginzberg: Dr. Evans' comment underscores one of the basic problems facing the industry. We are dealing with two forces that appear to be on a collision course. The reimbursement agencies, especially the state governments, are having difficulties in coming up with the money that hospitals say they need. At the same time, as Dr. Evans points out, we are caught in a cost spiral: the hopsitals and the physicians would like to spend more, the technology forces large expenditures, the trade unions are more powerful, and so on. What do you see as a likely resolution of this problem?

Mr. L. Hill: The *New England Journal of Medicine* recently reported that a patient who stayed in a surgical intensive care unit for six days or longer at a cost of $500 per day has only a 21 percent chance of being alive within ninety days. The public policy question in my mind is staggering; I cannot see a congressman or a state legislator walking up to that question, because he would be walking home without a job. I'm not sure that I have the wisdom to know how to handle it, and certainly not on a day-to-day basis when the patient presents himself at the hospital.

Dr. Blanpain: If it is true that a number of cost-ineffective procedures cannot be directly tackled by your politicians, then you would gain by examining the European negotiating mechanism which mediates between the medical profession and the government at the national level. In the United States there is a missing link between those committed to cost containment and those interested in the rising of costs. I have the impression that, in Europe, with the long tradition of struggle between insurance funds and the professional providers, the negotiating mechanism provides that link. Without it, the politician is confronted with both the issues and the profession, and he cannot avoid a fight.

❋ Chapter 10

Wrap-up Session: Summary Remarks

Gordon K. MacLeod

The many issues, arguments, and proposals which have been developed over the past two and a half days clearly and positively reflect upon the backgrounds and qualifications of the conference participants. This conference has brought together an unusually wide range of health related interests which have given rise to vigorous and far-reaching debate. I shall highlight only a few of the issues as they relate to government regulation, tax policy, reimbursement mechanisms, and the role of physicians.

The American health care system has been responsive to opportunities for expansion, even in the face of increasing governmental regulation. To the extent that health care legislation has been intended to increase the production of health services, even to the point of excess capacity, it has been successful. Such legislation has not been designed as an incentive for cost-efficiency. The inability of the government or the private sector to regulate the industry should serve as a mandate for reshaping the format for delivery of health care. Appropriately sized markets of approximately one million people can be considered to promote the efficient delivery of clinical services and cost effectiveness. Incentives for equity, for avoiding provider monopoly, and for using competition to promote the accessibility to services can easily be applied to a population of this size.

Another seeming deficiency of government regulations has been the emphasis on alleged costs rather than on relative prices. Full disclosure of price scales would tend to stimulate competition, thus channeling investment funds into the most efficient modalities.

Reconsideration of federal tax laws would be beneficial to any program that is aimed at cost containment. Tax reform could be used both to stimulate the economy and to correct present inequities. Proposals range from the removal of tax exemptions on health insurance to a guaranteed annual wage/negative income tax.

There was a general indictment of current reimbursement mechanisms which were faulted for not adequately addressing capital expenditures, for not encouraging cost-efficiencies and for not using capital levers for primary and ambulatory care to compete with inpatient care. Cost-plus and fee-for-service reimbursement mechanisms only contribute to inflationary trends. Reimbursement mechanisms could be used to improve the medical care delivery system by linkages, as with nursing homes to hospitals and with home health services to in-patient care, providing incentives for the most efficient utilization of resources within each sector of the health care system.

Some aspects of the public utility model could generally comply with many of the capital needs of the health care industry. The basis of the utilities' rate structure is return on assets, a method which can cover depreciation. Applied to the health care industry, this would help to correct at least that aspect of present reimbursement inadequacies and could encourage increased investment.

With respect to physicians, there was a clear call for improving the organization of services, containing the number of services, reducing the rate of increase in the number of physicians, developing cost effective and health outcome measures, and for the review of monopolistic practices resulting from PSRO and malpractice legislation.

ANALYSIS

This is an appropriate time to undertake an analysis and synthesis of the data presented at this conference. In such a study, serious questions are raised about the effectiveness of short-term cost control in contrast to continuing flexibility of the system, and about misdirected incentives within the health care system and their impact upon both quality and productivity in the system. The issue of regulation must be weighed against some degree of reliance upon the market-place. In both the public and private sectors, traditional and legal sanctions may be invoked either through regulatory mechanisms of government or through freedom of choice and competition.

As the conference proceedings indicate, there is no question that health care delivery and financing are still dynamic and responsive to economic manipulation but may be growing less flexible as a result of government regulation. It has been shown by the speakers that the cost to the public can be contained through cost control efforts in the short run. However, there is little evidence that these costs can long remain at acceptable levels without the give and take of the mar-ketplace. A more subtle question is whether those perverse incentives, leading to overutilization of diagnostic and acute care services, can be more manageable in order to contain costs and to promote utilization of preventive and rehabilitative services.

First, let us look at bricks and mortar capital formation. Inflation, recession, and cyclical interest rates have been both a challenge and an opportunity for astute managers within the health care delivery system. Capital funding sources have expanded in the face of demand. Unfortunately, the major thrust of capital funds has been diverted toward hospital construction that is directed primarily at inpatient services.

Capital funding of high technology equipment has proven to be a particularly perverse problem. Standard radiographic equipment has increased in cost some 80 percent in the past ten years. Similar increases have occurred in laboratory costs. Ever-increasing rates of obsolescence have halved the financial life of much medical equipment and have brought about a serious cash flow problem. Both labor and other capital costs are compounded by the need for trained personnel to operate this complex technical equipment. Unplanned obsolescence plagues depreciation predictions and, necessarily, results in underutilization of equipment. At the same time, unnecessary overutilization of high technology equipment further compounds the cost/price issue and contributes substantially to the rising cost of health care services. Central to these perplexing problems is the critical issue of defining appropriate incentives to stimulate and guide cost consciousness with respect to the application of technological developments.

Containment of operating capital can provide the most comprehensive control of the health care delivery system. Total control of operating capital—if this were possible—whether lodged in the Blues, in the private insurance companies, or with the government can yield the same results that monopolies have obtained in the nonhealth sector.

With respect to human capital, we have not yet found a way to get the public to accept less sophisticated health professionals in place of the highly trained specialists that it demands. We must devote increasing attention to the number of professionals entering the field and the impact that the expansion is expected to have on the cost spiral. The human capital issue is further complicated by monopolistic practices, tradition, maldistribution, and the lack of success in educating consumers to utilize health care personnel effectively. Any attempt to deal with these problems must include careful demographic studies. The use of collective bargaining is often mentioned as a method of negotiation between and among a variety of professional, as well as nonprofessional, groups in the health field. The complexity of these issues underscores the growing need for a concerted program to produce qualified managers trained specifically to deal with the special personnel problems of the health care industry.

It is fair to say that, in the absence of rigid government control, each of these four constituents of capital financing of health care can be used to increase flexibility in an otherwise rather rigid sector of the economy. Investments in facilities, technology, and manpower must be integrated and balanced. Any stratified or artificial categorical approach to any one of these capital areas, without awareness of its impact on the others, has contributed, and will necessarily do so, to inefficiency and the misallocation of resources which then result in cost overruns and escalation.

SYNTHESIS

The synthesis or combination of the elements of capital financing as studied at this conference offers us a useful measure by which to evaluate group practice and other kinds of prepayment plans as an alternative to traditional fee-for-service reimbursement.

Despite the likelihood of some inefficiency resulting from several patterns or modalities of health care delivery existing side by side, we must preserve a degree of flexibility to improve and strengthen the system in the future. The traditional fee-for-service reimbursement pattern has proven workable and, in the main, satisfactory to providers and patients alike, although subject to criticism in recent years for its inflationary tendencies. HMO prepayment plans, with some fifty years of experience, offer a clear alternative to the traditional pattern; the availability of such an alternative has many implications for capital financing. Because the HMO model has yet to be shown to be a sufficient stimulus to competition in all areas, competing health insurers, Health Care Alternatives, must also be looked to for leadership in reshaping the delivery system and expanding consumer choice. Employee and employer interest in containing health insurance costs, if properly exploited, is a powerful potential force against professional resistance to altering the configurations of the health care system.

Whichever modality of service is selected by consumers, it is proposed that this conference recommend and endorse the disclosure of all financial and organizational arrangements by professional groups receiving funds from federal, state, or local governmental health care sources. These data would be of great help in conducting further studies with an eye to future planning. Such disclosure should be as free as possible from other controls, to the extent that recipients of government funds comply with legislation and regulations. The idea, of course, is to encourage variety, competition, and innovation at the grass roots level rather than to impose a set of standards and constraints, other than honesty, integrity and candor, on only one sector of the economy.

If both freedom of choice and open disclosure are examined in the light of each of the four kinds of capital problems discussed at this conference, we can inspect the alternative available to each of them. Consideration must also be given to the separate philosophies which underlie the difference between fee-for-service and prepayment in capital expenditures.

First, bricks and mortar capital involves the acquisition, construction, and replacement of health care facilities. In hospitals, the traditional pattern of philanthropy and government subsidies is giving way to debt financing. Capital resources have been directed primarily toward inpatient services, with ambulatory services receiving short shrift. By contrast, the Kaiser-Permanente hospital-based group practice prepayment plan and other HMOs have not been able to rely on philanthropy and government subsidies, their funds being usually derived instead from a balance of accumulated earnings and debt financing. One guideline proposed for further capital expansion of existing HMOs is for total debt not to exceed net worth. The ready availability of ambulatory and preventive services in HMOs necessarily makes the entire operation more efficient than fee-for-service.

Full disclosure of mechanisms used in raising capital as well as cost should be made available to existing planning agencies whichever modality is in search of capital funds.

Second, high technology capital remains a problem for each system, especially in the light of burgeoning costs for laboratory and X-ray diagnostic equipment; both suffer from high costs resulting from technological obsolescence. However, differences between the two emerge most clearly in the areas of utilization of services and personnel cost. Under fee-for-service reimbursement, there is a tendency to overutilize diagnostic tests which, of course, contributes to increased costs for clinical pathology and radiology services. In the case of health maintenance organizations, there is little incentive to overutilize these procedures.

Again, full and open disclosure of the capital needs, sources, and use of any high technology equipment by hospitals, HMOs, and other vendors who are remunerated from government funds should be available to the public to point up the efficiency and effectiveness of these various approaches.

Third, operating capital has been subject to intense variation due to inflation, recession and fluctuation in interest rates. The diminished significance of voluntary contributions of time and effort by religious groups, physicians, and other health workers has affected the need for working capital. Health, a labor intensive industry, has experienced enormous growth in numbers of workers and in incomes at all levels, along with increasing specialization in institutional settings. The diversion of operating capital to meet increasingly burdensome regulations affecting the life safety code in hospitals has become a fact of life in capital investments in the traditional fee-for-service pattern as well as in the alternative modality of the health maintenance organization.

Disclosure of operating capital resources is, in effect, an audit in either modality. Audit standards for both patterns are still embryonic. Accountability under such audits should necessarily reflect upon quality in each modality of service, so as to include preventive and rehabilitative medical care.

Last, but by no means least, is the issue of human capital. With respect to the issue of free choice of career pattern, the HMO offers an attractive alternative to American physicians. At the same time, the principle of dual choice, now mandated for qualified HMOs under the Health Maintenance Organization Act of 1973, requires an employer of more than twenty-five persons to offer the HMO as an alternative wherever one is available. The choice between a fee-for-service reimbursement system and an HMO is enhanced by offering a choice of HMOs such as between a prepaid Individual Practice Association (IPA) or a Group Practice Plan. Human capital resources within an HMO are distributed in a significantly different fashion from those in the fee-for-service pattern both in physician numbers and in utilization by specialty. While the impact of HMO physician distribution has not yet been felt by society as a whole, such utilization has clearly shifted manpower practices within the HMOs themselves.

Still, a problem remains vis-à-vis the distribution of health manpower in medically underserved areas. One inducement might be through an extension of the Health Professions Education Assistance Act of 1976, whereby students who are indebted to the government for educational loans would repay their indebtedness through assignments in medically underserved areas for a period of two years. While completing this assignment, direct capital subsidies for ambulatory care such as office construction, for equipment purchase, and for operating capital could be made available through deposits in local banks, and with built-in incentives for the development of group practices in these areas.

Ongoing surveillance of capital sources, as well as of capital expenditures, and full disclosure to the public, are bound to promote freedom of informed choice between prepayment plans and fee-for-service. These surveillance and disclosure functions might be best administered by a modified form of Health Systems Agency or, perhaps, by insurance companies with elected consumer/subscriber representation on their boards of directors. These would also have the power to assign local priorities to new capital needs for health care delivery.

Finally, it must be recognized that, to date, neither cost-efficiency nor cost-limitation has been a high priority consideration in the operation of the system. Government regulations, taxes and various kinds of public subsidies have distorted the growth of specific components of the health care system without consideration being given to the overall effects. It is hoped that the dialogue begun here between health financiers and health care providers can serve as a springboard to future attempts to balance the various elements of the health care industry into a feasible, integrated system designed to provide needed services at reasonable cost.

Summary Remarks
Session Chairmen

Dr. Blendon: I would like to outline the important points that were brought out in the session that I chaired. They relate to the practical implications of the material.

The first point deals with our historical discussion of capital formation. We traced the sources of financing from philanthropy and government grants to operational earnings and borrowed capital. In our quick overview, the implications of that shift in capital sources were understated, and I would like to point them out. Capital from external sources is given to an institution based on perceived need, whereas internally generated capital and mortgages are given to a facility based on the ability to make payments. If capital is internally generated, need is measured along different criteria than if its source is philanthropy or grants. I make no case for either, but I want to draw your attention to the fact that the source of capital significantly changes how need is defined.

The second point is that this shift has a substantial effect on the federal policy-making process in particular. After Hill-Burton, capital formation decisions went to the finance committees, and yet the Public Health Service and the finance committees rarely dealt with each other. The problem of forming capital through tax policy as opposed to capital formation in the budget is that the implications of the former do not become visible until years later, while the latter has decisions that must be faced before the appropriation is passed. It is important to understand that we now have a process where the finance committees, years afterwards, are looking at the impact of their positions on capital formation. In addition, the main sources of capital formation have again become the tax committees; the so-called health finance committees are also the committees which determine tax policy. Tax policy is relevant here for two issues in capital formation. One, it provides an incentive for philanthropic giving while also setting some restraints on how the funds can be used. Two, it provides the mechanism whereby insurance becomes a tax benefit to the employer.

One of the most important issues of our discussion—and this came out again and again—was that the demand for capital is determined by the supply of professionals. I want to stress that this will be very difficult to explain to the public.

I would also like to discuss briefly the argument between service insurance benefits and indemnity benefits. Let me remind you that prior to 1967, there was a big debate about whether or not we should insure health with a voucher system. The unions and others were concerned with providing full cost benefits and, in fact, a great many of the providers, particularly the physicians and the private insurance companies, wanted something similar to the proposals of Lave and Lave. That is, you hand out vouchers and let the market go to work.

Let's turn now to the issue of regulation in the health field. Health is a regulated industry; I don't think that is an argument here. I think that the argument is whether we want to encourage private capital to enter this field on a large scale and whether we want it to compete. The ideological question is very real here. We want competition, we talk about the quality of management and, yet, many of the regulatory strategies are concerned with rate of return and safety of investment. We believe in HMOs, but in the discussion of the bill, the ideology got in the middle, with the result that capital to this field has been cut off by regulations that do not guarantee the quick returns or stability needed to attract high levels of investment.

The last point that I want to make concerns the issue of ideology and pragmatism. Pragmatism in the debate about health policy has become the umbrella under which we fight our ideology. People in very conservative blue suits argue their pragmatism around an ideological framework. It is important to mention that pragmatic people accept what is here and deal with it appropriately. However, pragmatists turn ideological when you talk about the future, and capital formation is the future.

These are some of the implications of our historical experience. It is going to be tougher to deal with these issues because we are in a more ideological world, and how capital is generated is the basis of many of these ideological debates.

Dr. White: My mother-in-law used to say that this is the season when Thanksgiving and Christmas have us by the throat again! Dr. MacLeod has given us quite a feast of roast turkey and Dr. Blendon has given us cold turkey, but we have turkey hash and turkey croquettes and turkey soup that the rest of us will be glad to place before you, and then we have the bones. I don't know what I can really add to this. I will essentially say the same things, perhaps from a somewhat different perspective. Let me give you the issues that we have identified.

The first is with respect to human, fiscal, and physical capital. We are talking about whether it is going to be determined largely on the supply side or on the demand side. Heretofore, it has been largely determined on the supply side, without any particular group being at risk—that is to say, the physicians, the public, the hospital administrators, or the boards of trustees. The only group that can be said to have been at risk, generally, without having had much of a voice in the whole exercise, has been the public, although it has expressed its views and expectations through the political process. It has been largely an aggregated forum that decided on the supply side.

Now, the alternative question is the extent to which it should be guided and determined on the demand side. In other words, should demand be determined by some enterprise, firm or the government with respect to the size and scale of the health care enterprise? If so, the enterprise will determine the mix of resources, the kinds of services to be provided, and the risks to be assumed by the physicians, administrators, managers, trustees, and other groups. The aggregated position set forth by Dr. Ginzberg shows the effect of contributions on the supply side. Dr. Evans' interpretation is that everybody just wants to make a living and that the sky is the limit. There is also the view that, with controls on the demand side, there are a fixed number of resources and services and mixes of facilities and personnel and capital that are required to meet the needs of the market that is determined by a set of people.

The next issue contrasts need to demand, and it is hard to distinguish between them, but whose needs are we talking about? I think that we have to be fairly precise here. The needs of the public have been only feebly articulated, while the needs of the physicians and the needs of the hospital administrators and the trustees have been very precisely articulated. Is it the need of the physician for a particular type of workshop, a particular type of activity, a particular set of support systems? Is it the need of the hospital administrator to meet and service his debt, to keep his occupancy rates high, to use the equipment that he has in order to justify its purchase? Or should we consider the needs of people for the kinds of services and the kinds of problems that they present? This is again a marketing perspective, an epidemiological perspective, if you like. It is a different perspective from the traditional notion that anything that the health enterprise does is necessarily good and beneficial and in the best interests of the people. That is the second assumption that needs to be examined.

The third issue relates to whether all of this concern makes any difference. Are there actual benefits, and what is the efficacy of a whole range of diagnostic, preventive, therapeutic and rehabilitative procedures and pills, potions and elixirs? To what extent are they, in fact, shown, on the basis of scientific evidence, to be more useful and beneficial than harmful or useless? There is increasing concern in the Congress, and perhaps in NIH and the DHEW Health Resources Administration about who is to decide whether current and new procedures are beneficial. If so, there must be a determination of how beneficial they are and to whom. It is not clear how and where these assessments are to be carried out.

The whole issue of efficacy is upon us, and related to this concern for making these determinations is the information vacuum in which we operate. We have had a series of disparate bodies of information generated by the federal government and the National Center for Health Statistics on the distribution of problems in communities and societies, nationally and regionally for the most part, with very little information on small areas. Dr. Ginzberg stressed the need to compare small areas with one another and to see variations in different practices and different outcomes. At the other end of the spectrum, we have the projections for capital need and the rising volume of debt in the hospitals in relation to other sources of financing and, particularly, the reduction in funds derived from internal operations. This whole concern, this whole decision-making process is being conducted in an information vacuum. The need to put the pieces together came out of the discussion.

Another concern that emerged is what to do with the differences between revenues and expenses. This is where, somehow or other, the capital has to be generated, has to be paid for, has to be serviced, depending upon what modality you use, or has to be justified in the case of philanthropy. There are here enormous implications for the future, as Dr. Blendon pointed out, depending upon whether you generate capital from internal operations, from retained earnings, and have the capacity to innovate, or whether you incur long-term debt and become locked into a particular position. This problem, in turn, has implications with respect to taxation policy on the one hand and with respect to reimbursement policies on the other, and it all needs very critical examination. Both of these have enormous implications for the shape of the health care system in the future and the extent to which it is going to be determined on the supply side and on the demand side, as well as the extent to which it is going to be flexible and have the capacity to innovate and change.

Then there is the issue of the scale of operations and the scale of thinking. What, essentially, we have had is either rather small thinking or extremely global thinking. We have either thought about the country as a whole and the large aggregations of manpower, and the large aggregations of debt mounting, and so on, or we have thought about the individual entrepreneur, the sole physician practicing by himself. The matter of scale comes up in considering the Kaiser-Permanente approach—not so much the idea, but the scale of its operations. It comes up with respect to the distribution of problems in the community. There are groups of problems that involve everybody, and they occupy the full time of one to three physicians who serve perhaps one to three thousand people. There are some very rare problems that require a larger population in order to justify keeping a particular subspecialty active, content and busy. These are marketing problems that can be determined and measured.

Within this framework it is important to identify recent legislation and the impact that it is going to have. The Planning Bill implies that planning will take place on a geographic basis. The implications of the Manpower Bill are substantial, both with respect to the mix of manpower and primary care physicians versus specialists, and with respect to the training of managers and people who will help to guide the entire enterprise. These have to be worked into any consideration of the problems and issues that we are tackling.

We need to think bigger in many ways with respect to the scale of enterprises, but not so large that we think we're running the whole country. We need to identify capable people and bring them into the enterprise to examine some of these issues and to set forth the options that are to be considered by the political decisionmakers, both at the national and the local level. For my own part, I think that it is extremely important to decide whether or not we want to retain the options for diversity, competition, and choice, and to determine how these can be protected and maintained in order to maintain the kind of flexibility that characterizes this country. I believe that unless some of these issues are addressed rather smartly, the option may no longer be with us.

Dr. Carley: Let me comment briefly on the discussion following Mr. Hill's paper on the private sector. I think that the larger question that went unaddressed in the papers was whether there is room for profit-oriented business in the health care field, and, if so, how we are going to help it.

Mr. Terenzio's paper on philanthropy talked about the usefulness of philanthropy with regard to capital formation. The question implicit in our discussion was cost efficiency of the philanthropic dollar. Dr. Evans mentioned Paul Ginsburg's paper and Dr. Blendon mentioned some other studies that are being prepared. It is hoped that those papers, when produced, might be addenda to this conference.

Dr. Morreale will discuss the policy proposals touched on during the session.

Dr. Morreale: Regarding the issue of government regulation, it was pointed out that the sharp increase in hospital costs will probably lead to direct controls, which will mitigate against the profit sector because the control will be set for the predominately nonprofit sector. Even so, we can expect that there will be a questionable effect on nonprofit capital investment and, of course, profit capital investment or private capital investment will decline. The other possibility is a radical change in government policy which would impose arbitrary ceilings and, in that case, you would get a depression of investment in both nonprofit and profit firms.

Another possibility is the alteration of the insurance system. One suggestion was that we could have a comprehensive national health care plan, using the Medicare reimbursement system as a model. It was felt that this would dry up equity and borrowed funds in the industry and, that in fact, investment would decline. Another suggestion was made to reform the insurance system by having greater coinsurance for middle and upper income groups and to remove the tax subsidy on health insurance. That would lead to greater diversity of hospital care and health care institutions, which should lead to an expansion of opportunities in the private sector. The implications for the nonprofit sector are unclear, but if the profit sector does prove to be more efficient, we should see a decline in the nonprofit sector.

Finally, there were several suggestions about reimbursement incentives. One was that we could have a new type of incentive reimbursement system which would allow present existing hospitals to maximize their return on investment, and that should increase capital financing. The effect should be an increase in the nonprofit sector but it could also spill into the profit sector if the yields increase sharply enough. The other possibility that was raised was to have cost reimbursement on a regional scale, allowing competition. That should provide more flexibility in capital funding, and it should lead to more private investment.

Turning to philanthropy, it is clear that if you adopt a do-nothing policy, philanthropy will continue to decline in importance. Three options were laid out for increasing the role of philanthropy. One is that you could increase government seed money and matching fund programs to increase philanthropic giving which, in turn, would raise capital investment. Another possibility is to build a greater sense of social responsibility from the corporate side since it has a tremendous amount of capital to work with. That would increase philanthropy, which would, at the same time, increase capital. The third suggestion was that you have actual tax credits for philanthropic contributions, not tax deductions, but credits—so that a dollar given in contribution would be a dollar less paid in taxes. That would stimulate more general public giving.

In terms of increasing the role of philanthropy, or reversing its decline, there were two particularly important points raised. One was accountability. It was pointed out that the people who provide large donations or large contributions are often involved in the health planning process and should be made more accountable to the public. Giving should be tied in with the health care needs of the population through public planning.

Another point raised was having philanthropic organizations involved with innovations in the health care industry. Philanthropic dollars as venture capital could promote innovations and new arrangements in organizations of health care delivery. Philanthropic organizations could get involved in analyzing human capital needs and they could get involved in financing nontraditional medical care facilities. The options discussed were fairly clear.

It is obvious that we are faced with some very important choices, which you can see from all of these diverse policy proposals.

Mr. Miller: I thought that I would take a minute to remind you of the thrust of the discussions in the two panel sessions under my guidance. We brought out the fact that capital expenditures for health care had increased markedly in the last ten years and could be expected to increase further at a rate of about 6 or 7 percent over the next five years. We concluded that capital markets seem to be able to meet the needs at the present time, and will probably be able to meet the larger demands in the future. However, it was observed that the adequacy of expected revenue streams is, and in the future will be, keyed to the response of capital markets to capital needs as they evolve. This highlights the desirability of assuring, in one way or another, that reimbursement policies recognize and make explicit and sufficient provision for the cost of capital as a part of operating expenditures.

The future substantial growth in capital for health care will likely come from the area of tax-exempt revenue bonds. Further, it was brought out that, by 1981, debt financing might account for as much as 80 percent of total capital outlay, and that the financial soundness of some health care institutions might be endangered thereby.

Now let me turn to the issues and concerns. I think that all of us know what they are because, in the largest sense, they run as a continuous thread through the whole of this conference, to whit: Can reimbursement methods and overall regulation, now and as they develop further, be devised to assure the consistency and continuity of appropriate revenue streams and not impede the process of securing capital and applying it efficiently? This is clearly a major concern from the point of view of the capital users as well as of the capital investors and the capital market.

The other big issue is: How can we be assured that the capital which is invested will be employed efficiently? This relates to the broader question of national health policy, which we don't seem to have well defined at present. The need for capital and capital expenditures must be an integral part of what we determine as our national health policy. Then, and only then, can the process of planning and the types of regulation which constitute the framework for carrying out the nation's health policies be evolved.

A question was raised on the propriety of using tax-exempt bonds to so large an extent. The argument was made that their favorable tax treatment represents a hidden, rather than direct, subsidy which, therefore, fails to be included, as it should be, along with other health care costs. The widespread use of revenue bonds also tends to have a distorting effect on the capital market as a whole.

It was argued that loan guarantee programs have the effect of lessening the investor's interest and involvement once a loan has been made. The guarantee, by removing the investor's risk, reduces the investor's incentive to take a strong hand in assuring the continuing effective management of the investee's operation. It was suggested that the subsidizing of interest rates would keep the investor at risk while achieving the same purpose as the guarantee programs.

Concern was also expressed over the ability of the health care industry to develop adequate numbers of trained managers capable of dealing with the increasingly complex situations with which they are being faced. In particular, there are the additional complexities of financing capital needs and arranging operations so that they can be anticipated and dealth with appropriately.

And lastly, sounding a note that I think was mentioned earlier, the papers developed by Kelling and Williams and by Clapp and Spector broke new ground in that they brought together, for the first time, we believe, figures showing what capital needs were and will be, what kinds of capital are being employed, and where the money is being used. We end, therefore, with a concern over the need for the compilation of similar data on a regular basis in the future so that the dimensions of this aspect of health care financing will be suitably defined for policy and operational considerations.

Discussion

Dr. Ginzberg: These are my ten reflections on the conference:

1. We haven't talked at all about capital for the nonaffluent areas and the complete failure of the market to be responsive to that dimension.

2. As far as I can see, we are very sensitive to the market return problem yet know very little about the appropriateness of proposed projects. We have a gross discrepancy, then, between social planning and the flow of dollars in this field.

3. The lack of flow of capital to HMOs ought to be an issue of very deep concern. One cannot reach this late point in the conference without asking what is behind their failure. What is really going on beneath the surface?

4. It is quite clear that our reimbursement policies are not viable.

5. There is little money flowing to significant innovation. The HMO is an example; capital is not flowing there. We have a colossal industry with no experimental monies available.

6. We have no system for closing out excess capital. We don't let hospitals fail, which keeps the pathology in the system, and that drives the costs up.

7. We're still without any leverage whatever on the control of high technology, which we all admit is a major factor on the cost end, but we don't have the faintest idea what to do about it.

8. I don't believe that the market, as here defined by my colleagues, the economists, is a serious alternative to the inherently controlled nature of the system, and the increased controls that appear to be inevitable, given the tremendous amount of public money that is flowing into the system.

9. We paid inadequate attention to what it means to change physician behavior and supply. That is what drives the system as far as I can see.

10. I don't think that we are yet at a total cost level, so I expect this business to "schlepp" along.

Mr. Terenzio: We have to concentrate a great deal more on the provision of capital for the sources of health care delivery and prevention. We haven't addressed ourselves to ambulatory care, primary care, home care, preventive medicine, or health education. I think that we really haven't given enough thought to those aspects of the delivery system.

Mr. Ubell: As long as reimbursement continues in much the same fashion as it has been going, there is no problem for capital formation for the traditional facility. Such capital formation for traditional facilities is going to knock out the possibility of building nontraditional facilities, and something has to be done to take care of that situation. If the current capital formation continues, with the current debt financing, it will lock out nontraditional, nonmedical measures for the improvement of the health of the population and, at the same time, knock out the ability to deal with serious diseases which are current in our society. For example, we have an epidemic of gonorrhea in this country and a very high level of syphilis which the current nonsystem does absolutely nothing about. As long as it keeps chewing up the money that is available, I'm afraid that there will be no resources left to deal with these very serious disease questions which remain in the population.

Mr. Hess: There seems to be a general consensus that we have to pay more attention to the issues of primary and ambulatory care and to the problems of underserved populations. I have not heard much discussion about what interim leverages there could be on the capital side that would move us in a direction that everybody agrees we want to go. We ought to address ourselves, in the short term, to readjusting the reimbursement formulae and the capital incentive to provide those interim leverages.

Mr. Hernandez: I think that the problem in the present system is not of overcapitalization but of improper capitalization. We must examine very carefully what the opportunities are for getting excess capital out of the system, or shifting it from an improper place to a proper one. It seems that we generally agree—certainly the people who are operating hospitals can tell you, and the data suggest—that there is not a recognition in the present system of what the true cost of capital is. Now there is one caveat here and one opportunity. The caveat is that you would have to recognize and tie capital-related sources to capital-related uses. This is really just an extension of the funded depreciation concept. If you have excess funds, you can turn them around and engage in innovative techniques for improving the efficiency of the system. That would not go so far as to change fundamental behavior patterns such as physician behavior, which is a separate and very interesting question that seems to belong in the public sector. But I think that an opportunity does exist to improve the present system if you look at what you can do with the amounts of capital that you have.

Dr. Ruhe: I want to say a word in defense of the physician who is said to be driving this system, the implication being that it is an unfortunate situation. I would like to say that it would have been a good idea to have more physicians at the conference. There are certain points of view and problems that should have been included.

Mr. Brindle: It seems to me that tackling the institutional end of this is not nearly as effective as using controls and incentives to confront the issue of the organization and containment of physician services. The organized systems of physician care have demonstrated that here is a place for cost containment out of all proportion to anything that we might do with capital financing.

Dr. White: It is very important to distinguish between capital for facilities and capital for services. It is also important to focus on the person served, the customers, the market, rather than on the volume of services provided. It doesn't really matter how busy the doctors are; the question is, how much is provided for the patient? It doesn't matter how many hospital days are consumed if people are not benefiting from the experience. Capital should be directed toward services.

Dr. Ruhe: There has been virtually no discussion of the capital expenditures in the establishment and expansion of medical schools. We paused at 114 medical schools a few years ago, two more have opened their doors this year, and there are at least ten more waiting in the wings. What is interesting about those ten is their location. I don't know enough about economic theory or practice or business practice to understand fully the implication of this, but the new medical centers that are going to be established over the next five or ten years are going to be located in what would have been considered very unlikely places a short time ago. The fact is that all of this has taken place, not because of any orderly or planned procedure, but, rather, because of the demand of local populations for what they perceive as institutions which would enable them to have more physicians in their area and, presumably, better health care. These social forces tend to override all of our best planning and all of our regulations.

Mr. Ball: We have been trying very hard to find places where there can be freedom of choice and competition in what, I think most of us now accept, is a heavily regulated industry with a clear prospect of being much more heavily regulated. We are not having an argument about real dependence on the market versus dependence on regulation; we are searching for places where there may be some freedom of choice, some use of competition. Let's look at the places where regulation has failed, and deal with the question of how we can make it better within a context that leaves competition and freedom of choice carefully delineated as to the places where it makes sense. I find that the idea of consumer choice and competition is a pretty weak reed to rely on for our restraint.

Dr. Enthoven: We must search for a rational model for creating incentives for equity and cost effectiveness in the allocation of medical care resources. We must reconsider the basic economic structure of the industry and much of what we have been talking about is irrelevant detail. We must try to create a financial framework in which consumers and physicians have an incentive to consider the cost and the effective use of resources, and in which efficient producers can generate capital. I want to see competition so that the providers will have to serve the people with accessible, cost-effective service while they are controlling total spending. What I'm afraid of, with many of the regulatory approaches—is that we will move from one form of provider monopoly to another, where the physicians will be worshipping their cobalt machines and their CAT scanners instead of taking care of sick people.

Dr. Eichhorn: I would like to suggest the following method as a solution for financing, planning and control in the health care field:
   1. The central government should determine the framework for the financing of health care services.
   2. All particulars of planning and control should be decentralized and negotiated on an interim level between the suppliers of health services, on the one hand, and the social and/or private health insurance companies on the other. The associations of self-government in the health care field (doctors or medical associations, hospital associations, social and private health insurance associations) would then take the lead but would also accept the responsibility for planning and control. The associations' range of action would be limited by the total expenditure predetermined by the government.

Ms. Miller: There is one issue that I don't think this conference has gone into quite as much as we might have, and that is the nursing home industry. It deserves further discussion from two points of view, the first of which is, of course, politics. Secondly, from a systems point of view, we should talk about the interrelationship of the nursing home industry to the hospital sector. We must look for trade-offs to make the systems more organized and to relate the sectors to each other.

Mr. Havighurst: I would like to have some attention given to the question of tax law. People tend to write off the possibility of changing the tax law a little bit too quickly. I would propose to a new administration that it entertain this possibility: Switch from a system of deductions and exclusions from income to a system of limited tax credits for health insurance premiums paid and give everyone a 100 percent subsidy for some premiums. The amount of the credit could be tailored to the income, if you wish to make sure that it is larger for people in the lower income brackets, and there are many other ways of fine-tuning it. It would be quite easy to couple this with a tax reduction to stimulate the economy, particularly for lower and middle income people and tax increases for the upper income people who now get the maximum subsidy under the tax system using deductability. This would put people back into the position where they care how much money they are spending out-of-pocket for health insurance. That would be a change that has almost no adverse consequences and a good number of positive ones.

Considering the Future of American Health Care Capital Funding October 1975 Steering Committee Working Paper

Mark Perlman
Gordon K. MacLeod

The purpose of this report is to provide a basis for discussion by the steering committee for a future conference on alternative methods of health facility funding. We have been charged with examining several problems relating to the capital funding of the health care industry. For this effort there are several reasons. One is the repeated fear that the medical care industry is, in some significant senses, overcapitalized, particularly in regard to hospital beds. Another is that there is repeated fear that the United States economy, as a whole, is facing a period of chronic capital shortage. A third is the concern that hospital facilities for the urban poor can no longer be adequately supported by the traditional benefactors or by tax sources. The fourth is that the pace of technological changes in the medical care industry shows few signs of slackening—obsolescence repeatedly occurs long before planned depreciation has been realized. Finally, with the effective elimination of the present pattern of expenditures under the Hill-Burton Act, a by now accustomed source of capital funding for hospitals is drying up; need it be replaced, and, if so, how should it be replaced?

The invitation for establishing the committee came to Nathan Stark, Esq., Vice Chancellor of the Health Professions, University of Pittsburgh, from Dr. Kenneth Endicott, Administrator of the Health Resources Administration (HRA), U.S. Department of Health, Education and Welfare (DHEW). Dr. Endicott's views have been communicated to us by a variety of people (besides himself); that group includes Mr. Edgar Duncan, Dr. William Lybrand, Dr. Thomas McCarthy, Dr. Gerald Rosenthal, Mr. Eugene Rubel, and Mr. Daniel Zwick.

THE GOAL

The ultimate object of this total effort (i.e., a conference and the presentation of a report, buttressed by expert papers) is identifying for HRA (DHEW) alternatives and recommendations for harnessing the economic aspects of the health care industry. Economically harnessing the medical care industry means diverting it from its present tendency toward higher prices, possibly inappropriate medical care delivery to many groups, and an ever increasing (relative) share of the gross national product (GNP).

This steering committee has been selected to offer both "new" expertise with regard to the problems to be solved and "new" voices to urge its recommendations. The present steering committee members, consequently, consist of only a cadre of individuals, many of whom traditionally have not been known for their public expressions on the topic. In addition to this cadre, there will later be a larger group conference of people who have a broad understanding of the financial implications of the American Health Care Delivery system and of the supply and demand aspects of various classes or types of capital funding.

The steering committee's initial exercise is to define the directions which it is likely that the conference's products will take. After such determination, particular research papers would be identified and commissioned. These papers are to be presented at the three- to four-day conference to be held November 19-21, 1976. While the conference will involve critical considerations of each paper and thorough discussion of the spectrum of feasible programs, its principal purposes include the selection of health facility financing priorities, the development of some kind of formal proposal, and the organization of a formal report (preferably in book form), that report to be delivered in Washington before the first of September of 1977. Yet, in spite of that postelection date, it is quite possible that the basic ideas will become known earlier.

AN ASSUMPTION ABOUT LEGISLATION

It is probably useful to articulate some assumptions regarding the state of national health care legislation immediately after the 1976 presidential election. The current consensus is that the status of national health insurance in December of 1976 will be pretty much what it is now, although it is possible that legislation may be enacted (a) to establish a national program for catastrophic medical expense insurance, (b) to introduce some reforms in the administration of the Medicare/Medicaid programs, and (c) to provide for more standard reporting of third party carrier administrative activities. That same consensus suggests that none of the more comprehensive legislative programs will be enacted into law. Specifically, no one of the other proposals being considered by the House Ways and Means or the Interstate and Foreign Commerce Committees or the Senate

Finance or the Labor and Public Welfare Committees will be either the law of the land or will have a high probability of enactment in the 94th Congress.

CRITERIA FOR INDEXING HEALTH CARE EFFECTIVENESS

Anyone interested in health care legislation must have concern with the problems of measuring output. All perceptions of cost effectiveness ultimately require some perception of output/input ratios. A crisis has come because no one has devised a widely acceptable direct or indirect measure of health care output, be it a result of preventive or therapeutic activities. It is now commonplace to remark that neonatal mortality rates and life expectancy rates do not reflect well-being, let alone the quality of life. Likewise, there is much current criticism of "days lost from work" or "doctor-patient contacts" as an index of illness.

Nonetheless, no committee, charged as this one is, can neglect the opportunity to try to improve health care output measures. Indeed, one specific charge for the steering committee is to outline the details of a reporting system. What follows, therefore, is simply an argument that, *in addition* to making a renewed effort to develop health care output measures, we believe that this committee should consider whether the readily available economic indices could be linked in some sense to the efficacy of the present organization and/or allocation of scarce medical care resources. Not only should a general index be used, but precise prices in the health care complex can be regularly examined to see which are rising most rapidly. With knowledge of these price changes, one can infer what is happening, at least ordinally, to medical care capacity utilization, even if one cannot come directly to grips cardinally with the question of what these changes mean about health care delivery.

Recently, *Standard and Poor* issued a study which noted, with alarm, the growth of the medical care industry in terms of its share of the gross national product. This macroeconomic measure is, at best, a derived signal; nonetheless, it, too, indicates the direction in which allocation of other resources in this country's whole economy seems to be moving.

It is almost intuitively obvious that the time has come to study closely the economic signals being sent out by the American health care sector, and to use those signals, along with whatever information we can develop through better health care indices, both to judge the performance of the American health care industry and to predict the areas of probable imminent crisis.

PROGRAMS FOR AFFECTING MEDICAL CARE COSTS

We have reviewed both the recent literature on this problem, including testimony before the 92nd and the 93rd Congresses, as well as a spectrum of opinions of

members of the steering committee and of many expected conference participants. This present report represents, quite obviously, our synthesis of the many
views which were encountered and which seem to be trenchant to this steering
committee's function. When anyone synthesizes the positions taken by many
parties, the parties themselves often fail to recognize their own interpretations;
one immediate effort therefore, is to make sure that, in the process of general-
izing for this discussion, we have not significantly distorted individual positions.

The specific capital areas are, of course: (1) construction of hospitals: (a)
municipal, (b) private but not-for-profit, and (c) proprietary; (2) extended care
facilities, including nursing homes; (3) ambulatory health care centers; and
(4) teaching institutions. The kinds of capital involvement are (a) construction
costs, (b) equipment costs, (c) working capital costs (particularly important
where bank rates of interest are high), and (d) costs of "human capital" (investing
in people's skill).

Let us turn to a discussion of general policy directions. Of these there are two;
they are discussed *ad seriatim.*

PRINCIPAL POLICY CHOICES

There are essentially two kinds of policies in the capital funding area where the
future federal role might be used to improve the quality of health care output.

Involving Further Establishment of Federal Standards

One way is the use of the pattern of presently enacted legislation which involves sanction of need or certification of social necessity.

Certification. Here the idea has been to set up, within states, district certifi-
cating authorities which can lend "legitimacy" to what is socially needed. The
implication is that the local district authority will employ federal guidelines to
which it will adhere efficiently and within which it will operate disinterestedly.
Any institution receiving a sanction of necessity would have access to certain
kinds of institutional advantages. These might include:

1. generous allocation of Medicare/Medicaid "depreciation funds";
2. reasonably easy access to tax-free local bonds;
3. access to taxable bonds issued by state building authorities;
4. access to federally established operating capital balances against which charges
   may be drawn *in advance* of the first level of auditing;
5. allowances for third party carriers to be more flexible in relating to institutional pecuniary needs.

In sum, the threat of certification denial or nonrenewal can be the "stick";
those lacking certification would be hurt thereby, while those having such sanc-

tion would enjoy explicit economic benefits or "carrots." In a free society, no responsible institution should be forced out of the health care industry because it lacks certification, but the implication is that those having sanction should be able to outcompete those lacking it.

Health Districts. Recently, several states have experimented with the creation of hospital or health care regions, an approach which parallels virtually all states' experiences with school districts. In most instances, school districts do have taxing power as well as the right to issue bonds against estimates of future tax revenue. The relevant argument is that if local hospital or medical care regions are willing to meet federal standards, the federal government should be willing to match, according to some formula, the revenue collected and/or the bonds issued. The logic is simply one of community self-interest which could parallel school districts' governance through the *election* of consumer majorities to serve on health boards. If the electorate of a particular district or community is willing to assign so high a priority to health care delivery as to tax itself, the federal government can then judiciously offer some kind of federal support. Generally, reluctance of the community to tax itself keeps the federal government from rushing to pour in national tax funds.

Federal Investment in the Geographic Distribution of Human Capital. Another possible area of continued, or even expanded, federal activity goes directly to the question of possible regional shortages of different kinds of health care personnel. Physicians could be encouraged, by direct capital subsidies, to practice in "shortage" or what we call "listed" areas (so called because they would be *listed*, as designated by the Secretary of Health, Education and Welfare). Individuals, particularly foreign medical graduates, might be induced to practice in these areas or communities by allocating funds to purchase, or to build, the necessary physical facilities, to buy the necessary equipment, and to use as cash deposits in banks for working capital purposes. The object is to provide both American and foreign trained physicians a margin of incentive when it comes to the choice between (1) taking jobs at high, personal pecuniary costs and practicing in areas not suffering relative shortage, or (2) taking a position with easy federal funding for anyone willing to take up work or practice in "listed" areas. Almost every industrialized nation faces serious problems with maldistribution of physicians, yet no nation has thus far tried this double inducement. There is no reason why, with suitable manipulation, nurses and occupational therapists, anesthestists, dental technicians, optometrists, podiatrists, and other specialists would not respond to the same kind of incentives. The program requires that the secretary of HEW make wise determinations regarding "listed" areas and that the incentives be readily available and sufficient.

It is particularly important to realize that the same kind of incentive program, adequately modified, could work to increase the supply of hospital managers, ambulatory medical center managers, and nursing home managers. In this instance, the secretary might thus be asked to designate "listed" *specialties* or *professions* as well as areas. Moreover, the kinds of expenditures involved might be relatively small—relatively inexpensive fellowships combined with job or "residency" stipends in listed areas or specialties.

Summary. This approach, involving increased reliance upon federal standards, employs federal capital as the incentive for achieving, where needed, an increased supply and/or geographical redistribution of medical care facilities and personnel.

Involving Increased Reliance upon Citizen Choice or Preference

The second general approach shifts emphasis from the establishment of federal standards and the expansion of federal responsibility to reliance upon the operation of the normal market mechanisms. Here, the belief is that increased reliance upon state (as distinct from federal) regulation of business and professional practices (the normal police power) can combine with normal economic incentives. Such a combination can be used to reallocate medical care service in order to achieve a better program. In this case, the health care institution, as provider, would be required to rely on the marketplace[a] for the necessary money to support the four kinds of capital involvement that were mentioned previously. The idea is to place the consumer and the provider in an environment of noncontrols where each must rely on knowledge, priorities, intuition, and efficiency for survival.

Relying upon the market mechanism involves reconsideration of what has occurred to obtain relatively free choice by informed consumers and relatively free access to the market by different kinds of responsible producers. Consumer interest could be heightened by extension of the pattern of substantial consumer participation in HMO governance to include fee-for-service reimbursement schemes.

Policed Market Alternatives. In this instance, the idea is that federal legislation should be targeted to provide a *choice* for all Americans between individual or family reliance upon (1) a fee-for-service reimbursement system, and (2) a prepaid individual practice association (IPA) or group practice plan now known as health maintenance organization (HMO). Under optimal conditions, individuals or families should be able to choose any one of a group of fee-for-service reimbursable plans or any one of several HMOs (either of the group practice or the IPA type). There might well have to be a rather profound reconsideration of some of the federal tax laws and regulations in order to make the usual market

[a]Government might be considered as a capital provider of last resort or even, under special circumstances, the provider of services.

self-interest incentives work. Specifically, so long as an employer is willing and able to compensate his employees with tax-exempt medical care plans, neither he nor his employees have any particular interest in seeking controls over the cost of the program. On the other hand, if employees are taxed on the amount of income augmentation that is afforded them by their employer's payments to a health plan, the employees might raise the question of whether they might want that much coverage or prefer the cash.

Similarly, if the employer were charged on the basis of actual experience rating in terms of the precise services provided to his employees by the carrier (third party payer), the employer might begin to wonder whether the plan which he offered for his employees necessarily represents the optimal use of his payroll-oriented, but not payroll-disbursed, expenditures.

In any event, the act of offering a choice between a fee-for-service reimbursed system and a prepaid (HMO) system involves a recognition that a market system makes sense if there is adequate disclosure of full costs and full (no tax shelter) prices. With adequate disclosure and consumer participation in governance, there results no need to prohibit profit-making or even to establish detailed federal standards anent fees for specific medical services. The carrier, be it a fee-for-service reimbursed plan or a group of physicians at risk practicing in HMOs (the traditional medical group or IPA modalities, the latter being systems where the patient prepays all of his medical expenses but the individual physician is likewise at risk since he is reimbursed out of prepaid premiums on the basis of specific services provided) operates according to the normal market system. If it makes a profit, it can pocket the profit, reduce prices in the future, or decrease its costs by paying its personnel more and/or by increasing the quality of the services that are offered. If the HMO engages in fraud, its officers should be punished according to state felony laws.[b]

It is clearly obvious that both fee-for-service reimbursement schemes and HMOs can add to their individual contract charges reserves for reinsurance in the case of catastrophic expense. In the case of both fee-for-service reimbursement schemes and HMO schemes, some effort can be made to limit demand for certain types of medical care coverage, in the former case through reliance upon coinsurance based on a significant proportion of a small share of the insured's annual income and in the latter case by nominal copayments.

The coinsurance or nominal copayment programs make initial contact with the system of some pecuniary cost to the patient. One argument might well be that the patient, as in the case of the fee-for-service reimbursement scheme, would have to pay one-quarter of the total bill up to 15 percent of the family annual income. Thereafter, it might well be a public policy that the scheme should be designed to meet a much lower share of the cost (3 percent). In the case of the

[b]Because of inherent difficulties, some states may want to experiment with an ombudsman.

wealthy, this should not be much of a problem. In the case of the poor, it becomes a problem only if the family involved has little discretionary income.

The general problem of how to provide medical care to the relatively impecunious probably leads to a reconsideration of the usefulness of the guaranteed annual wage/negative income tax proposal. That proposal, buried in the 92nd Congress, could be resurrected and reexamined. The real question is whether it can be modified to provide services for those who cannot wisely handle government-derived cash flow. The problem may well involve making those individuals who cannot handle cash flow wisely, "wards of the government" and relieving them of both the responsibilities of trying to handle decisions which experience indicates that they cannot and the opportunity to shape social policy. It may well be that the era, which encouraged those who benefited from a generous social policy to make the social policy with scant consideration for those who had to pay for it, is coming to an end. If that is the case, certainly the ingenuity of the legislators should prove equal to the task.

The Medical Tax Exemption. Finally, now is probably the time to consider what are the advantages and disadvantages of continuing the present policy of federal income tax exemption on amounts spent on medical care in excess of 3 percent of the gross taxable (before deductions) income. Against the obvious advantages of providing a release for those heavily hit by major medical expenses there is the equally obvious disadvantage of encouraging individuals who have met the 3 percent deductible law and who are in high tax brackets to share somewhat enthusiastically the costs of medical luxury with the federal government. The 1973 tax returns indicated that amounts approximating $11 billion were claimed in such deductions. That tax loss must have been considerably more than $4 billion.

Summary. This second approach, emphasizing reliance on market operation, also has the likely impact of returning all aspects of health care planning, organization and delivery to the state governments where the police power constitutionally exists. In that way, the artificial distinction between financing medical care delivery and the legal consequences of it is partly erased, and the same state legislatures which have to cope with the legal side of the problem can begin to worry about all other regulatory aspects.

PROPOSED STUDIES

Each of the following topics is to be assigned to one or more authors with a recommendation, wherever feasible, for consideration of the impact of various kinds of facilities (inpatient care, ambulatory care and teaching institutions) upon the construction costs, upon the cost of equipment and upon working capital costs.

Topics

1. An examination of the stated purpose (as seen in the literature) in consequence of principal health legislations since 1946: "Yesterday's Incentives Become Today's Perverse Incentives."

2. A study of the American capital market and its relationship to the capital needs of the health care field, being a survey of the current outlook of the capital market with regards to bonds and equity, with due consideration being made for specified changes in federal and state policies.

3. Medical care and prices, share of the gross national product; the tax loss problem; and arguments for policy reconsideration, with research and data requirement implications.

4. Investment in human capital in the medical care field; past experience, current considerations.

5. Current political and tax impediments to private investment in three of the four areas of the medical care industry (excluding the human capital area).

6. Private venture and other forms of capital investment in the HMO modality, including the risk to physicians for the effective delivery of health care services.

✳ *Appendix B*

Participants Capital Investment Conference November 19–21, 1976

Chairman

Nathan J. Stark, J.D.
Vice Chancellor of Health Professions
University of Pittsburgh
President of the University Health
    Center of Pittsburgh
Pittsburgh, Pennsylvania 15261
Steering Committee Chairman

Albert C. Baker
Deputy Director
Government Relations
Federation of American Hospitals
Suite 310
1101 17th Street, N.W.
Washington, D.C. 20036

Robert Ball
Scholar in Residence
Institute of Medicine
2101 Constitution Avenue, N.W.
Washington, D.C. 20418

Karl D. Bays
Chairman of the Board

American Hospital Supply
    Corporation
1740 Ridge Avenue
Evanston, Illinois 60201
Discussant

Elizabeth Berman
Director
Outpatient Administration
Rehabilitation Institute of Chicago
345 E. Superior Street
Chicago, Illinois 60611

Howard J. Berman
Vice President of Research and
    Development

Blue Cross Association
840 North Lake Shore Drive
Chicago, Illinois 60611
Discussant

Thomas Bice, Ph.D.
Professor of Sociology
Box 1113, Department of Sociology
Washington University
St. Louis, Missouri 63130

Jan Blanpain, M.D.
Director
Program and Hospital Administration
    and Medical Care Organization
School of Public Health
University of Leuven
102 Vital Decosterstraat
Leuven 3000, Belgium

Robert J. Blendon, Sc.D.
Vice President
Robert Wood Johnson Foundation
P.O. Box 2316
Princeton, New Jersey 08540
Steering Committee Member
Session Chairman

Barry Bosworth, Ph.D.
Research Associate
Brookings Institution
1775 Massachusetts Avenue, N.W.
Washington, D.C. 20036
Discussant

Norman A. Brady
President
Norwalk Hospital
24 Stevens Street
Norwalk, Connecticut 06856

James Brindle
Professor
Health Services Administration
School of Allied Health Professions
State University of New York
Stony Brook, New York 11790
Discussant

Harry Cain, II, Ph.D.
Director
Bureau of Health Planning and Re-
    sources Development
Room 1105, Parklawn Building
5600 Fishers Lane
Rockville, Maryland 20852

Virgilio C. Canlas, M.D.
Associate Professor
Institute of Public Health
University of the Philippines
625 Pedro Gil, P.O. Box EA460
Ermita, Manila, Philippines

L. David Carley, Ph.D.
President
Medical College of Wisconsin
561 N. 15th Street
Milwaukee, Wisconsin 53233
Steering Committee Member
Session Chairman

H. Robert Cathcart
President
Pennsylvania Hospital
Eighth and Spruce Streets
Philadelphia, Pennsylvania 19107
Discussant

David C. Clapp
Vice President
Goldman, Sachs Company
55 Broad Street
New York, New York 10004
Coauthor

Darryl Clemmens
News and Publications
Representative of the Health
    Professions
University of Pittsburgh
1117 Scaife Hall
Terrace and DeSoto Streets
Pittsburgh, Pennsylvania 15261

William J. Copeland
Vice Chairman of the Board

Pittsburgh National Bank
Pittsburgh National Building
5th Avenue & Wood Street
Pittsburgh, Pennsylvania 15222

Robert M. Cunningham, Jr.
Consultant
2126 N. Dayton Street
Chicago, Illinois 60614

Edgar N. Duncan
Director
Office of Regional Operations
U.S. Department of Health, Education
 and Welfare
Room 1747, Parklawn Building
5600 Fishers Lane
Rockville, Maryland 20852

Siegfried Eichhorn
Professor
German Hospital Institute
Tersteegenstrasse #9
D 4000 Dusseldorf, West Germany

Kenneth M. Endicott, M.D.
Administrator
Health Resources Administration
U.S. Department of Health, Education
 and Welfare
Room 1005, Parklawn Building
5600 Fishers Lane
Rockville, Maryland 20852

Alain C. Enthoven, Ph.D.
Marriner S. Eccles
Professor of Public and Private
 Management
Stanford University
Stanford, California 04305
Discussant

Robert G. Evans, Ph.D.
Associate Professor
University of British Columbia
2085 Restbrook Place
Vancouver, Canada V6D 1W5
Discussant

Martin Feldstein, Ph.D.
Professor of Economics
Harvard University
1737 Cambridge Street, Room 403
Cambridge, Massachusetts 02138
Discussant

Marian Fox
Special Assistant
Health Resources Administration
U.S. Department of Health, Education
 and Welfare
Room 1011, Parklawn Building
5600 Fishers Lane
Rockville, Maryland 20852

Clifton R. Gaus, Ph.D.
Director
Division of Health Insurance Studies
U.S. Department of Health, Education
 and Welfare
Room 9-14, Universal North Building
1875 Connecticut Avenue, N.W.
Washington, D.C. 20009

Eli Ginzberg, Ph.D.
Director
Conservation of Human Resources
Columbia University
525 Uris Hall
New York, New York 10027
Author

Charles R. Goulet
Executive Vice President
Health Care Services Corporation
P.O. Box 1364
Chicago, Illinois 60690

Winters Hames
Acting Director
Division of Facilities Development
U.S. Department of Health, Education
 and Welfare
Room 414, Federal Building
9000 Rockville Pike
Bethesda, Maryland 20014

Clark Havighurst, J.D.
Professor
Duke University Law School
Durham, North Carolina 27706
Discussant

Arthur Hess
Director
Commission on Public General
    Hospitals
1001 Connecticut Avenue, N.W.
Washington, D.C. 20036

Michael D. Hernandez
Vice President
Kidder, Peabody, Inc.
10 Hanover Square
New York, New York 10005
Discussant

John Hill
Chairman of the Board
Hospital Corporation of America
1 Park Plaza
Nashville, Tennessee 37203
Author

Lawrence A. Hill
Executive Director
New England Medical Center Hospital
171 Harrison Avenue
Boston, Massachusetts 02111
Discussant

George A. Huber, J.D.
Lecturer, Health Services Administra-
    tion, Graduate School of
    Public Health
University of Pittsburgh
Special Assistant to the President for
    Legal Affairs
University Health Center of Pittsburgh
Pittsburgh, Pennsylvania 15261
University of Pittsburgh Faculty
    Support

Jeffrey Human
Acting Associate Director of Program
    Operation
Bureau of Health Planning and Re-
    sources Development
Health Resources Administration
U.S. Department of Health, Education
    and Welfare
Room 1105, Parklawn Building
5600 Fishers Lane
Rockville, Maryland 20852

Thomas Joe
Consultant
Lewin and Associates, Inc.
470 L'Enfant Plaza
Suite 4100
Washington, D.C. 20024
Coauthor

Robert S. Kelling, Jr.
Vice President
Originations Department
John Nuveen and Company, Inc.
209 S. LaSalle Street
Chicago, Illinois 60604
Coauthor

Ronald M. Klar, M.D., M.P.H.
Acting Deputy Director
Office of Policy Development and
    Planning
U.S. Department of Health, Education
    and Welfare
Room 17A40, Parklawn Building
5600 Fishers Lane
Rockville, Maryland 20852

James Klingensmith
Department of Health Services
    Administration
Graduate School of Public Health
University of Pittsburgh
Pittsburgh, Pennsylvania 15261
University of Pittsburgh Student
    Support

L.F. Krystynak, Ph.D.
Senior Scientific Advisor
Health Resources Administration
U.S. Department of Health, Education
   and Welfare
Parklawn Building, 5600 Fishers Lane
Rockville, Maryland 20852
Rapporteur

Robert J. Lampman, Ph.D.
Professor of Economics
University of Wisconsin
Social Security Building
Department of Economics
Madison, Wisconsin 53706
Discussant

Judith Lave, Ph.D.
Professor
Carnegie Mellon Institute
Pittsburgh, Pennsylvania 15213

Lawrence S. Lewin
President
Lewin and Associates, Inc.
470 L'Enfant Plaza, S.W.
Washington, D.C. 20024
Coauthor

Seymour Martin Lipset, Ph.D.
Professor of Political Science and
   Sociology
Senior Fellow
Hoover Institute
Stanford University
Stanford, California 94305
Discussant

William A. Lybrand, Ph.D.
Associate Administrator
Health Resources Administration
U.S. Department of Health, Education
   and Welfare
Room 1005, Parklawn Building
5600 Fishers Lane
Rockville, Maryland 20852

Thomas McCarthy, Ph.D.
Deputy Associate Administrator
Office of Scientific Affairs
Health Resources Administration
U.S. Department of Health, Education
   and Welfare
Parklawn Building, 5600 Fishers Lane
Rockville, Maryland 20852
Project Officer

Gordon K. MacLeod, M.D.
Chairman and Professor
Department of Health Services
   Administration
Graduate School of Public Health
University of Pittsburgh
Pittsburgh, Pennsylvania 15261
Steering Committee Member and
   Project Director

Harry M. Malm
President
Lutheran Hospital
Home Society of America, Inc.
70 North 5th Street
Fargo, North Dakota 58102
Steering Committee Member

Harold Margulies, M.D.
Deputy Administrator
Health Resources Administration
U.S. Department of Health, Education
   and Welfare
Room 1005, Parklawn Building
5600 Fishers Lane
Rockville, Maryland 20852

Ida C. Merriam, Ph.D.
Former Director of Research
Social Security Administration
Room 1121
1875 Connecticut Avenue, N.W.
Washington, D.C. 20009
Discussant

Libby D. Merrill
Acting Director

Office of Policy Coordination
Bureau of Health Planning & Resources Development
Health Resources Administration
U.S. Department of Health, Education and Welfare
Room 1127, Parklawn Building
5600 Fishers Lane
Rockville, Maryland 20852

Judith Miller
Director
Health Staff Seminar
George Washington University
Suite 3305
1901 Pennsylvania Avenue, N.W.
Washington, D.C. 20006

Morton D. Miller
Vice Chairman of the Board
Equitable Life Assurance Society of the U.S.
1285 Avenue of the Americas
New York, New York 10019
Steering Committee Member
Session Chairman

Joseph C. Morreale, Ph.D.
Assistant Professor
Health Services Administration
(Health Economics)
Graduate School of Public Health
University of Pittsburgh
Pittsburgh, Pennsylvania 15261
Rapporteur

John Moscato
Associate Administrator for Division of Legislation
Health Resources Administration
U.S. Department of Health, Education and Welfare
Room 10A43, Parklawn Building
5600 Fishers Lane
Rockville, Maryland 20852

Jack Needleman
Consultant
Lewin and Associates, Inc.
470 L'Enfant Plaza, S.W.
Washington, D.C. 20024
Coauthor

Monte Nichol
Deputy Director
Division of Operations
Health Resources Administration
U.S. Department of Health, Education and Welfare
Room 10A22, Parklawn Building
5600 Fishers Lane
Rockville, Maryland 20852

Walter K. Palmer
Vice President of Finance
Kaiser Foundation Medical Care Program
Ordway Building, Kaiser Center
Oakland, California 94666
Coauthor

Mark Perlman, Ph.D.
The University Professor of Economics
University of Pittsburgh
P.O. Box 7230
Oakland Station
Pittsburgh, Pennsylvania 15213
Steering Committee Member

M. Allen Pond
Professor
Health Services Administration
Graduate School of Public Health
University of Pittsburgh
Pittsburgh, Pennsylvania 15261
Rapporteur

Wesley W. Posvar, Ph.D.
Chancellor
Room 107 Cathedral of Learning
University of Pittsburgh
Pittsburgh, Pennsylvania 15260

Paul Rettig
Staff Director
U.S. Senate Subcommittee on Health
412 House Office Building Annex 1
Washington, D.C. 20515

Dorothy Rice
Director
National Center for Health Statistics
Health Resources Administration
U.S. Department of Health, Education
and Welfare
Room 805, Parklawn Building
5600 Fishers Lane
Rockville, Maryland 20852

H. MacDonald Rimple, M.D.
Regional Health Administrator
U.S. Department of Health, Education
and Welfare
3535 Market Street
Room 4311
Philadelphia, Pennsylvania 19101

Collin C. Rorrie, Jr., Ph.D.
Deputy Director
Bureau of Health Planning & Re-
sources Development
U.S. Department of Health, Education
and Welfare
Room 1107, Parklawn Building
5600 Fishers Lane
Rockville, Maryland 20852

Richard N. Rosett, Ph.D.
Dean
Graduate School of Business
University of Chicago
5836 S. Greenwood Avenue
Chicago, Illinois 60647
Discussant

C.H. William Ruhe, M.D.
Senior Vice President
American Medical Association
535 N. Dearborn Street
Chicago, Illinois 60610

John T. Ryan, Jr.
Chairman, Board of Trustees
University Health Center of Pittsburgh
c/o Mine Safety Appliance & Company
400 Penn Center Blvd.
Pittsburgh, Pennsylvania 15235

Paul Schwab
Scientific Advisor for Data Policy
Coordination
Health Resources Administration
U.S. Department of Health, Education
and Welfare
Parklawn Building, 5600 Fishers Lane
Rockville, Maryland 20852
Rapporteur

D. Eugene Sibery
Executive Vice President
Blue Cross Association
840 North Lake Shore Drive
Chicago, Illinois 60611
Discussant

Arthur B. Spector
Senior Associate
Goldman, Sachs Company
55 Broad Street
New York, New York 10004
Coauthor

Charles Storrs
Multi Family Program Specialist
U.S. Department of Housing and
Urban Development
451 Seventh Street, S.W.
Room 6141
Washington, D.C. 20410

Richard J. Stull
President
American College of Hospital
Administrators
840 North Lake Shore Drive
Chicago, Illinois 60611

William J. Swanson
Financial Advisor
1860 Oak Knoll Lane
Menlo Park, California 94025
Steering Committee Member

Joseph V. Terenzio
President
United Hospital Fund of New York
3 East 54th Street
New York, New York 10022
Author

John F. Tomayko
Assistant to the President
United Steel Workers of America
5 Gateway Center
Pittsburgh, Pennsylvania 15222

Earl Ubell
Director
NBC Television News
30 Rockefeller Plaza
New York, New York 10020

Lyman Van Nostrand
Associate Administrator
Division of Planning
Health Resources Administration
U.S. Department of Health, Education
   and Welfare
Parklawn Building, 5600 Fishers Lane
Rockville, Maryland 20852

James A. Vohs
President
Kaiser Foundation Medical Care
   Program
Ordway Building, Kaiser Center
Oakland, California 94666
Coauthor

Stanley Wallach, Ph.D.
Deputy Assistant Director for Health
   Income Assistance and Veteran
   Affairs
Congressional Budget Office

Room 3404, HOB Annex 2
Second and D Street, S.W.
Washington, D.C. 20515

Kerr L. White, M.D.
Director Institute for Health Care
   Studies
United Hospital Fund of New York
3 East 54th Street
New York, New York 10022

Paul C. Williams
Assistant Vice President
Originations Department
John Nuveen & Company, Inc.
209 S. LaSalle Street
Chicago, Illinois 60604
Coauthor

Richard Williams
Treasurer
American Hospital Supply
   Corporation
1740 Ridge Avenue
Evanston, Illinois 60201
Discussant

Claus A. Wirsig
Executive Director
University Teaching Hospital
   Association
1300 Yonge Street, Suite 704
Toronto, Ontario, Canada M4T 1X3

Irwin Wolkstein
Associate Director
American Hospital Association
Washington D.C. Office
1 Farragut Square
Washington, D.C. 20006
Author

Diane Wolman
Program Analyst
Bureau of Health Planning and Re-
   sources Development

U.S. Department of Health, Education
and Welfare
Room 1105, Parklawn Building
5600 Fishers Lane
Rockville, Maryland 20852

Mary A. Wrenn
Vice President
Investment Banking Division
Merrill Lynch, Pierce, Fenner &
Smith, Inc.
1 Liberty Plaza
165 Broadway
New York, New York 10006
Discussant

John D. Young
Assistant Secretary
Comptroller
U.S. Department of Health, Education
and Welfare

Room 5760 HEW Building North
330 Independence Avenue, S.W.
Washington, D.C. 20201

Bernard C. Ziegler
Chairman of the Board
B.C. Ziegler and Company
215 Main Street
West Bend, Wisconsin 53095
Steering Committee Member

Daniel Zwick
Associate Administrator
Office of Planning, Evaluation and
Legislation
Health Resources Administration
U.S. Department of Health, Education
and Welfare
Parklawn Building, 5600 Fishers Lane
Rockville, Maryland 20852

Index

About the Editors

Gordon MacLeod is a Professor and Departmental Chairman of Health Services Administration in the Graduate School of Public Health at the University of Pittsburgh. He spent five years on the faculty of the Yale University School of Medicine where he was an Associate Clinical Professor of Medicine and Public Health and Director of the Yale Diagnostic Clinic. While in New Haven, he was instrumental in establishing an HMO affiliated with Yale and was both an incorporator and charter member of the HMO's Board of Directors. Dr. MacLeod was the first Director of the Health Maintenance Organization Service in the Department of Health, Education and Welfare. In 1974, he conducted a study on the role of consumers under national health insurance in several European countries under the auspices of the Ford Foundation. Dr. MacLeod is the author of numerous publications in the field of Health Services and Health Financing. He served as consultant to the World Health Organization in Manila to assist in restructuring the teaching and research programs in public health administration at the University of the Philippines. He also has served as consultant to the Ford Foundation, German Marshal Fund of the United States and the National Planning Association.

Mark Perlman is the University Professor of Economics and Professor of Economics in Public Health at the University of Pittsburgh. He has served on the faculties of the University of Hawaii, Cornell University and Johns Hopkins University. In addition to writing articles and essays on health and economic development, he is editor of the *Journal of Economic Literature*. He was a Senior Fulbright Lecturer in Melbourne in 1968 and served as co-chairman of the 1973 International Economic Association Conference on Economics of Health in Industrialized Nations in Tokyo. He is editor of *Economics of Health and Medical Care* and is the co-author of *Health Manpower in a Developing Economy*.